# DISABILITY AND WAR IN THE LATE MIDDLE AGES

**WAR AND CONFLICT IN PREMODERN SOCIETIES**

**Further Information and Publications**

www.arc-humanities.org/series/book-series/

# DISABILITY AND WAR IN THE LATE MIDDLE AGES

## BECOMING, SURVIVING, MANAGING

Edited by

**NINON DUBOURG** and
**CHRISTOPHE MASSON**

ARC HUMANITIES PRESS

**British Library Cataloguing in Publication Data**
A catalogue record for this book is available from the British Library.



ISBN (Hardback): 9781802701647
e-ISBN (PDF): 9781802703948
e-ISBN (EPUB): 9781802703931

**www.arc-humanities.org**

Printed and bound in the UK (by CPIGroup [UK] Ltd), USA (by Bookmasters), and elsewhere using print-on-demand technology.

**Publisher (manufacturer) details:** Arc Humanities Press, 14 Clifton Moor Business Village, James Nicolson Link, York YO30 4XG, United Kingdom.

**EU Authorized Representative details (for GPSR purposes):** Amsterdam University Press, Nieuwe Prinsengracht 89, 1018 VR Amsterdam, The Netherlands. www.aup.nl

# CONTENTS

List of Illustrations .......... vii

Preface .......... x

Introduction. Disability and War: Becoming, Surviving, Managing
**NINON DUBOURG and CHRISTOPHE MASSON** .......... 1

Chapter 1. The Recidivists: Healed Cranial Trauma from Conflicts in the Late Medieval Period
**CHRISTOPHER J. KNÜSEL** .......... 29

Chapter 2. Disability and Trauma in Battle in the Medieval Icelandic Sagas
**YOAV TIROSH** .......... 57

Chapter 3. Hungry for Love: Disabling the Knightly Body and Mind through Starvation in Sir Thomas Malory's *Le Morte Darthur*
**KRISTINA HILDEBRAND** .......... 79

Chapter 4. A Vulnerable Military Masculinity: Soldiers and Disability in Late Medieval Pardon Letters (France, England, and the Low Countries)
**QUENTIN VERREYCKEN** .......... 99

Chapter 5. Traumatic Repercussions: Warfare and Disability in the French Countryside
**ALEKSANDRA PFAU** .......... 121

Chapter 6. Investigating the Lifecycle of the Medieval English Soldier: Disability, Mental Trauma, and Medicine in Connection with War in Late Medieval English Records
**WENDY J. TURNER** ........ 143

Chapter 7. "What pain I suffered at that time, anyone can well imagine": Experiences of War, Injury, and Pain in Fifteenth- and Sixteenth-Century Germany and Switzerland
**BIANCA FROHNE** ........ 165

Chapter 8. Mechanism/Organism: The Premodern Iron Hand as Conceptual Interface
**JOHN GAGNÉ** ........ 193

Chapter 9. After Combat: War Wounds, Soldiers' Benefits, and Dynastic Policies in the Burgundian-Habsburg Armies (1363–1506)
**MICHAEL DEPRETER** ........ 211

Select Bibliography ........ 239

Index ........ 243

# LIST OF ILLUSTRATIONS

## Chapter 1. The Recidivists — *Christopher J. Knüsel*

Figure 1.1. A copper-based metallic fragment embedded in the right *os coxae* of Towton 42.. 35

Figure 1.2. Sharp-force weapon trauma of Towton 32. 36

Figure 1.3. The left occipital of Towton 8, showing concentric, comminuted fractures of blunt force trauma. 37

Figure 1.4. A small-diameter perforation of the left frontal bone of Towton 40. 37

Figure 1.5. Endocranial view of the bevelled fractures around a penetrating wound of the inner table of the cranium of Towton 8. 38

Figure 1.6. Lingual view of the deeply penetrating wound on the left side of the mandible, with a mid-line ante-mortem fracture of the chin of Towton 16. 40

Figure 1.7. The ante-mortem fracture of the left side of the mandible of Towton 16.. 41

Figure 1.8. Facial reconstruction of Towton 16, with scarring of the mandibular wound and loss of muscle tone and retraction at the left corner of the mouth.. 41

Figure 1.9. The extent of Towton 16's perimortem injuries after cranial reconstruction from fragments, with comminution (crushing) of the left side of the face. 42

Table 1.1. Number of individuals with perimortem wounds and number of individuals with antemortem (healed) cranial wounds. 44

Figure 1.10. Superior view of the cranium of Towton 41. 44

**Chapter 2. Disability and Trauma in Battle in the Medieval Icelandic Sagas — *Yoav Tirosh***

Figure 2.1. Recreating Klaufi's weaponized-head scene in the Svarfdaela saga set in North Iceland, April 2013. ......................64

Figure 2.2. Yoav Tirosh (@RealMundiRiki), "Ruðolf the Red-Nosed-Viking." ................................................66

Figure 2.3. Yoav Tirosh (@RealMundiRiki), "A Talking Human." .............66

**Chapter 6. Investigating the Lifecycle of the Medieval English Soldier — *Wendy J. Turner***

Figure 6.1. Details from the lower marginalia in the Luttrell Psalter. London, British Library, Additional MS 42130, fol. 208v................ 151

Figure 6.2. The man with the prosthetic hand. Detail from London, British Library, Additional MS 42130, fol. 208v. ............... 152

Figure 6.3. A warrior attempting to continue to fight even while disabled. New Haven, Yale University, Beinecke Rare Book & Manuscript Library, MS 229, fol. 257v...................................... 163

**Chapter 7. "What pain I suffered at that time, anyone can well imagine" — *Bianca Frohne***

Figure 7.1. Hans von Gersdorff, *Feldbuch der wundtartzney* (Strasbourg: Schott, 1517), fol. 18v......................................... 166

Figure 7.2. Hans von Gersdorff, *Feldbuch der wundtartzney* (Strasbourg: Schott, 1517), fol. 38r. ......................................... 175

**Chapter 8. Mechanism/Organism — *John Gagné***

Figure 8.1. "Prosthetic Hand." Ambroise Paré, *Dix livres de la chirurgie, avec le Magasin des Instrumens necessaires à icelle* (Paris: Jean Le Royer, 1564)........ 194

Figure 8.2. The interior of the "Paré hand" during its restoration in 2000. Paris, Musée de la médecine........ 198

Figure 8.3. Interacting with the Cambridge, Fitzwilliam Museum hand, ca. 1550........ 199

Figure 8.4. Two views of the iron hand fashioned by Ulrich Wagner for Ulrich Wyss, 1476. Fribourg, Musée d'Art et d'Histoire, MAHF 7611........ 200

Figure 8.5. "Portrait of Andreas Vesalius," in Vesalius' *De humani corporis fabrica libri septem* (Basel: Johannes Oporinus, 1543)........ 203

Figure 8.6. Christian von Mechel, *Die eiserne Hand* (Berlin: Decker, 1815), Plate II........ 206

Figure 8.7. "Strongly and bravely." The iron hand of Marcus Sergius in Geffrey Whitney's *Choice of Emblemes* (Leiden: Plantin, 1586)........ 207

# PREFACE

THE CONJUNCTION OF medieval disability and war studies was conceptualized by Ninon Dubourg (disability historian) and Christophe Masson (military historian) when their paths crossed at the University of Liège. This shared vision emerged from a profound recognition of the need to bridge these two disciplines, uncovering new perspectives on how medieval societies understood and navigated the interplay between disability and conflict. Their collaboration marked the beginning of an interdisciplinary journey which resulted in the present volume.

This vision materialized through an ambitious series of events, starting with an online workshop that brought together specialists from a variety of fields, including (bio)archaeology, literature, and history, to engage in vibrant discussions. Held from February 2023 to April 2024, this series of public events provided a dynamic platform for exploring the nuanced ways in which disability and warfare intersected during the later Middle Ages. The culmination of these efforts was a two-day closed workshop in November 2024, where contributors gathered at the University of Liège to deepen their analyses and establish the foundations for this volume.

Such an undertaking would not have been possible without the generous support and collaboration of several institutions. We extend our heartfelt gratitude to the Fund for Scientific Research (F.R.S.-FNRS), the University of Liège (through RISE—Research, Innovation, Support and Enterprises and the Faculty of Philosophy and Letters), and the Research Unit "Transitions. Moyen Âge et première modernité" for their funding and unwavering encouragement. Their support not only facilitated the organization of these events but also ensured the successful realization of this book, which stands as a testament to the power of interdisciplinary dialogue.

This volume represents the collective efforts of scholars dedicated to shedding light on a complex and often-overlooked aspect of medieval history. It is the editors' hope that the insights and discussions contained within will inspire further exploration and dialogue, enriching both disability studies and war studies in ways that honour their interconnected histories.

Introduction

# DISABILITY AND WAR

## BECOMING, SURVIVING, MANAGING

NINON DUBOURG and CHRISTOPHE MASSON

WAS THERE A better place for sustaining permanent injuries than the battlefield? Was there a worse place for a disabled person than a battlefield? These two questions seem inescapable when we consider the intersection between warfare and disability. Yet, they partly derived from the assumption that no one would dare to yield a sword or fire a bombard if not in entire control of their physical or mental capacities. This may explain why scholars often overlook this intersection. If some valuable studies provide a solid foundation for us to develop our own analyses, they mostly came either from disability historians happening to address a martial context because of their sources, or from military historians who came across injured or disabled warriors while reading chronicles or account books. The aim of this volume is to foster a dialogue between specialists of both topics and to open new interpretative paradigms and research questions. This dialogue first took place in the form of a monthly webinar, hosted by the two editors, where contributors to this book presented their research.[1]

1 Unfortunately, Giulia Morosini (whose presentation was entitled "The Limping Captain: Injuries, Wounds, and Scars between Praise and Mocking in Renaissance Italy") could not take part in the editorial process of this volume. The editors have nonetheless relied on her oral presentation to support the present text.

**NINON DUBOURG** is an Alexander von Humboldt Fellow based at the University of Cologne. Her research interests revolve around old age and physical, sensory, and mental disabilities within the framework of material, cultural, and social medieval history. Her first monograph, *Disabled Clerics in the Late Middle Ages: Un/suitable for Divine Service?* (2023), delves into the relationship between the church and disability.

**CHRISTOPHE MASSON** is Permanent Researcher for the Fund for Scientific Research–FNRS based at the University of Liège. His work addresses the social, cultural, institutional, and technical dimensions of late medieval warfare.

They subsequently convened at the University of Liège for an in-person workshop designed to ensure the publication's cohesive nature.

This volume specifically addresses the Latin later Middle Ages, understood as a period ranging from the fourteenth century to the 1530s. On a military level, this whole period expressed the same common patterns. While gaining in size, armies did not consist of more than a few thousand men. Gunpowder weapons appeared in the 1320s in Western Europe, but they did not drastically change the face of battle before the second part of the sixteenth century, when the number of portable firearms significantly increased. Martial culture remained relatively coherent, emphasizing the social importance of chivalry and honour in the conduct of war. In a similar manner, it appears that these centuries did not witness any shift in the perception of disability and disabled people. The following chapters argue for a more relevant division between combatants and non-combatants, instead of the more traditional distinctions between nobles, non-nobles, warriors, soldiers, feudal levies, and standing armies. A wide variety of military scenarios/tactics/operations, such as sieges and razzias (i.e., ambushes and raids) involved individuals who were lacking formal training and had to fight and defend themselves with weapons that, in many cases, were improvised. This commonly resulted in severe injuries. Finally, this volume argues that warfare should not be regarded exclusively as an open and widely publicised confrontation between two major lords focused on political domination or geographical expansion. Rather, it should be considered as a context of organized and sustained violence involving structured groups of individuals. This violence encompassed various forms, including pitched battles, destruction of property or theft, ambushes, and guerrilla tactics, ranging from small-scale local feuds to major continental conflicts.

## State of the Art

In contrast to war, the definition of which did not drastically change since the medieval period, disability is a modern concept crafted by recent scholarship.[2] The 1980s were a period of significant progress for the disability rights movement, with paralleling developments in the interest of historians and other humanities and social scientists in researching disability as a subject.

---

**2** See Daniel Blackie and Alexia Moncrieff, "State of the Field: Disability History," *History* 107 (2022): 789–811. When not linked to one of the chapters of this volume (indicated by the author's name in brackets), references to sources and secondary literature are provided by Ninon Dubourg and Christophe Masson.

In this understanding, disability encompasses a multitude of definitions, including economic, social, political, cultural, religious, legal, philosophical, artistic, moral, and medical interpretations, thus establishing itself as a polysemous subject. This compelled historians to contextualize and define the term "disability" as a concept prior to its utilization.[3] In this regard, historians have benefited from the conceptual frameworks developed by activist movements, particularly within English-speaking contexts. Within these movements, the issue of accessibility became a matter of immediate concern: organized groups, such as the UPIAS (Union of the Physically Impaired Against Segregation), provided the foundation for the development of an analytical framework known as the "social model of disability."[4] This model highlights a distinction between impairment (as defined in the "medical model," which looks at individual and biomedical aspects) and disability (as a disadvantage or restriction of activity fostered by the social organization exerting its power over individuals on the grounds of "objective" physical or mental limitations).[5] In this definition, which is largely utilized within the academic domain, disability is no longer considered to be intrinsic to the individual. Rather, it is understood to be shaped by the challenges encountered within the individual's social and physical environment.

However, activists and academics soon called for a renewal of the social model, which proved notably inadequate for analyzing past societies.[6] This led to the emergence of the cultural model, also referred to as "social constructivism," which offered greater flexibility than the social model and took into account individuals' experiences in the definition of dis/ability.[7] It allowed for

---

**3** Catherine J. Kudlick, "Disability History: Why We Need Another 'Other,'" *The American Historical Review* 108, no. 3 (June 2003): 763–93.

**4** See Carmelo Masala and Donatella Rita Petretto, "From Disablement to Enablement: Conceptual Models of Disability in the 20th Century," *Disability and Rehabilitation* 30, no. 17 (2008): 1233–44.

**5** Len Barton and Michael Oliver, "Introduction: The Birth of Disability Studies," in *Disability Studies: Past, Present and Future*, eds. Len Barton and Michael Oliver (Leeds: Disability, 1997), i–v.

**6** Tom Shakespeare and Nick Watson, "The Social Model of Disability: An Outdated Ideology?," in *Exploring Theories and Expanding Methodologies: Where We Are and Where We Need to Go*, eds. Sharon N. Barnartt and Barbara M. Altman (Bradford: Emerald, 2001), 9–28, notably p. 13.

**7** See Bianca Frohne, "Heutige Modelle von Dis/Ability—tauglich für die Vormoderne?: The Cultural Model," in *Dis/Ability History der Vormoderne: Ein Handbuch = Premodern Dis/Ability History: A Companion*, eds. Cordula Nolte et al. (Affalterbach: Didymos, 2017), 61–63.

the consideration that a phenomenon like disability is not confined to physical conditions and does not have a fixed existence; rather, it changes depending on the period and culture under study.[8] Researchers employing this model redefine concepts such as ability, health, or normality, examining how societies construct their own norms regarding disabled bodies.[9] This analytical framework proposes a holistic approach to disability and impairment as cultural phenomena. While historical sources often describe physical impairments, such descriptions must be distinguished from retro-diagnoses, which risk imposing modern medical categories on historical documents that do not address them in such terms.[10] Thus, impairment and disability are no longer viewed as opposite, but both as constructed concepts. Both thereby enable the study of power structures through the lens of multiple identities (such as gender and disability), which are used to describe social processes.[11]

The 2000s witnessed a proliferation of publication on disability in the Middle Ages.[12] This has resulted in a series of recent publications that *synthesize* prior research and *build on* the knowledge produced over the past two decades.[13] These publications illustrate the shift from a social history of marginality, poverty, and impairment as a physical anomaly to the construction of analytical models, and, among these, from the long-preferred cultural model—insofar as it highlights the changes and evolution of the concept

---

**8** Ian Hacking, *The Social Construction of What?* (Cambridge, MA: Harvard University Press, 1999), 38. See also Mark Priestley, "Constructions and Creations: Idealism, Materialism and Disability Theory," *Disability & Society* 13, no. 1 (1998): 75–94; and Tom Shakespeare, "Cultural Representation of Disabled People: Dustbins for Disavowal?" *Disability & Society* 9, no. 3 (1994): 283–99.

**9** Sharon L. Snyder and David T. Mitchell, *Cultural Locations of Disability* (Chicago: University of Chicago Press, 2006).

**10** Jenni Kuuliala, *Childhood Disability and Social Integration in the Middle Ages: Constructions of Impairments in Thirteenth and Fourteenth-Century Canonization Processes* (Turnhout: Brepols, 2016), 33–34.

**11** Ange-Marie Hancock, "When Multiplication Doesn't Equal Quick Addition: Examining Intersectionality as a Research Paradigm," *Perspectives on Politics* 1 (2007): 63–79.

**12** Cordula Nolte, ed., *Homo debilis: Behinderte — Kranke — Versehrte in der Gesellschaft des Mittelalters* (Korb: Didymos, 2009); Joshua Eyler, ed., *Disability in the Middle Ages: Reconsiderations and Reverberations* (Farnham: Ashgate, 2010).

**13** Christian Krötzl, Katariina Mustakallio, and Jenni Kuuliala, eds., *Infirmity in Antiquity and the Middle Ages: Social and Cultural Approaches to Health, Weakness and Care* (Farnham: Ashgate, 2015); Jonathan Hsy et al., eds., *A Cultural History of Disability in the Middle Ages* (London: Bloomsbury, 2020).

across both time and space—to a variety of alternatives.[14] The focus shifted more towards the concept of fluidity[15] and variability,[16] exploring the impact of lived and social environments on disabled individuals. This shift in focus served to debunk the myth that no one cared for disabled individuals before the modern era and that oppression was the only possible answer to disability.[17] In all these cases, medievalists primarily seek today to gain insight into the living experiences of disabled people in the medieval period.

In the field of disability studies, the subject of war emerged as a research topic through the question of the body in battle, first investigated through papers and then through collective volumes, such as the 2015 *Wounds and Wound Repair in Medieval Culture* directed by Kelly DeVries and Tracy Larissa.[18] The main focus has since shifted towards a more comprehensive consideration of mental health issues, taking the history of emotions into account.[19] The first step was towards courage and fear.[20] Amongst the first and few to be involved in the intersection of the history of disability and war, Wendy J. Turner published "Mental Incapacity and the Financing of War in Medieval England" in a volume dedicated to the Hundred Years' War published in 2008.[21] In this paper, she analyzed the mental state of

**14** Wendy J. Turner, "Models of Disability: Connecting the Past to the Present," *Zeitschrift für Disability Studies* 1 (February 2022): 1–18.

**15** Bianca Frohne and Klaus Peter Horn, "On the Fluidity of 'Disability' in Medieval and Early Modern Societies," in *The Imperfect Historian: Disability Histories in Europe*, eds. Sebastian Barsch et al. (Frankfurt am Main: Lang, 2013), 17–40.

**16** Chris Mounsey, "Introduction: VariAbility: Beyond Sameness and Difference," in *The Idea of Disability in the Eighteenth Century*, ed. Chris Mounsey (Lewisburgh: Bucknell University Press, 2014), 1–29.

**17** Ninon Dubourg, "European Medieval Disability History: An Overview," in *Handbook of Disability: Critical Thought and Social Change in a Globalizing World*, eds. Marcia H. Rioux et al. (Singapore: Springer, 2022), 89–106.

**18** Katie K. Walker, "Peril, Flight and the Sad Man: Medieval Theories of the Body in Battle," in *War and Literature: Essays and Studies*, eds. Laura Ashe and Ian Patterson (Cambridge: Brewer, 2014), 21–37; Kelly DeVries and Tracy Larissa, eds., *"His brest tobrosten": Wounds and Wound Repair in Medieval Culture* (Leiden: Brill, 2015).

**19** Donna Trembinski, "Comparing Premodern Melancholy/Mania and Modern Trauma: An Argument in Favour of Historical Experience of Trauma," *History of Psychology* 14 (2011): 80–99.

**20** As encouraged by Chelsea Grosskopf, "Fear and Loathing in *Eyrbyggja Saga*: Combat Trauma in Medieval Iceland," in *Combat Stress in Pre-Modern Europe: Mental Health in Historical Perspective*, eds. Owen Rees et al. (London: Palgrave, 2022), 151–69.

**21** Wendy J. Turner, "Mental Incapacity and the Financing of War in Medieval

English fighters returning from France after campaigning. In the 2013 volume of the same book series, Aleksandra Pfau also focused on the question in her paper entitled "Warfare, Trauma, and Madness in French Remission Letters of the Hundred Years' War."[22] This focus on trauma—defined as a psychological response to extremely stressful events, both physically and mentally—has been illustrated by publications such as *Trauma in Medieval Society*, edited by Wendy J. Turner and Christina Lee in 2018,[23] and *Combat Stress in Pre Modern Europe* to quote another publication from 2022, edited by Owen Rees, Kathryn Hurlock, and Jason Crowley.[24] In addition to addressing subjects such as facial wounds and burn victims (by Patricia Skinner), and mental and physical health (by Michael Livingston), these books deal with the subject of trauma (thanks to papers from Christina Lee, Robert C. Woosnam-Savage, and Kelly DeVries).[25] This growing focus on mental disabilities is reflected in the present volume. Kristina Hildebrand, Sasha Pfau, and Wendy J. Turner indeed chiefly address this issue, while other contributors consider it alongside physical disabilities. Despite the absence of the term in medieval sources, and even though retroactive diagnoses are most often unreliable, the concept of "trauma" has proven to be useful as a tool of inquiry. It facilitates a more profound exploration of our sources, thereby enabling a more precise understanding of the impact of warfare on social groups and individuals. In this theoretical framework, situated at the intersection of emotions and mental disabilities, the issue of a medieval Post Traumatic Stress Disorder (PTSD) remains.[26]

---

England," in *The Hundred Years War (Part II): Different Vistas*, eds. L. J. Andrew Villalon and Donald J. Kagay (Leiden: Brill, 2008), 387–466.

**22** Aleksandra Pfau, "Warfare, Trauma, and Madness in French Remission Letters of the Hundred Years War," in *The Hundred Years War (Part III): Further Considerations*, eds. L. J. Andrew Villalon and Donald J. Kagay (Leiden: Brill, 2013), 437–54.

**23** Wendy J. Turner and Christina Lee, eds., *Trauma in Medieval Society* (Leiden: Brill, 2018).

**24** Rees et al., eds., *Combat Stress in Pre-Modern Europe.*

**25** See also Thomas Kristian Heebøll-Holm, "Apocalypse Then? The First Crusade, Traumas of War and Thomas de Marle," in *Denmark and Europe in the Middle Ages c. 1000–1525: Essays in Honour of Professor Michael H. Gelting*, eds. Kerstin Hundahl et al. (London: Routledge, 2014), 237–54; Maurizio Paciaroni and Valentina Arnao, "Neurology and War: From Antiquity to Modern Times," in *War Neurology*, eds. Laurent Tatu and Julien Bougousslavsky (Basel: Karger AG, 2016), 1–9; Catherine Clarke, "Signs and Wonders: Writing Trauma in Twelfth-Century England," *Reading Medieval Studies* 35 (2009): 55–77.

**26** Kathryn Hurlock, "Was There Combat Trauma in the Middle Ages? A Case for

This shift in focus from the body to the mind prompted an examination of the concept of "ableism" in the context of determining an individual's suitability for the role of a warrior. As researchers continue to examine disability across various cultural and temporal contexts, the pivotal role of defining normality in delineating otherness becomes increasingly evident.[27] From this perspective, studies on disability highlight a certain fluidity between disability and normality,[28] with the emphasis seemingly being placed on the warrior's practical value, a matter of paramount importance in pre-industrial eras.[29] In a meticulous examination of Sir Thomas Malory's *La Morte d'Arthur*, Tory V. Perman has demonstrated that in this romance, combatting knights were expected to sustain both physical and mental injuries in order to prove their valour and enhance their reputation.[30] This demonstrates that, although potentially painful and debilitating, a physical or mental limitation did not necessarily preclude an individual from continuing to fulfil their social role, even when this role involved combat.

A number of studies have focused on the aftermath of physical disability. It was not uncommon for soldiers surviving the battlefields to sustain injuries that resulted in amputation of a limb or other injuries. Confraternities such as the one funded by blind veterans of the 1212 Battle of Las Navas de Tolosa could support for impaired soldiers, as evidenced by José Luis Fernández Fernández Iglesias.[31] The social interactions of the newly impaired are highlighted in the *Eyrbyggja Saga* in which Onund "Tree Leg" explained how he was affected by the loss of his leg during the Battle of Hafrsfjord, following the analysis of John P. Sexton.[32] These insights have prompted significant

---

Moral Injury in Pre-Modern Conflict," in *Combat Stress in Pre-Modern Europe*, eds. Rees et al., 124–31.

**27** Kudlick, "Disability History."

**28** Frohne and Horn, "On the Fluidity of 'Disability.'"

**29** Timothy E. Jones, "'A lame man can ride…a deaf man can kill…a dead man is of no use to anyone': When Was a Deformity not a Disability in Early Medieval Europe?," in *Disability and Impairment in Antiquity*, ed. Rupert Breitwieser (Oxford: Archaeopress, 2012), 131–35.

**30** Tory V. Pearman, *Disability and Knighthood in Malory's Morte Darthur* (London: Routledge, 2018).

**31** José Luis Fernández Fernández Iglesias, "Historia, discapacidad y valía," in *La imagen social de las personas con discapacidad: Estudios en homenje a José Julián Darriga Dravo*, ed. Juan Antonio Ledesma (Madrid: CINCA, 2009), 177–210.

**32** John P. Sexton, "Difference and Disability: On the Logic of Naming in the Icelandic Sagas," in *Disability in the Middle Age*, ed. Eyler, 149–63; see also John P. Sexton,

discussions about the social implications of war injuries, prompting us to further explore how they were perceived and managed in military contexts and their aftermaths. Moving forward, a deeper examination of disability on the battlefield from the perspective of the history of war can shed new light on the experiences of injured soldiers and the evolving responses to their needs.

From the perspective of a military historian, the traditional and outdated model of medieval warfare fails to explain the part taken by disabled people. It is regularly emphasized, especially in the Western Middle Ages, that waging war was the privilege of strong white men. The disabled, just like the old, the youngster, the woman, and the cleric had no part to play in it. However, we also know that this clear-cut division was never fully enacted. During sieges, a large part, if not all, of the population participated in the defence efforts. This participation could take many forms, including throwing stones at the besiegers, feeding the defenders, and maintaining and repairing weapons and fortifications.

It was not until relatively recently that military historians began to consider disabled persons as research subjects. While John Keegan's *Face of Battle*[33] and Philippe Contamine's *War in the Middle Ages*[34] have been instrumental in propelling researchers towards a more embodied approach to military matters, both paid little attention to "marginal" fighters. Military historians initially approached the subject of disabilities through the question of wounds. Their initial concern was to understand how one can hurt and be wounded while fighting.[35] This approach entailed the utilization of literary and, more broadly, textual sources, as well as archaeological evidence. The focus on battlefield archaeology has led to significant collaborative efforts among historians, archaeologists, and forensic scientists, particularly within the context of the Anglo-Saxon world, as evidenced by the studies conducted on the battles of Towton (1461), Visby (1361) and, to a lesser extent, Othée (1408).[36] On a global scale, the primary focus was on the experience of injury

---

"Atypical Bodies," in *A Cultural History of Disability in the Middle Ages*, eds. Jonathan Hsy et al. (London: Bloomsbury, 2020), 19–34.

**33** John Keegan, *The Face of Battle* (New York: Viking, 1976).

**34** Philippe Contamine, *War in the Middle Ages* (Oxford: Blackwell, 1985 [first French edition: Paris, 1980]).

**35** See for example Alain Mounier-Kuhn, "Les blessures de guerre et l'armement au Moyen Âge dans l'Occident latin," *Médiévales* 39 (2000): 112–36.

**36** Veronica Fiorato, Anthea Boylston, and Christopher Knüsel, *Blood Red Roses: The Archaeology of a Mass Grave from the Battle of Towton AD 1461*, 2nd ed. (Oxford: Oxbow, 2007); Bengt Thordemann, *Armour from the Battle of Visby, 1361*, 2 vols.

and death in medieval battles, as opposed to the experience of living with a disability. This was a plausible consequence of reflections on the highly debated question of the lethality of medieval wars and its effects on human behaviour on the battlefield.

Conversely, historians of medicine approached the question the other way. The military context was selected for study due to its provision of a wide variety of examples of medical practices. However, in this instance as well, the focus was not on the disabled or injured individuals themselves, but rather on gaining insights into the techniques employed in the management of injuries, and on their relative efficiency. This also served to complement the knowledge about hospital practices, which may have been less documented. Secondly, several studies highlighted the careers of the healers active in armies, with eminent figures such as Henri de Mondeville.[37] From this perspective, the disabled were, perhaps unconsciously, disregarded or marginalised as unworthy of the researchers' attention.

The shift towards examining both the consequences of permanent injury to fighters and the potential for disabled individuals to fight alongside able-bodied individuals is very recent. It may be a delayed consequence of the social approach that renewed the military history from the 1960s onwards, as put forward by scholars such as, in France, André Corvisier and Philippe Contamine. This has led scholars to redirect their attention from elite fighters to actors who have traditionally been considered marginal. Following on from the consideration of the roles of women and clerics, the focus has now shifted to the disabled. Obviously, we all know of John the Blind of Luxemburg, King of Bohemia, who died during the Battle of Crécy in 1346 where he was led by fellow knights guiding his horse with chains and possibly warning him where to defend himself or to strike.[38] We also know that he did not survive the day, and despite the fact that numerous other French combatants lost their lives on that occasion, modern authors, including historians, have frequently

---

(Stockholm: Almqvist och Wiksell, 1939); Yves Charlier, "Un charnier à Othée," *Activités du SOS Fouilles* 5, 86 à 87 (1988): 232–33; Françoise Cornet, "Étude anthropologique des ossements découverts au lieu-dit Al Savatte à Othée," *Activités du SOS Fouilles* 5 (1988), 228–31; and Jean-Marc Léotard, "Inhumation collective au lieu-dit Al Savatte à Othée," *Activités du SOS Fouilles* 5 (1988), 225–28.

**37** Rabah Ali Bacha, "Les blessures de guerre à la fin du Moyen Âge," 3 vols. (PhD diss., Université Lille 3–Charles de Gaulle, 2010); Jon C. Clasper, "The Management of Military Wounds in the Middle Ages," in *Wounds in the Middle Ages*, eds. Anne Kirkham and Cordelia Warr (Farnham: Ashgate, 2014), 17–39.

**38** Jean le Bel, *Chronique*, vol. 2, eds. Jules Viard and Eugène Deprez (Paris: Renouard, 1905), 108.

associated his fate with sheer folly. This anachronistic common sense posits John the Blind as the quintessential example of why one should not engage in combat if disabled. In a sense, this interpretation reinforced an unconscious inclination towards "ableism" that has for a long time hindered research in this area. However, John probably saw things in a totally opposite way. It has been convincingly argued that his decision to participate in the battle despite being blind was a means of restoring his honour.[39] One month earlier, at the Battle of Vottem, he had been present alongside his son Charles of Luxembourg, who had recently been elected "King of the Romans" but did not participate in the combat. The battle culminated in a crushing defeat for the prince-bishop of Liège against the rebel towns of Liège and Huy, even though he was supported by an impressive troop, which included German knights. The fact that John's honour was to be restored implied that the contemporary expectations were to have him joining the episcopal forces, despite being blind. Following this line of thought, it seems more interesting to look at "disabled" or blind people—notwithstanding the fact that medieval authors also used this last adjective to mean partially sighted—who survived battles. In fact, sources are less silent on the subject than what might initially be presumed. In 1325, a local battle was fought in the Liège countryside, involving several hundred nobles from two rival lineages. According to sources, at least two men were honoured with knighthoods prior to the commencement of the fight. The first of these, Guillaume Wilkar d'Awans, was blind. The second one, Alexandre de Saint-Servais, had two hands and a foot *afoleis*, to quote the Middle French word meaning "[more or less largely] broken.[40] "As a chronicler specifically attested, thanks to the effective and purposeful protection of their fellow knights, none of these newly anointed knights perished during the course of the battle.[41] They fought, nonetheless.

In the same vein, the fate of disabled combatants has already attracted attention from early modernists. The existence of such institutions as the French *Hôtel des Invalides*, along with the archival documentation available,

**39** According to Andrew Ayton, "The Crécy Battle: Context and Significance," in *The Battle of Crécy, 1346*, eds. Andrew Ayton and Philipp Preston (Woodbridge: Boydell, 2005), 25, no. 103.

**40** Monique Haas, "Affoler (2)," in *Dictionnaire du Moyen Français (1330–1500)*, http://zeus.atilf.fr/dmf/, accessed December 21, 2024.

**41** Jacques de Hemricourt, "Le traité des guerres d'Awans et de Waroux," in Jacques de Hemricourt, *Œuvres*, eds. Alphonse Bayot and Camille de Borman (Bruxelles: Kiessling, 1931), 3:45–46.

has evidently attracted researchers' interest.[42] Since such institutions did not exist during the Middle Ages, medievalists have historically paid little attention to this question, up to this day.[43] Nonetheless, this raises the important question of the development of the state's protective role, both in favour of its military servants and of its subjects who feared the herds of vagrant veterans. Current research suggests that during the Late Middle Ages, this was not a primary concern for rulers and their officers, except for some clearly delimited cases. Even if the latter were then involved in the "Genesis of the Modern State," they did not feel compelled to provide protection to individuals who had been injured in service. The fact that permanent armies only emerged in the second half of the period considered in this book implies that contracts between soldiers and their rulers were mostly temporary. The former may thus rely on other support tools once demobilized or unable to continue to engage in combat, leaving the state or the ruler unencumbered with the responsibility of providing such support.

As demonstrated by these examples, specialists in premodern military and disability studies integrated or exploited diverse disciplinary contributions: history, archaeology, literature, and modern medicine. This combination provides compelling evidence that future research in the field of Disability and War must be interdisciplinary and comparative in nature. At a heuristic level, the papers gathered in this volume argue for the utilization of a wide variety of sources. Although narrative and literary sources are the most readily available, scholars have demonstrated for a long time that they are not enough to support proper research in military or disability history. Their preoccupation with exceptionality and their socially and politically biased interpretation of the events they recall poses significant challenges. Sources more concerned with day-to-day management prove essential to overcome this obstacle. Account books and normative and judicial texts offer regular insights into the attitude towards disability. We discover the methods by which payments of wages or the hiring of surgeons were pursued (sometimes with the mention of the results of their actions), as well as how warriors were selected. Finally, material artefacts—that is to say, bones, prostheses and, although not discussed in this book, adapted weapons—shed light on the lives of people

**42** Jean-Pierre Bois, "Les soldats invalides au XVIII^e^ siècle: Perspectives nouvelles," *Histoire, économie et société* 1 (1982): 237–58.

**43** They mostly address this question in passing, as did Christophe Masson in *Des guerres en Italie avant les Guerres d'Italie: Les entreprises militaires dans la Péninsule à l'époque du Grand Schisme d'Occident* (Rome: École française de Rome, 2014), 423–26.

expected to have become disabled but who continued to engage in warfare despite their sometimes severe injuries. In this perspective, interdisciplinarity must be associated with a wide range of primary materials.

## Through Warriors' Lives: How Injuries Became Disabilities, or Not

Building on the findings of previous research, this volume is structured around three key themes. *Becoming disabled* focuses on how medieval society labelled battlefield injuries and trauma suffered by warriors as disabilities. *Surviving (Heavy) Injuries* highlights the ways in which people physically or mentally marked by their war experience were integrated into their communities, contributed to society at large, and shaped their identities, revealing their agency in the process. It also sheds light on the responsibility of deeming one eligible for campaigning, and the institutional process by which this happened. Finally, *Managing Disabilities* examines the strategies employed by disabled individuals to navigate their post-injury lives, as well as the social and institutional (including religious[44]) supports that allowed them to endure in a challenging environment. These three themes correspond to pivotal moments in the lives of medieval soldiers: the experience of being injured in warfare and combat, the personal and social reaction to such injuries, and the societal management of wounded and traumatized veterans.

### Becoming Disabled

A number of pivotal instances were identified that either precipitated the transition from injury to disability, or impeded such a transition from occurring on a systematic basis. First and foremost, a recurring trend in warfare

**44** While religion undoubtedly shaped medieval conceptions of the body and suffering, this volume does not aim to apply the "religious model" of disability (as developed by Edward Wheatley, *Stumbling Blocks before the Blind: Medieval Constructions of a Disability* [Ann Arbor: University of Michigan Press, 2010]) as such. As recent scholarship has shown, theological interpretations were often flexible, situational, and coexisted with other social logics; but people were also able to act and "ascribe new meaning to pain, suffering, and marginalization through their own lived religious experience" (Karen McCluskey, Louise St. Guillaume, and Daniela Da Silva, "Ability and Disability in the Pictorial *Vitae* of Beata Fina in Fifteenth-Century San Gimignano," in *The Routledge Companion to Disability and Art*, eds. Keri Watson and Timothy W. Hiles (London: Routledge, 2022), 94–114, esp. 95). The essays collected in this volume approach disability as embedded in broader contexts (legal, medical, literary, and material) where religious meaning may be implicit but not necessarily dominant in shaping the treatment of impaired soldiers or their lived experience.

is the care taken in the selection of warriors. Regularly, archival documents thoroughly recorded who was deemed fit to fight (i.e., the "able-bodied" individuals), and who was not. Commanders were allowed to dismiss warriors they deemed disabled, before or during campaigns, as documentation testifies. Such a concern is illustrated by early thirteenth-century normative sources. In 1215, the Fourth Lateran Council reinforced the conditions for fulfilling vows, while in the meantime Innocent III enunciated the reasons for being deemed incapable of fighting when authorizing to commute a vow of—armed—pilgrimage to the Holy Land.[45] A few decades later, by a letter issued on May 31, 1265, Pope Clement IV granted Count Bouchard V of Vendôme the money paid by those deemed "unfit" to join the fight in the Near East, which allows us to understand who they were:

> We, moved by your supplications, in order for you to more easily and effectively fulfil your vow, cede to you as a gift, as a financial compensation for the said tithe, the legacies destined to support the said Holy Land and the subsidies coming from certain persons—that is to say elderly people, clerics, sick persons, women, and others who are unfit to fight—who cannot or do not want to personally come to the Holy Land to rescue it, but who nonetheless desire through sending certain sums of money [to be] participants of the indulgence granted by the general council in aid of the said Holy Land.[46]

In this context, with the exception of clerics and women, one was seen as unable to fight when old, sick, or (physically) impaired (as we believe the word *inhabiles* refers to this last situation), which left open the possibility to fight with injuries. As crusades were holy wars, and not mere pilgrimages, and since the Council of Lateran IV in 1215 and Pope Innocent III's decision

**45** On the Crusaders' vows, see Alain Demurger, *Croisades et croisés au Moyen Âge* (Paris: Flammarion, 2011), 70–71.

**46** Our emphasis. Vatican City, Archivio Apostolico Vaticano (AAV), Reg. Vat. 32, fol. 14r. Edouard Jordan, ed., *Les registres de Clément IV (1265–1268): Recueil des bulles de ce pape* (Paris: Thorin, 1893), 20, no. 80: "Nos itaque tuis supplicationibus inclinati, ut facilius et efficacius exequi valeas votum tuum, in recompensationem predicte decime tibi auctoritate presentium indulgemus, ut redemptiones et legata hujusmodi predicte terre sancte subsidio deputata, et obventiones a quibuscunque provenientes, personis videlicet senibus, clericis, valitudinariis, mulieribus, et personis aliis, que sunt inhabiles ad pugnandum, queque non possunt nec volunt in prefate terre sancte succursum personaliter proficisci, desiderant tamen, mittendo illuc certas pecuniarum summas, participes fieri indulgentie que subvenientibus predicte terre sancte in generali concilio est concessa." The addressee of the letter did indeed go on the Eighth Crusade of 1270 alongside Louis IX. He died of the plague in Tunis in 1271. Dominique Barthélemy, *La société dans le comté de Vendôme: De l'an mil au XIVe siècle* (Paris: Fayard, 1993), 820.

promised salvation to the crusaders through the full remission of their sins,[47] they implied a penitential dimension.[48] The pontifical administration thus had to clearly delineate who could enjoy a full indulgence for past sins despite not actually fighting in the Holy Land. The petition (*petitio*) was the foundational process, where individuals humbly sought the pope's benevolent intervention, acknowledging their own incapacity or weakness. As a hegemonic cultural practice, supplication reinforced papal authority while allowing petitioners to shape their own identities through their appeals. Thus, this substitution process of financial rather than personal support highlights a conception of incapacity linked to physical ability and not associated with economic or social criteria. On the contrary, when unable to fulfil the initial vow to fight the infidels, one purchased crusading vows to secure the indulgence promised to those who go to battle. Consequently, they became advantageous to the crusade, despite their incapacity to engage in combat, as the financial resources were utilized to support the war effort. This was so extensive that the income from the commutation of the crusade vow resulted in numerous monetary transactions and the establishment of the "indulgence trade," as asserted by Alain Boureau.[49] These questions about the "functionality" or "usefulness" of the impaired person are also found in other religious traditions, notably in the Quran, where the person viewed as "unable/disabled" is exempted from going to battle.[50]

It is thus even more striking that normative military sources—as opposed to pontifical decrees regarding indulgences and customary practices—paid no attention to disability. Historians have long recognized the exhaustive nature of the Burgundian ordinances issued in the 1470s by Duke Charles the Bold, through which he established the core of a standing army. However, not a single line of these sources was dedicated to physical or mental status, not to mention disabilities, of the men-at-arms, footmen, and archers whose equipment was so meticulously described.[51] The earlier French ordi-

**47** Jean Richard, "L'indulgence de croisade et le pèlerinage en Terre Sainte," in *Il Concilio di Piacenza e le crociate* (Piacenza: Tip.Le.Co, 1996), 213–23, especially p. 220.

**48** Demurger, *Croisades et croisés*, 132–33.

**49** Alain Boureau, "Le vœu, la dette et le contrôle pontifical des échanges au début du XIIIe siècle," *Annales: Histoire, sciences sociales* 67, no. 2 (2012): 417–49.

**50** Henri-Jacques Stiker, *Corps infirmes et sociétés: Essais d'anthropologie historique*, 3rd ed. (Paris: Dunod, 2005), 22, citing Sura 24, verse 60, and Sura 48.

**51** Fabien Delpu, "Aux sources d'une armée permanente: Édition critique et commentaire des ordonnances militaires de Charles le Téméraire (1471–1476)" (Thèse, École des Chartes, 2013).

nances—specifically those of 1439 and 1445—exhibited a consistent pattern, although the former was never implemented in full, with only certain provisions being adopted.[52]. This pattern was also evident in late medieval Icelandic literature (Tirosh) or German autobiographies (Frohne). Similarly, we note that fifteenth-century noble Castilian authors writing about warfare did not mention disabled fighters. This does not mean that they did not exist, but that their physical peculiarities counted less than their ability to fight. However, it also appears that the same writers celebrated the fact of dying "intact." They also despised the ones who survived injuries and were unable to perform military duties because of the consequences of surgical interventions, such as amputation.[53] More generally, as the cases of Renaissance Italy testify, critics who assimilated injured warriors to incapacitated leaders or fighters were predominantly non-combatants or individuals hostile to the leaders or fighters about whom they spoke or wrote. From their bearers' point of view, it was imperative that an injury was recognized as such, without any superfluous stigmatizations.

The fundamental question pertains to the precise interpretation of the term "intact." It seems clear that medieval warriors boasted of their injuries, first to emphasize their experience, but also because facing and overcoming risks constituted an integral aspect of their identity. Fifteenth-century Italian captains exhibited wounds as proofs of valour.[54] The man known as "Towton 16," thanks to Christopher Knüsel's work, exhibited through a considerable part of his life the marks of an impressive blow on the left side of his face. Despite the possibility that the individual previously had a beard or subsequently grew one in order to conceal it, the mark was nonetheless unmistakable.[55] This helps us to understand and confirm the veracity of the otherwise intriguing habit of medieval chroniclers to recall the participation

---

**52** *Construire l'armée française: Textes fondateurs des institutions militaires*, vol. 1, *De la France des premiers Valois à la fin du règne de François Ier*, ed. Valérie Bessey (Turnhout: Brepols, 2006), 88–105, and Stéphane Péquignot, "De la France à Barcelone: Une version catalane de 'l'ordonnance perdue' de Charles VII sur les gens d'armes (1445)," *Revue historique* 317, no. 4 (2015): 824–28.

**53** Daniel Baloup, *L'homme armé: Expériences de la guerre et du combat en Castille au xve siècle* (Madrid: Casa de Velázquez, 2022), 244.

**54** We owe these last two elements relating to Italy to Giulia Morosini's webinar presentation. On her work, see Giulia Morosini, "Manly Virtues, Emotions, and Scars: Competition among Italian Renaissance Soldiers through Bodily Practices," in *Gender and Status Competition in Pre-Modern Societies*, eds. Martha Bayless et al. (Turnhout: Brepols, 2021), 79–107.

**55** Even though the beard was quite negatively considered at the time. Jean-Marie

of warriors who previously lost the use of an eye, an arm, or a leg. In addition to proving their experience to their peers, it asserted that they were capable of overcoming what would be "disabling" for less worthy people and that they had retain their ability to fight.[56] The fact that the sums of money given/paid by Burgundian princes to veterans was proportionate to the financial losses incurred by their disabilities highlights the pivotal role that the capacity to fulfil one's duty played in the conceptualization of disability (Depreter). There was thus an evident desire to distinguish oneself from the rest of the population, implying that the latter was less worthy and strong (and thus less masculine?) and more closely associated with the masses than with the military elite (Verreycken).

We argue that medieval warriors, irrespective of their rank, consciously did not associate serious injuries with disability. This also means that they had a clear understanding of what disability was, and that this understanding was precisely why they took great care to describe it as rarely as possible. For the nobility, gentry, and more largely for the commoners who regularly went to war, the quintessential definition of disability was the inability to fulfil one's rank. It was imperative to demonstrate one's ability, regardless of the nature and number of obstacles encountered. Premodern armies allowed a wide range of profiles to join them. This changed with the advent of modern armies, which were built on the principle of efficiency, essentially fuelled by uniformity. Pain and prosthesis were thus admissible if they enabled the overcoming of physical deficiencies. We witness the same kind of reasoning in pardon letters. Supplicants emphasized how much they suffered in the service of their prince, while defending the idea that a proper warrior must be able to overcome anything. Cynically enough, we could also consider that by systematically mentioning that they were attacked and did not initiate the fight for which they asked pardon, supplicants not only complied with court expectations but also demonstrated their ability to overcome assaults and injuries.

---

Le Gall, *Un idéal masculin: Barbes et moustaches, XV^e–XVIII^e siècles. Suivi de "Le barbu ou Dialogue sur la barbe" d'Antoine Hotman* (Paris: Payot, 2011).

**56** This follows a common pattern of fear management, see the papers of Benjamin Deruelle, "Contrôler l'incontrôlable: Perception et contrôle du sentiment de la peur au combat chez les hommes de guerre du XVI^e siècle," and Christophe Masson, "Des chevaliers irréfléchis: Peur et témérité dans les traités d'art militaire (c. 1330–c. 1530)," in *Le feu et la folie: L'irrationnel et la guerre de la fin du Moyen Âge à 1920*, eds. Marion Trévisi and Laurent Vissière (Rennes: Presses universitaires de Rennes, 2016), 101–12, and 113–31.

Another point to address is the permanence of disability. The knight Thibaud de Beloczac, who took an active part in Brittany's fourteenth-century civil war, is said to have remained severely and incurably wounded in his shinbone by an enemy sword for twenty years, before being healed by the miraculous intervention of a deceased—yet on his way to canonization—Charles of Blois in 1367. Thibaud might not have had a disability, as his injury and its consequences are not mentioned in his statement gathered in the canonization process.[57] However, medieval authors underlined how fear, as well as chronic or intense pain, may have caused disabilities (Frohne).

Medieval warriors made a significant distinction between their body and soul. While they recognized that any part of the former could be hurt—which could lead to permanent disabilities—they regarded the latter as a completely different matter. As Kristina Hildebrand records, mad knights did not become so because of traumatic battles, but because of love sorrow. A great number of sources have attributed the love-madness experienced by warriors to harsh captivity, rather than to physical injuries. Morally and physically induced disabilities were considered as different, as Honorat Bovet stated clearly in his *Arbre des batailles* (Turner). Most remission letters that argued that war had been a catalyst for mental disturbances referred to cases of non-combatants (Pfau). This implicitly suggests the existence of a specific cultural trait. A warrior should not be moved by what he experiences on a regular basis—i.e., martial context and its accidents—as this would go against his identity and deprive him of his social status. Additionally, one may consider that his social milieu, within which he was intended to share his experience of warfare, could have played a role in processing the events experienced. This difficulty in sharing traumatic experiences within one's family is indeed indicated as one of the elements explaining the high rates of veterans suffering from PTSD in modern times.[58] It is noteworthy that chroniclers placed significant emphasis on the role that military stress and the discomfort of wearing armour played in the first of Charles VI of France's mental crises (Pfau). This possibly served to reinforce the argument for the sovereign's unfitness, particularly in light of his pronounced predilection for chivalric culture. Additionally, human interventions—that is military or knightly solidarity—was to cure the mental distress caused by love, or dramatic social interactions (Hildebrand). On the other hand, in the event of a

---

**57** Jenni Kuuliala, "Nobility, Community and Physical Impairment in Later Medieval Canonization Processes," in *Infirmity in Antiquity and the Middle Ages*, eds. Christian Krötzl et al. (Farnham: Ashgate, 2015), 67–82.

**58** Pauline Maucort, *La guerre et après…* (Paris: Les Belles-Lettres, 2017).

warrior (i.e., a dominant male) becoming "insane," he was required to relinquish his "natural" authority over his family and earthly possessions, as well as his political and judicial powers, as their legitimacy was questioned on account of the social disturbance that it caused. This explains why the English crown (Turner) and other princely powers acted to protect such landholders from the thirteenth century onwards.[59] Mental disability dissolved the community of warriors on campaigns, social organization "at home," and even threatens the kingdom when striking the ruler.[60]

Disability was a divisive marker between combatants and non-combatants that contributed to re-establish a social division that the sole possession of a feudal title could no longer generate.

## Surviving (Heavy) Injuries

The juxtaposition of these contrasting situations enables us to understand, and not only from the silence of the sources, that determining who was fit to fight was also a decision made on an individual level. For instance, a papal bull dated January 28, 1306, reveals that Clement V granted Robert, Count of Clermont-en-Beauvaisis (present-day Clermont-sur-Oise), a dispensation from his vow to undertake a pilgrimage to the Holy Land, citing his inability to do so as the reason for the dispensation.[61] Robert was the sixth son of Louis IX and Marguerite of Provence. He suffered from dementia from 1279 onwards, following a blow to the head.[62] Although he could still manage his duchy, Robert still suffered from evident aftereffects, as evidenced by his decision to avoid tournaments and his inability to lead campaigns. He was no longer able to compete with the ideal of crusades that his father, Louis IX, had so fervently promoted. Therefore, he sought to change his vow while

---

**59** Maud Ternon, *Juger les fous au Moyen Âge dans les tribunaux royaux en France: XIV^e^–XV^e^ siècles* (Paris: Presses universitaires de France, 2018), 107–12.

**60** See Bernard Guenée, *La folie de Charles VI, roi bien-aimé* (Paris: Perrin, 2004), who nonetheless underscored how a king's madness could be and have been used to strengthen the State.

**61** In exchange, the supplicant must pay ten thousand livres of "good money" to those who will fulfil his vow in his place. Paris, Archives nationales de France, P $1377^1$, no. 2760; AAV, Reg. Vat. 52, fol. 106r: Clement V to Robert, Count of Clermont, January 28, 1306 (abstract in *Regestum Clementis papae V* [Rome: Typographia Vaticana, 1885], 111, no. 610).

**62** Jules Roy, "Corrections et additions à l'histoire de Robert de Clermont, sixième fils de Saint Louis, tige de la maison ducale et royale de Bourbon," *Annuaire de l'École pratique des hautes études* 32, no. 1 (1899): 5–20.

lamenting his inability to contribute to the liberation of the Holy Land from Muslim rule.[63]

The papal chancery proved to be as systematic with granting indulgences and spiritual benefits to those dispensed from going to the Holy Land as it was with addressing the resulting impact on the bodies of combatants who fought for the Christian faith. This is particularly evident in the case of Laurence de Beaumont [*Bellomonte*], a cleric of the diocese of Viviers, who received a letter from the Avignon pope Clement VII, (most probably ante-) dated from November 29, 1378:

> *Item* Laurence of Beaumont, a cleric of the Diocese of Viviers—who lost his left hand and one eye while fighting against the Saracens, enemies of the Catholic faith, alongside certain Christian nobles in the overseas territories, as testify letters of witnesses he held with him—is unable to support himself, nor be properly maintained, nor be promoted to sacred orders due to the loss of his hand, having no temporal property from which he can be provided with what he needs. He therefore requests an ecclesiastical benefice without cure of souls, either complete or divided, collated by the archbishop, the dean, the chapter, as well as by each of the canons individually, or the *personatores* of the [Cathedral] Church of Sens, even if this means a hospital, a Maison-Dieu, or a leprosarium, notwithstanding the mutilation of his hand and the loss of his eye. Like above [for the papal agreement procedure and the issue date].[64]

The violence of the confrontations and their impact on the bodily integrity of combatants appear to be a frequent cause of disability. Indeed, the brutality of war led to numerous injuries, approximately a quarter of which affected the upper limbs, as in the case of Laurence, who also lost an

---

**63** On the importance of the crusade in nobles' memoirs, see Nicholas Paul, *To Follow in Their Footsteps: The Crusades and Family Memory in the High Middle Ages* (Ithaca: Cornell University Press, 2017).

**64** AAV, Reg. Suppl. 55, fol. 223v: "Item Laurencius de Bellomonte, clericus Vivariensis diocesis, qui dudum in societate quorumdam nobiliorum Christianorum in partibus ultramarinis exitus contra Sarracenos, fidei catholice dimicos, debelerando manum sinistram et occulum amisit, ut apperet per litteras testimoniales quas secum defert, propter quod victum suum acquerere non potest, nec alias commode sustentari, nec ad sacros ordines promoverit propter amissionem manus predictam, cum in bonis temporalibus non habeat unde sibi necessaria possit ministrari; quot sibi de beneficio ecclesiastico sine cura, specialiter communiter uel divisis, ad collationem etc. archiepiscopi, decani et capituli singulorumque canonicarum et per[sonnatorum] ecclesie Senonensis, ectiam si sit hospitale vel domus Dei seu leprosaria dignari providere, non obstantibus dicta sue manus mutilacione et dicti sui oculi amissione ac cum allis non obstantibus, ut supra."

eye.[65] These mutilations represented serious conditions according to medieval surgeons, who found regular descriptions of treatments for injuries in the literature they consulted. As noted earlier, the incapacity of *bellatores* rarely appears in historical works. The sources used to discuss nobility often overlook their disabilities, focusing instead on their war exploits. In the example above, as well as in general, the papal chancery is interested in the daily consequences of injuries, in this case of a person who, despite being associated with nobles, does not appear to belong to the wealthiest strata of lay society. For those who were neither noble nor wealthy, a disability could diminish or even suppress their sources of income. In this case, as the mutilation occurred during a crusade or at least a "saintly expedition," the cleric sought to recover a stable and sufficient source of income to ensure his daily subsistence thanks to the intervention of the papal chancery.[66] After an assessment of Laurence's injury, the pope authorized him to receive an income without *cura animarum*, meaning he would not be able to celebrate Mass, but would still have a source of revenue to live with his disability without having to beg for his living.[67] The pope could not admit that a cleric would tarnish ecclesiastical dignity by begging and thus permitted the institution to assimilate individuals who would typically be marginalized within its own ranks.

Upon closer examination of this phenomenon, medieval written sources reveal a preponderance of individuals who, despite having experienced partial or complete healing, continued to engage in military engagements. The veracity of such assertions is corroborated by the findings of archaeology. The capacity of biological anthropologists and bioarchaeologists to differentiate between injuries sustained prior to death (ante mortem) and those that result in fatality (lethal) has been significantly enhanced. This advancement

---

**65** These figures are based on the works of Alain Mounier-Kuhn, "Les blessures de guerre et l'armement au Moyen Âge," and Pierre-André Sigal, "Les coups et blessures reçus par le combattant à cheval en Occident aux XIIe et XIIIe siècles," in *Le combattant au Moyen Âge: XVIIIe congrès de la SHMESP (Montpellier, 1987)* (Paris: Publications de la Sorbonne, 1987), 171–83.

**66** On clerical disability from the point of view of the papal chancery, see Ninon Dubourg, *Disabled Clerics in the Late Middle Ages: Un/suitable for Divine Service?* (Amsterdam: Amsterdam University Press, 2023).

**67** On the physicians' role in the implementation of pontifical graces, see Ninon Dubourg, "*Expertis medicis videatur*: Legal Medical Expertise in the Assessment of Personal Injury Damages by the Apostolic Chancery during the Avignon Period (1309–1378)," in *Art of Illness: Malingering and Inventing Health Conditions*, ed. Wendy J. Turner (London: Routledge, 2023), 207–44.

is evidenced by the analysis of corpses discovered in the vicinity of a battlefield or in burial sites (Knüsel). However partial they were, pardon letters tend to elicit the supposition that the majority of the injured warriors who were still active were the ones with minor injuries. Those afflicted with more severe conditions are significantly less represented in these sources, meaning they may have been excluded from active social life, and thus from these documents. Consequently, a high degree of caution should be exercised when considering the proportion of warriors who became disabled, despite the narratives presented in the majority of sources. Although it may have appeared to contradict the ideals of noble appearance and strength, for medieval people, an injury was not a disability in the context of warfare, even if it might have been seen as such in other social contexts, such as in relationships with family members, neighbours and strangers.[68]

This observation aligns with the fact that the military or the knightly identity was above all determined by social agreement. Rejecting one man because of injuries anyone could suffer during the next battle would put the whole "military body" at stake, as it would have meant renunciation of the cohesive solidarity amongst warriors. Paradoxically enough, while Icelandic literature has almost no specific vocabulary to denote the injured warriors fighting, it exhibits a preoccupation with men who used physical differences to fight, such as a (fake) hunchback relying on his peculiar back to strike his adversaries (Tirosh). It seems that as soon as they allowed their "owner" to fulfil his social role or aspirations, physical peculiarities did not exclude them from the society to which they belonged; on the contrary, they ensured their continued inclusion within it. This situation is comparable to that of prosthesis bearers. Documented by physical evidence only from the fifteenth century onwards, but most probably older, prostheses were not exclusively the privilege of high-ranking individuals. This question of the interface between prostheses and the human body to which they are attached remains to be the subject of more thorough exploration. Scholars have highlighted that middle class warriors who had lost a hand could be equipped with iron hands that prolonged their ability to continue fighting, or to at least appear "complete" in public events, if they could not play a functional role. They could even be painted to evoke skin and flesh helping their bearers maintain their role and identity within the martial community (Frohne, Gagné). Even though medievalists work on sources which rarely openly address gender,

68 Irina Metzler, *A Social History of Disability in the Middle Ages: Cultural Considerations of Physical Impairment* (London: Routledge, 2013), 37–40.

the latter mostly recall male combatants. Their injunction towards overcoming both physical and visual physical limitations to remain able to fight is more likely to be linked with the definition of masculinity. This appears to be a trend common to most of the martial literature of the time, uniting authors such as the fourteenth-century French nobleman Geoffroy de Charny and the early sixteenth-century *landsknechts* (Frohne). Additionally, fighting despite injuries is a statement of one's emotional self-control, a trait that late medieval writers frequently ascribed to men, and more specifically to knights. Conversely, failure to fulfil one's duty was perceived to diminish a man's masculinity (Verreycken).[69] Finally, the social environment for individuals could, for a number of reasons, fail to "cure" disability (Hildebrand) or even exacerbate it (Pfau).

On a comparable level, the chapters of this volume echo another social dimension of warfare. The ability to fight despite being blind, having broken limbs, or exhibiting physical limitations was not exclusive to elite warriors, nor was inability linked to social inferiors. Figures such as Charles VI or Hörðr (Pfau, Tirosh) are two perfect examples of that. This phenomenon is most likely connected to the notable openness exhibited by late medieval military society towards newcomers, provided they aligned with the prevailing chivalric values. In some cases, this went as far as allowing for the literary or actual knighting of commoners.[70] This relative openness also applied to solutions to overcome the consequences of injuries. As the military society apparently recognized the legitimacy and use of prostheses, it promoted a new perception of the body as a machine that could be "restored" through instruments like iron hands (Gagné). This ultimately evokes the mechanization of human behaviour in warfare, a phenomenon which would not be theorized until in the early modern period.

The habit of going into battle when wounded was not proof of sheer folly; it translates the serious concern and interest in one's own health and cures, both before, during, and after a campaign. The Kampen (Overijssel, Netherlands) priest Geert Kuynretorff advised fellow pilgrims in 1520 that "before

---

**69** See for example Kim Berqvist, "Performing Chivalric Masculinity: Morality, Restraint, and Emotional Norms in the *Libro del Cavallero Zifar*," in *Affective and Emotional Economies in Medieval and Early Modern Europe*, eds. Andreea Marculescu and Charles-Louis Morand Métivier (Basingstoke: Palgrave, 2018), 227–46.

**70** Christophe Masson, "Dire l'homme d'armes du XV^e^ siècle: L'exemple des mémoires et biographies chevaleresques franco-bourguignonnes," in *Les mots du militaire*, vol. 3, *Dire et se dire militaire en Occident (XV^e^ –XIX^e^ siècle): De la guerre de Cent ans à l'Entre-deux-guerres*, eds. Benjamin Deruelle et al. (Paris: Publications de la Sorbonne, 2020), 19–34.

[sailing] from Venice, [they should] go to an experienced physician, who can examine [their] condition properly. And [to] let him prescribe [them] various pills and potions, so that [their] constitution may be armed against whatever fever or diarrhoea, or any constipations may befall [them]."[71] The consequences on the crusaders' bodies could vary. In another account dated from 1485–1486, Georges Lengherand tells us that: "because of the great heat that day, the pilgrims were so weakened, faint, and thirsty that most of them fell ill, so much so that, upon [the] arrival at Rames, three hours later, two Germans there gave up their spirits to God."[72] This also applied to warriors. In preparation for his crusade, Duke Philip the Good of Burgundy commissioned two surgeons to compile a comprehensive inventory of surgical instruments and medicinal remedies intended to address the potential diseases that crusaders could face during their undertaking.[73] More largely, retinues usually comprised one or several practitioners, who joined campaigns equipped with their own arsenal of treatments (Knüsel).

## Managing Disabilities

Previous examples show that the determination of one's fitness for combat or pilgrimage in the Middle Ages was closely tied to physical ability and social status. Papal decrees allowed those physically unable to fight, such as the elderly or disabled, to fulfil their Christian duties through financial contributions. This practice ensured their place in Christian society, recognizing a form of spiritual utility despite their physical limitations. The church adapted its expectations to accommodate these individuals, offering alternatives such as the commutation of vows and the granting of absolution and indulgences, ensuring that they could take part in the collective religious effort even if they could not physically engage in combat. Simultaneously, the church could also provide avenues for maintaining dignity and livelihood

---

**71** Geert Kuynretorff, *Jerusalemsche Reyse, soe in verganghen Jaren gheschiedt is* (Kampen: Peter Warnersen, 1555), 27 (kindly translated by Maja Perić, University of Zagreb).

**72** *Voyage de Georges Lengherand, mayeur de Mons en Haynaut, à Venise, Rome, Jérusalem, Mont Sinaï et le Kayre, 1485–1486*, ed. Godefroy Ménilglaise (Mons: Masquillier et Dequesne, 1861), 115.

**73** Rabah Ali Bacha and Laurie Baveye, "Le mauvais côté de la croisade? À propos d'un document établi par les chirurgiens de Philippe le Bon," in "La face noire de la splendeur. Crimes, trahisons et scandales à la cour de Bourgogne aux XIV<sup></sup>e et XVe siècles," eds. Werner Paravicini and Bertrand Schnerb, special issue, *Revue du Nord* 91, no. 2 (2009): 491–510.

through ecclesiastical benefices for those who were injured in battle and left unable to sustain themselves, even when their physical disabilities prevented them from performing full priestly duties. In this way, the church integrated disabled individuals into its institutional fabric, recognizing both their spiritual contributions and the social implications of their disabilities.

The pontifical institution not only included them but also offered them spiritual compensation for taking part in the hostilities. Indeed, those who managed to reach the Holy Land, after a long and perilous journey, earned spiritual benefits in exchange for their travels. Letters called "letters of absolution *in mortis articulo*" (at the point of death) offered plenary absolution from the most serious sins.[74] In most cases, they contain no mention of the petitioner's disability, illness, or old age. The request for absolution is made in a concise manner. However, some of these letters go into detail, revealing the petitioners' concerns about their own salvation. The stakes are high, as these indulgences allow the recipients—living or dead—to quickly save their souls without performing any penance.[75] They were used by the papal chancery to strengthen its ties with the most powerful laymen but also to allow them to die peacefully. These letters could be individual or collective, as in the following case for crusaders dying in the Holy Land. The letter, sent by Urban V to the Hospitallers of St. John of Jerusalem on July 17, 1363, states:

> Inclined to your supplications, [we grant] that a confessor [will] be elected to give full remission of all sins at the point of death, to any of you and your benefactors, slaves, and paid men who are in the same region as you, as well as to other believers in Christ who shall be wounded, or otherwise bruised, and maimed, or crippled, or killed by the hands of unbelievers, in defending their lands and places and property, or in persecuting and attacking such unbelievers, or elsewhere in lawful warfare, public or private, against them.[76]

---

**74** Michel Mollat, *La vie religieuse aux XIV^e^ et XV^e^ siècles* (Paris: Les cours de Sorbonne, 1962), 195.

**75** Arnaud Berard, "L'indulgence jubilaire," *Revue thomiste* 100 (2000): 423–68.

**76** AAV, Reg. Vat. 261, fol. 42v (Reg. Av. 155, fol. 469r), analyzed by François Avril et al., eds., *Urbain V (1362–1370): Lettres communes analysées d'après les registres dits d'Avignon et du Vatican* (Paris: Bibliothèque des Écoles françaises de Rome et d'Athènes, 1954), no. 6 419, of which we give the transcription from the register: "Vestris supplicationibus inclinati ut confessor quam quilibet vestrum ac eorumdem donatorum, servitorum et stipendiariorum qui in eisdem partibus vos et alios christi fideles necnon vos et ipsorum fidelium terras ac loca et bona defendendo aut eosdem infideles persequendo et offendendo, aut alias in bello legitimo, publico vel privato cum infidelibus eisdem commisso vel etiam postea ex ipso tamen bello vulnerati seu alias lesi et debilitati seu infirmitati aut alias in manibus infidelium eorumdem

The letter has a broad penitential scope. It is addressed to the master and brothers of the order, as well as to *conversi* (lay brothers), servants, and warriors in their employ. We learn that they will automatically receive full remission from their sins if they are wounded in the Holy Land at the hands of infidels. The crusade then replaced the usual penances, allowing men, women, children, free or enslaved, to benefit from a broader salvation in exchange for their participation in the liberation of the Holy Land—whether through financial contributions or by making the journey in person and fighting to extend Christian influence in those lands.

This inclusive and "rewarding" attitude towards disability found resonance within secular governments. In 1425, a prince such as Philip the Good, Duke of Burgundy, could appoint an amputee veteran as castellan of Beveren to compensate for his inability to continue campaigning.[77] The question remains as to know to what extent these kinds of decisions were customary, and whether they depended on circumstances, such as being closely connected with a lord or being part of potent networks of power. Sources argue that the social and moral protection enjoyed by warriors during their service stopped as soon as the army—if it was not permanent—was demobilized. This is probably also because of those situations in which the petitioners asked for support from the prince after the end of a campaign (Verreycken). This also provides a framework for an inquiry into the self-perception of the state, the principality, or the prince. Did the officers and servants of the institution in question consider their responsibility to ensure the well-being of those who suffered while serving under their prince's authority? Did this care also serve to strengthen a sense of belonging, and thus contribute to the development of the "modern," centralized state that is often encountered in institutional developments?

To date, studies have emphasized that late medieval rulers did not organize extensive systems of care for injured fighters but did for injured artists, with the duke of Burgundy paying a pension to an artist because of *sa debilitacion et vieillesse* ("his disability and old age").[78] However, Wendy J. Turner

decesseritis seu decesserint duxerit eligendum omnium peccatorum vestrorum et ipsorum de quibus corde contrici et ore confessi fueritis seu fuerint semel tamen in mortis articulo plenam remissionem."

**77** Latin de Coninglant in 1425. Kevin Poschet and Bart Verwerft, "De Vlaamse burchtvoogd: Een grafelijke pion op het politieke schaakbord? Casus Beveren, Rupelmonde en Saaftinge (*ca.* 1300–1550)," *Revue belge de philologie et d'histoire* 100 (2022): 941–1004.

**78** Federica Veratelli, *À la mode italienne: Commerce du luxe et diplomatie dans les*

has emphasized the existence of a care system dedicated to certain former warriors in England, and Michael Depreter has highlighted how pensions could occasionally be granted to veterans, especially those belonging to the prince's hotel. Scholars usually attribute this situation to the incomplete nature of a medieval state which would not *yet* assume responsibility for the welfare of its citizens. This is probably too teleologic a view. One should bear in mind that medieval armies were micro-societies of their own. They were built to take care of themselves and their components. A captain's main duty was to keep the people serving him as fit and safe as they could be by ensuring they had access to food, drinks, pastoral care, and thus medical support. In accordance with this, it would make no sense for him to delegate the care of the injured and disabled to the prince he was serving. Additionally, following the conclusion of their military campaign, warriors returned to their regular occupations and social networks. This meant a return to solidarity systems, whether familial or professional. For instance, the Flemish guilds provided surgical care to their members to prevent fatalities and the onset of permanent disabilities, a system Duke Charles of Burgundy seemed to have wished to challenge (Depreter).

A further consideration is that medieval fighters were likely to be reluctant to acknowledge their own disability, even if this entailed their prince providing them with a pension. To a certain extent, it could be argued that a pension for injuries equated to a public mark for disability. This correlation between injuries and money could serve as a venue for future research into theories and practices of early modern disabilities. This was evidently concomitant with the fact that warriors were very much aware how slow princely treasuries could be in paying army wages. No pensions were awarded by princes to disabled warriors—with some exceptions, such as Burgundian or Venetian gunners because one did not wish to see their expertise going to a rival (Depreter, Gagné)—as responsibility for the disabled was considered to depend on guilds. One might consider that it was only once the armies underwent a steady rise in their size and were composed of an ever-larger proportion of commoners that captains had to let the state, or the principality, develop its own system of care for disabled warriors. On a parallel note, it is worth mentioning that archaeology has shed light on a trend towards blows that were deliberately lethal. The battlefields that have been scrutinized are quite rare and distant in place and time, which should preclude

*Pays-Bas méridionaux (1477–1530). Édition critique de documents de la Chambre des comptes de Lille* (Villeneuve-d'Ascq-Lille: Presses universitaires du Septentrion–Archives départementales du Nord, 2013), 306, no. 120.

excessive generalization. However, figures point toward a progressive diminution of infra-cranial injuries simultaneously with an increase in cranio-facial wounds. This phenomenon may be connected with the evolution of the late medieval "military society," which comprised an increasing number of non-noble combatants who could not be exchanged for ransoms and were therefore potentially perceived as more expendable than other individuals. Moreover, this may have led to an increase in mental trauma cases (Knüsel). This increased necessity for a care system may explain why such institutions appeared exclusively during the early modern period, and why their absence during the Middle Ages does not signify more rudimentary societal considerations for disability.

* * *

In order to foster dialogue between diverse case studies, we have chosen not to formally divide the volume into sections. It was impossible to assign each chapter to one of the three key themes outlined in the introduction, as all these themes emerge organically across the essays. The complexity of the lived experiences of medieval disabled soldiers rarely allows for the full reconstruction of an individual's life trajectory to be traced, from the event that caused the impairment to its aftermath and the ways they coped with it in daily life. The collection begins with an exploration of the physical evidence of combat injuries (Knüsel); moves into literary representations of disability in Icelandic sagas (Tirosh) and Middle English Arthurian romance (Hildebrand); and continues with an examination of criminal (Verreycken), historical, legal, and medical archives (Pfau, Turner). The final three chapters cover German-language traumatological and autobiographical narratives (Frohne); the visual, textual, and physical significance of the iron hand prosthesis (Gagné); and the support provided to veterans in the Burgundian Low Countries (Depreter). This arrangement allows for recurring motifs (visibility of wounds, negotiation of identity, role of institutions) to surface across disciplines and documentation. Indeed, by drawing on a wide range of sources (historical, archaeological, literary, legal, medical, and material), the essays collected here not only showcase the methodological diversity required to study war-related disability in the Late Middle Ages but also engage in a sustained conversation across disciplinary boundaries. The structure of the volume thus reflects our intention to foster this dialogue between military and disability history by allowing interpretative paradigms and research questions to emerge from the intersections and resonances between individual contributions, rather than by forcing a rigid thematic compartmentalization onto the subject.

Chapter 1

# THE RECIDIVISTS

## HEALED CRANIAL TRAUMA FROM CONFLICTS IN THE LATE MEDIEVAL PERIOD

CHRISTOPHER J. KNÜSEL

**Glossary:** *Antemortem wound/injury*: a traumatic injury preceding death with evidence of bone reaction related to bone remodelling (healing), a testament to survival after injury for a variable period of time.

*Perimortem wound/injury*: a traumatic injury sustained around the time of death, without signs of bone remodelling (healing) of the site of injury. Death may have occurred just before or immediately after receiving the wound, with the bone retaining its collagen (i.e., protein component) and thus its flexibility and capacity for remodelling even after death for a period of time.

*Post-mortem breaks/breakage*: breakage of bone that occurs when a bone has lost much of its collagen and thus which breaks based on its more rigid crystalline hydroxyapatite constituent. This type of breakage is also referred to as "recent" or "new" and occurs when the bone is said to be "dry," lacking in collagen, and occurs after death when collagen is no longer replenished and bone can no longer remodel.

**CHRISTOPHER J. KNÜSEL**, Professor of Biological Anthropology, Université de Bordeaux, addresses past social relations from a bioarchaeological perspective, specifically violence and warfare and activity-related skeletal changes. With Martin J. Smith, he is co-editor of, and contributor to, *The Routledge Handbook of the Bioarchaeology of Human Conflict* (2014); with Eline M. J. Schotsmans, he co-edited and contributed to *The Routledge Handbook of Archaeothanatology* (2022).
Christopher Knüsel thanks the EVODIBIO (Évolution et diversité biologique) research team, UMR 5199 PACEA, Université de Bordeaux, for financial assistance to attend the colloquium in Liège organized by the editors in November 2024.

ALTHOUGH HISTORY IS replete with violent encounters that often provide the framework for historical accounts, the physical evidence for conflict is rare. Moreover, due to their often unrecorded and unmarked state, human remains relating to violent encounters are often unanticipated and only comparatively few have received study to date. Even when studied, the remains are frequently only a part or one of several deposits of human remains excavated and analyzed from sites associated with violent encounters. The absence of physical evidence is also due to the complex nature of commingled remains, which have often lost their original skeletal integrity due to taphonomic changes that occur after burial and later disturbance. Incomplete recovery and former archaeological practices also play a role, especially for remains collected in the period prior to training in human osteology and bioarchaeology, a comparatively recent development of the late twentieth century (see, for example, Cunha and Silva 1997 for the Battle of Aljubarrota, Portugal, 1385).[1] Bones from older studies, typically more than thirty-five years ago, not only deteriorate through lengthy storage but are often sorted by element and individual skeletons are no longer discernible. This hinders research on wounds and, especially, wound patterning in individuals.

Stylized depictions of soldiery are common elements of treatments of warfare in the past, but these are often based on artistic renditions that postdate events by considerable time, more akin to the array of brightly coloured toy soldiers than reflective of the reality of war and its aftermath, including dead and wounded combatants. There are very few eye-witness battlefield depictions (although Hildebrand, in this volume, alludes to the potential impact of author Thomas Malory's presence at Towton on the text of *Le Morte Darthur*), paintings, drawings, or descriptions for the period up to the nineteenth century and the pioneering photographs of Alexander Gardner, an associate of the celebrated nineteenth-century photographer Mathew Brady. Gardner's photographs of the dead after the Battle of Antietam (September 1861), near Sharpsburg, Maryland, USA, were the first graphic battlefield images—complete with bodies—ever printed, appearing in *Harper's Weekly* on October 18, 1862,[2] the field of battle being deserted for a period of time prior to its eventual "cleaning up." There are no accounts of the state of the corpses and little notion of treatments until that time, these being

---

1 Eugenia Cunha and Ana Maria Silva, "War Lesions from the Famous Portuguese Medieval Battle of Aljubarrota," *International Journal of Osteoarchaeology* 7, no. 6 (December 2008): 595–99.

2 Mary Panzer, *Mathew Brady and the Image of History* (Washington: Smithsonian, 1997), 107–9, Figures 7.6–7.9.

associated with the work of individuals who rarely left accounts of their activities and treatments. The publications in the sixteenth century of Ambroise Paré, barber-surgeon to four French kings, remain shining exceptions.[3]

The nineteenth century marks a critical turning point in perspectives of war with the founding of the Red Cross inspired by the writings of Jean-Henri Dunant after the Battle of Solferino, June 24, 1859, a decisive encounter in Italy's Reunification under King Victor Emmanuel II. Dunant had been horrified by the sight of dead and dying soldiers left on the field of battle in its aftermath. It was these scenes of misery and neglect that inspired him to write *Un souvenir de Solferino*,[4] which culminated in the establishment of the Geneva Conventions and the founding of the Red Cross that mandated the humane treatment of the injured of war. Before this milestone, there were developments contributed by some literate and many more unnamed and illiterate practitioners that left their legacy in the form of healed injuries recorded in skeletal remains from the past. This contribution considers four medieval population samples dating from the High and Late Middle Ages, from three sites: two from the parish church-cum-monastery Fishergate site in York, England, another from the 1520 Långfredags-slaget (Battle of Good Friday), Uppsala, Sweden, that pitted a Swedish peasant army against a Danish mercenary garrison force of the Danish king Kristian II in Uppsala Castle, and the last from the 1461 Battle of Towton (Yorkshire, England), a defining encounter of the Wars of the Roses (see Table 1.1 below), previously studied for bodily injury patterning. The head (cranium and mandible) was clearly targeted, as attested by perimortem injuries (those inflicted around the time of death) from which only a minority recovered (Knüsel 2014). It is the latter, those that show evidence of survival in the form of healed wounds from these sites, that are the focus of this contribution.

A reflection of the increasing awareness of casualties of conflict later in the nineteenth century came with the publication of the Surgeon General of the United States of America Joseph K. Barnes's 1870 account *The Medical and Surgical History of the War of the Rebellion (1861–65)*, which forms another important milestone in the treatment of casualties of conflict. Based

**3** Philippe Bonnichon, Athénaïs Pion, and Marine Fontaine, "Ambroise Paré, père de la chirurgie française," *Histoire des sciences médicales* 5 (2023): 69–76; Christopher J. Knüsel, "The Unwritten History of Medical Treatment: Evidence for Ritual-healers and their Activities in the Pre-literate Past," *International Journal of Paleopathology* 34 (September 2021): 206–16; see also in this volume Gagné and Frohne for early orthopaedic innovations and Depreter for accounts originating from fourteenth- to the early sixteenth-century Burgundy.

**4** Henri Dunant, *Un souvenir de Solferino* (Paris: Croix-Rouge Française, 2014).

on numerous accounts of the treatment of the wounded by field medics before, during and after evacuation to hospitals, in addition to some follow-up medical information, this lengthy report provides a wealth of information on the types and the circumstances by which wounds were sustained, as well as detailed descriptions of injuries, the outcomes of remedial surgery and the extent of disabilities, physical and mental. At the time, the goal of these reports was both to determine the extent of pensionable disability and to better understand the efficacy of treatments and surgical procedures. It offers insights into the effect of injuries on behaviour and the mental health consequences of them, especially those affecting the head. These detailed accounts provide insight into the potential effects of weapon-related injuries in the deeper past and their consequences for the physical and mental health of the injured. The themes of this book, notably becoming disabled, surviving (heavy) injuries, and managing disabilities, can be addressed with variable success, the most tractable being survival of heavy injuries from the analysis of human remains and, in conjunction with texts, they provide a measure of insight into the extent and management of disability. More recent medical case studies provide insight into the physical and mental consequences of wounds that can be retrodicted into the past. This subject will be revisited in the conclusion.

## Perimortem (Unhealed) Wounds

Perimortem wounds, predominantly found on crania from the medieval study sites presented above—from 18 to as much as 89 percent of inflicted wounds—were often fatal, and survival was not a common outcome. Cranial wounds were especially deadly, and their repeated occurrence suggests lethal intent on the part of assailants. From a general survey of the injuries sustained, these indicate that training and targeting of specific parts of the body played a role in aggressive encounters in the medieval period.[5] From medieval fight-books, training manuals for aspiring warrior combatants using various specialized weapons, such as that of the fifteenth-century Master of Arms Hans Talhoffer,[6] the torso is the most often indicated tar-

5 Christopher J. Knüsel, "Courteous Knights and Cruel Avengers: A Consideration of the Changing Social Context of Medieval Warfare from the Perspective of Human Remains," in *The Routledge Handbook of the Bioarchaeology of Human Conflict*, eds. Christopher J. Knüsel and Martin J. Smith (London: Routledge, 2014), 263–81.

6 Hans Talhoffer, *Medieval Combat: A Fifteenth-Century Manual of Swordfighting and Close-quarter Combat*, ed. and trans. Mark Rector (London: Greenhill, 2000).

get (36 percent), with the neck (18 percent), cranial vault (17 percent), and face (10 percent) being next most represented.[7] This is also the case from analysis of the position of injuries gleaned from medieval literary accounts of violent confrontations. Mounier-Kuhn harvested textual sources to identify the weapons and types of wounds, with their severity gauged on deaths of named individuals, for the most part nobles.[8] He noted that although wounds affected all parts of the body, there was a preponderance of head and neck wounds, some forty-seven of 110 wounds affecting these anatomical areas, with smaller numbers affecting the limbs (thirty), thorax (twenty-four), and abdomen (twenty-four).[9] Although this type of exhaustive analysis provides good insights because they come from different encounters in very diverse historical circumstances in the medieval period, they are informative but also anecdotal in the sense that they cannot provide comparative frequency data and, moreover, there is no outcome information from treatments provided. Furthermore, neurological effects can only be suspected from the severity of head wounds, based on the penetrating depth of lesions. Although these figures could be seen as resulting from an intent to kill, they better reflect fatality and morbidity from wounds to these areas. Such seems to have been the case of Estienne Chatart, squire and breadmaster of the Habsburg Archduke Maximilian I (later Holy Roman Emperor), who survived and was compensated after receiving a head injury from a cross-bow bolt and another eventually crippling arquebus-inflicted upper limb injury at the siege of Calais in 1480, as reported by Depreter in this volume. For Mounier-Kuhn, longer-term neurological effects can only be surmised based on the location of head wounds and a penetrating depth of 20 mm or more, enough to impact the underlying brain.[10]

## Bone Trauma Responses

Bone is a plastic, thus malleable, material that deforms before breaking; once fractured, healing is identifiable as porous bone formation. The formation of a haematoma (clotted blood), porous fibre bone (from osteoblastic activity that forms reparative bone), develops from two weeks to a few months and

---

**7** Craig Wagstaffe, "Were Medieval Warriors Trained to Fight?" (Master's Thesis, University of Bradford, 2001).

**8** Alain Mounier-Kuhn, *Chirurgie de la guerre: Le cas du Moyen Âge* (Paris: Economica, 2006), 54.

**9** Alain Mounier-Kuhn, "Les blessures de guerre et l'armement au Moyen Âge dans l'Occident latin," *Médiévales* 39 (2000): 112–136.

**10** Mounier-Kuhn, *Chirurgie de la guerre*, 54.

commonly occurs during the second and third weeks post-injury in many cases.[11] This is followed by the formation of a bony lattice, called a callus. The porous fibre bone attests to survival of the injury for a time afterwards and a better organized, less porous callus to a longer but unspecified period of healing. Once the callus forms completely it is hard to estimate the amount of time required for its formation. One can, however, distinguish recent breakage of bone (post-mortem) from that which occurs around the time of death (perimortem) and both of these from more completely healed bone as porous bone is remodelled to form compact bone, which is indicative of full antemortem healing. This sequence distinguishes bone from other materials, such as ceramics, metals, and stone, for example, that do not possess the capacity for self-repair, and thus other materials provide no insight into the timing of breakage.

## Weapon Injuries

Weapon injuries form a sub-group of traumatic injuries distinguished by the type of force required to produce bone fracture. These include sharp-force trauma produced by a bladed weapon; blunt-force trauma identifiable as depressed bone fractures, especially evident in the cranium, is indicative of the use of club-like weapons; penetrating wounds from projectiles or pointed weapons;[12] ballistic trauma from bullets and musket balls, for example; and blast trauma from high explosives. The last of these refers to a compression and suction wave created by the detonation of high explosives from artillery that rupture blood vessels within internal organs, especially the lungs,[13] as well as the development of chronic neurodegenerative diseases, and cognitive and behavioural declines. These include psychiatric disorders such as Post Traumatic Stress Disorder (PTSD), depression, and anxiety as a result of even mild traumatic brain injuries,[14] in addition to basic problems of

---

**11** Lenore T. Barbian and Paul S. Sledzik, "Healing Following Cranial Trauma," *Journal of Forensic Sciences* 53, no. 2 (March 2008): 263–68.

**12** Christopher J. Knüsel, "The Physical Evidence of Warfare: Subtle Stigmata?," in *Warfare, Violence, and Slavery in Prehistory: Proceedings of a Prehistoric Society Conference at Sheffield University*, eds. Mike Parker-Pearson and I. J. Nick Thorpe (Oxford: Archaeopress, 2005), 49–65.

**13** Solly Zuckerman, "Experimental Study of Blast Injuries to the Lungs," *The Lancet* 236, no. 1604 (August 1940): 219–24.

**14** Heather R. Siedhoff et al., "Perspectives on Primary Blast Injury of the Brain: Translational Insights into Non-inertial Low-intensity Blast Injury," *Frontiers in Neurology* 12 (January 2022). https://doi.org/10.3389/fneur.2021.818169.

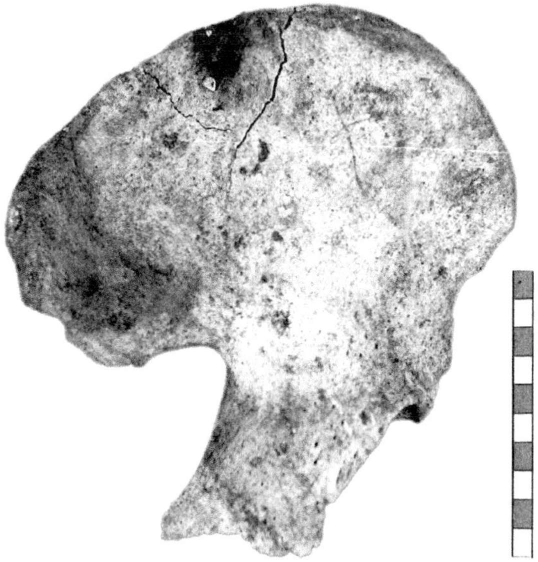

Figure 1.1. Right *os coxae* of Towton 42 showing dark staining on the upper left, below the iliac crest, in the vicinity of a copper-based metal fragment from the early use of firearms. Photograph courtesy of Dr. Jo Buckberry, Biological Anthropology Research Centre (BARC), University of Bradford, UK.

dizziness and balance.[15] Because blast injuries affect mainly soft tissue, it is not clear if and by what means they can be detected in skeletonized remains, but head injuries from both blunt and sharp force trauma, as well as ballistic trauma can also produce neurological sequelae due to brain injury.

Importantly, rather than being sustained as a result of accidents (for the most part), the use of weapons requires premeditation with an intention to injure. The advent of firearms and artillery in the late medieval period caused a number of historically recorded deaths of prominent individuals.[16] Ballistic trauma from early firearms can be anticipated in the form of embedded metal fragments. One example was found embedded in a right *os coxae* (hip-bone) among the remains from the Battle of Towton (1461, Yorkshire, England), one of the earliest examples, in Towton 42, found to date (figure 1.1).[17] Injuries from armed conflict do not necessarily affect the skeleton, although this changed with firearms, such as the hand-held arquebus,

**15** Jeffrey R Basford et al., "An Assessment of Gait and Balance Deficits after Traumatic Brain Injury," *Archives of Physical Medicine and Rehabilitation* 84 (March 2003): 343–49.

**16** Kelly R. DeVries, "Military Surgical Practice and the Advent of Gunpowder Weaponry," *Canadian Bulletin of Medical History* 7, no. 2 (Fall 1990): 131–46; Justin Barr et al., "'Through and Through' History: The Management of Gunshot Wounds From the 14th Century to the Present," *Annals of Surgery Open* 3 (July 17, 2023). https://doi.org/10.1097/AS9.0000000000000299.

**17** Shannan A. Novak, "Case Studies," in *Blood Red Roses: The Archaeology of a Mass Grave from the Battle of Towton AD 1461*, eds. Veronica Fiorato et al. (Oxford: Oxbow, 2000), 240–68.

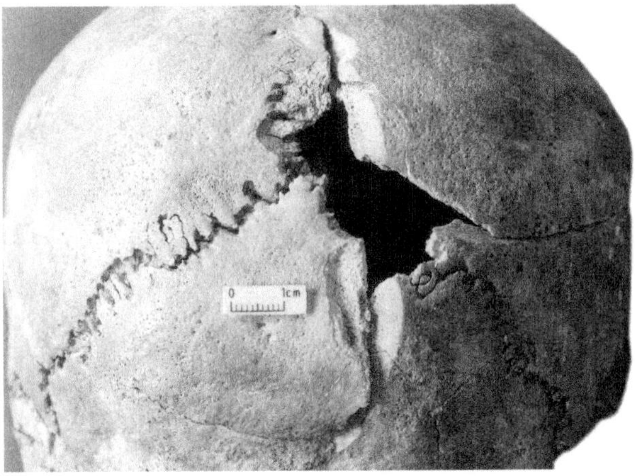

Figure 1.2. Sharp-force weapon trauma of Towton 32: a straight fracture outline to the right and a more irregular opposing outline to the left, with a sharp fracture margin and a smooth fracture surface on the right-hand side of the defect. © BARC (Biological Anthropological Research Centre), University of Bradford, UK. Used with permission.

a type of hand-held gun, from the fifteenth century, and present at Towton, probably in the hands of Burgundian gunners on the Yorkist side.

Sometimes the type of weapon responsible for an injury can be identified through matching cross-sections of particular skeletal lesions to specific types of weapons or tools,[18] which can be further augmented in replicative experiments based on objects suspected to have been used to inflict injuries, including specialized weapons from the past.[19]

Injuries and their types can be deduced from patterned changes in bones. Sharp-force weapon trauma has one elliptical or straight fracture

---

**18** See, for example: Christopher J. Knüsel, Adrien Thibeault, and Sébastien Villotte, "A Cranial Injury from the Earliest Gravettian at the Cro-Magnon Rock Shelter (Vézère Valley, Dordogne, Southwest France)," *Journal of Human Evolution* 177 (2023): 103329. https://doi.org/10.1016/j.jhevol.2023.103329; Novak, "Case Studies"; Hugh E. Berryman and Steven A. Symes, "Recognizing Gunshot and Blunt Cranial Trauma through Fracture Interpretation," in *Forensic Osteology: Advances in the Identification of Human Remains*, eds. Kathleen J. Reichs and William M. Bass, 2nd ed. (Springfield: Charles C. Thomas, 1998), 333–52; Philip L. Walker and Jeffrey C. Long, "An Experimental Study of the Morphological Characteristics of Tool Marks," *American Antiquity* 42, no. 4 (October 1977): 605–15.

**19** Miguel Angel Moreno-Ibáņez et al., "Was it an Axe or an Adze? A Cranial Trauma Case Study from the Late Neolithic and Chalcolithic Site of Cova Foradada (Calafell, Spain)," *International Journal of Paleopathology* 32 (March 2021): 23–30; MacKenzie Downing and Linda Fibiger, "An Experimental Investigation of Sharp Force Skeletal Trauma with Replica Bronze Age Weapons," *Journal of Archaeological Science: Reports* 11 (2017): 546–54; Eva Forsom and Martin J. Smith, "Getting to the Point: An Experimental Approach to Improving the Identification of Penetrating Projectile Trauma to Bone Caused by Medieval Arrows," *Journal of Archaeological Science Reports* 11 (January 2017): 274–86; Jason E. Lewis, "Identifying Sword Marks on Bone: Criteria for Distinguishing between Cut Marks Made by Different Classes of Bladed Weapons," *Journal of Archaeological Sciences* 35, no. 7 (July 2008): 2001–8.

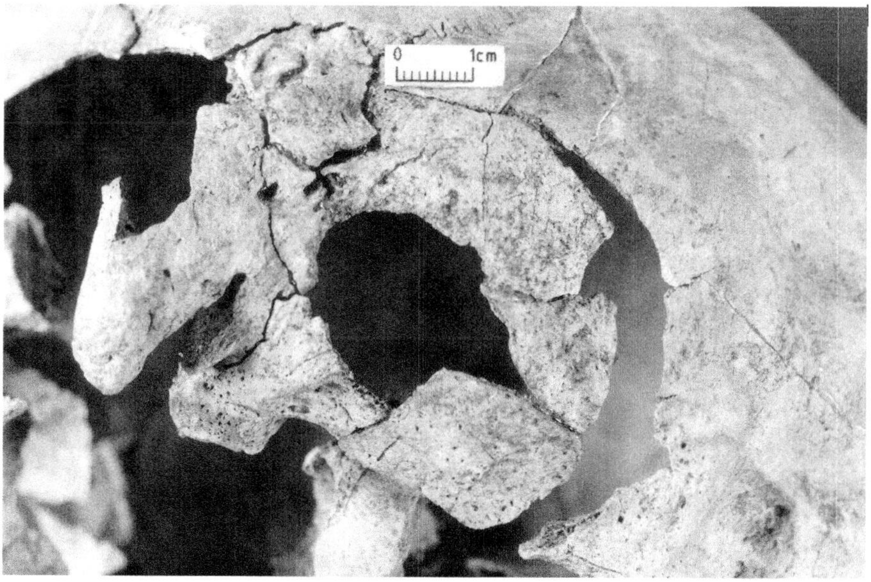

Figure 1.3. The left occipital of Towton 8, showing concentric, comminuted fractures (i.e., multiple broken fragments) of blunt force trauma with a penetrating central perforation that bears the shape of the penetrating weapon. © BARC (Biological Anthropological Research Centre), University of Bradford, UK. Used with permission.

outline and one opposing outline that is more irregular; a sharp fracture margin; and a smooth fracture surface (figure 1.2). The elliptical part of the fracture results from the entry of the weapon into the bone, while the opposite, irregular part relates to the removal of the weapon from the bone after it has become embedded and, in the process, producing small fractures of the margin. Blunt force trauma is characterized by crushing injuries that can produce comminuted fractures, those with multiple broken pieces (figure 1.3). Bladed weapons may also produce comminution depending on the weight of the striking weapon. Blunt-force fractures are identified by linear

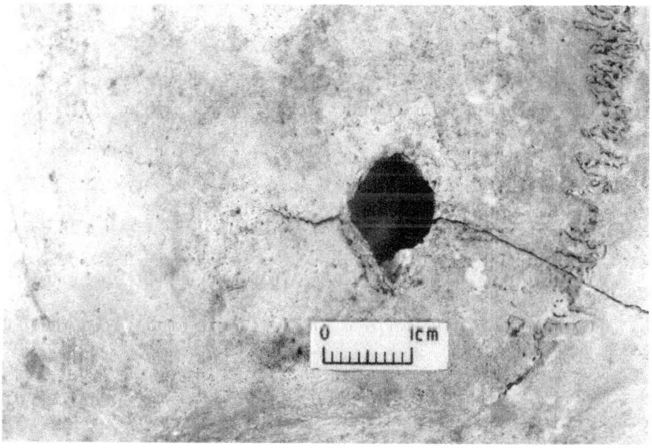

Figure 1.4. A small-diameter perforation of the left frontal bone of Towton 40, characteristic of penetrating trauma caused by a projectile (arrowhead), with linear fractures radiating from the site of perforation due to the weight and speed of the striking projectile. © BARC (Biological Anthropological Research Centre), University of Bradford, UK. Used with permission.

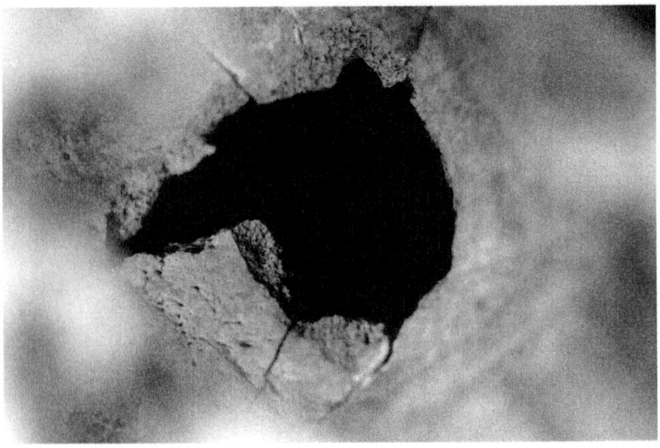

Figure 1.5. Endocranial view of the bevelled fractures around a penetrating wound of the inner table of the cranium of Towton 8. The external entry wound is thus smaller than this internal exit wound. © BARC (Biological Anthropological Research Centre), University of Bradford, UK. Used with permission.

fractures that radiate from the site of depression. Penetrating injuries are usually small-diameter perforations/punctures of bone with linear fractures that radiate from the site of perforation due to the weight and speed of the striking projectile (figure 1.4). All these fractures produce a bevelled fracture within the medullary canal of long bones and of the inner table of the cranium around the opening of the perforation (figure 1.5), which indicates that they had occurred in the perimortem interval, around the time of death, if unhealed. If the recipient survives the injury, these fractures may show signs of healing with rounded fracture margins and porosity among the earliest signs of healing. In addition, especially in the long bones of the body, perimortem injuries can be identified by spalls and larger splinters removed from the cortical bone surface. Splinters or spalls are produced when a hinged piece of bone breaks free from the cortical surface when an embedded weapon is withdrawn from the bone. Sometimes this is referred to as "peeling" because the resulting fracture resembles that of a broken green tree branch.[20] In essence, these are longitudinal fractures that run within the cortical bone laminae, those structures that give cortical bone its grainy appearance.

## Trauma Location and Patterning

Cranial trauma is considered to be the most life-threatening form of trauma, with often fatal or debilitating consequences for the recipient due to brain injury with both physical and mental consequences. The locations of healed trauma on crania are similar to the locations of perimortem trauma; mostly found above the hat-brim line,[21] it seems they resulted from the same intent

**20** Tim D. White, *Prehistoric Cannibalism at Mancos 5MTUMR-2346* (Princeton: Princeton University Press, 1992).

**21** Célia Kremer et al., "Discrimination of Falls and Blows in Blunt Head Trauma:

on the part of assailants. Although having been delivered with the same intent, the recipient survived in some cases, perhaps due to the buffering of blows by protective head coverings, misapplied strikes, luck, or owing to the robust health status and immune response of the individual to prevent subsequent infection, such as meningitis (blood poisoning). In the nineteenth century, Barnes referred to meningitis as a "formidable affection," being "one of the most common causes of death after gunshot contusion of the cranium."[22] It is also possible that after-injury treatment played a role in survival, but evidence of this requires explicit investigation, with treatments for head wounds being a specific focus of treatises written by practitioners more recently for violence-related casualties.[23] Perimortem wounds often involved penetration of the full thickness of cranial bone, leading to brain injuries, either directly or indirectly due to pressure from internal haemorrhaging and haematoma (blood clots). Minimally, antemortem injuries, i.e., fully healed or showing healing bone response to close the wound, attest to previous engagement in violent encounters and, in rare cases, access to remedial treatment.

Survival of especially head trauma is rare enough in the past that instances have been published as case reports,[24] as well as part of general surveys.[25] Healed cases are often associated with remedial procedures, such

---

Systematic Study of the Hat Brim Line Rule in Relation to Skull Fractures," *Journal of Forensic Sciences* 53, no. 3 (May 2008): 716–19; Célia Kremer and Anny Sauvageau, "Discrimination of Falls and Blows in Blunt Head Trauma: Assessment of Predictability through Combined Criteria," *Journal of Forensic Sciences* 54, no. 4 (June 2009): 923–26.

**22** Barnes, *The Medical and Surgical History of the War of the Rebellion*, 110.

**23** Barnes, *The Medical and Surgical History of the War of the Rebellion.*

**24** Knüsel et al., "A Cranial Injury from the Earliest Gravettian"; Holger Schutkowski, Michael Schultz, and Moritz Holzgraefe, "Fatal Wounds in a Late Neolithic Double Inhumation: A Probable Case of Meningitis Following Trauma," *International Journal of Osteoarchaeology* 6 (March 1996): 179–84.

**25** For example: Natasha Powers, "Cranial Trauma and Treatment: A Case Study from the Medieval Cemetery of St. Mary Spital, London," *International Journal of Osteoarchaeology* 15, no. 1 (January/February 2005): 1–14; Jochen Weber and Alfred Czarnetzki, "Brief Communication: Neurotraumatological Aspects of Head Injuries Resulting from Sharp and Blunt Force in the Early Medieval Period of Southwestern Germany," *American Journal of Physical Anthropology* 114, no. 4 (March 2001): 352–56; John Verano, "Trepanation in Prehistoric South America: Geographic and Temporal Trends over 2,000 Years," in *Trepanation: History, Discovery, Theory*, eds. Robert Arnott et al. (Amsterdam: Swets, 2003), 223–326; Matthew H. Kaufman, D. Whitaker, and J. McTavish, "Differential Diagnosis of Holes in the Calvarium:

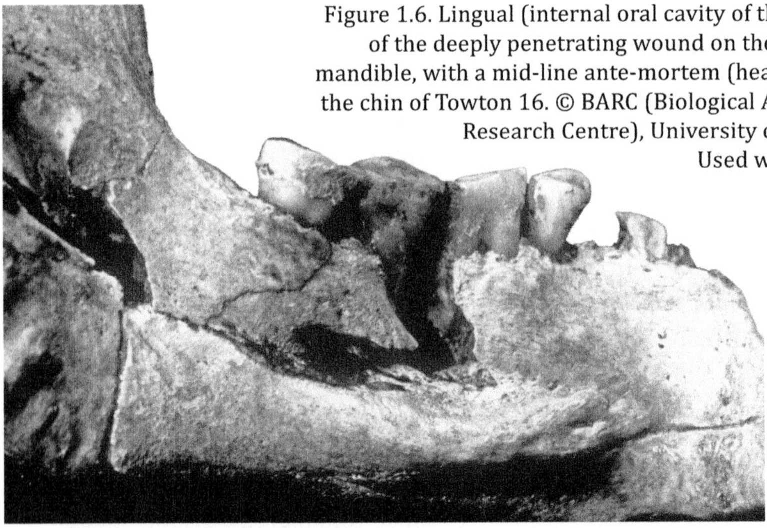

Figure 1.6. Lingual (internal oral cavity of the mouth) view of the deeply penetrating wound on the left side of the mandible, with a mid-line ante-mortem (healed) fracture of the chin of Towton 16. © BARC (Biological Anthropological Research Centre), University of Bradford, UK. Used with permission.

as trepanation (treatment of head wounds by this method is discussed by Turner and Frohne, in this volume, with respect to descriptions in the *Chirurgia* by Roger Frugard and in the *Feldbuch der Wundarznei* by Hans von Gersdorff, respectively), that aid survival by reduction of pressure from intra-cranial bleeding (haematoma) and abscessing from infection, and thus reveal awareness of the relationship between head injury, treatment, and improved chances of survival.[26]

## Towton 16

A good candidate for an individual receiving remedial medical treatment is Towton 16, whose deeply penetrating sharp-force wound on the left side of the mandible (that also produced a mid-line antemortem fracture of the mandible at the same time), cut through the distal apex of the distal root of the left first mandibular molar, leaving the mesial root of the second molar exposed (figures 1.6 and 1.7). This very severe wound shows both rounding of its edges indicative of longer-term healing and that the broken tooth root fragments had been removed. This action of debriding the wound performed

---

Application of Modern Clinical Data to Palaeopathology," *Journal of Archaeological Science* 24, no. 3 (March 1997): 193–218; Joseph K. Barnes, *The Medical and Surgical History of the War of the Rebellion (1861–1865)*, vol. 2 (Washington: Government Printing Office, 1870–1888).

**26** Graham Martin, "Why Trepan? Contributions from Medical History and the South Pacific," in *Trepanation: History, Discovery, Theory.*

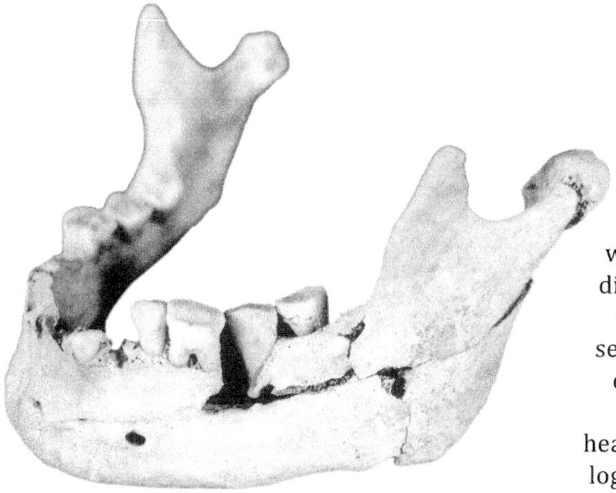

Figure 1.7. The healed (ante-mortem) fracture of the left side of the mandible of Towton 16, which removed the distal apex of the distal root of the left first mandibular molar, leaving the mesial root of the second molar exposed, with rounding of the edges of the wound indicative of bone resorption of longer-term healing. © BARC (Biological Anthropological Research Centre), University of Bradford, UK. Used with permission.

by an unknown person avoided the development of an infectious focus around the dead fragments of bone and tooth. More suggestive effects for this individual could have included damage to the mandibular branch of the trigeminal nerve and its branch to the mental nerve, which would have resulted in loss of sensation in the face and chin region, impaired facial expression, swallowing, and created problems with mastication and speech.[27] In Figure 1.8, this is represented in the loss of muscle tone and retraction at the left corner of the mouth. This treatment would have preserved this individual's life, if only to succumb in subsequent hostilities at Towton on Palm Sunday, March 29, 1461.

This facial injury would have made him visually distinctive and readily identifiable,[28] which may have occasioned the ten perimortem craniofacial injuries delivered to his head and face.

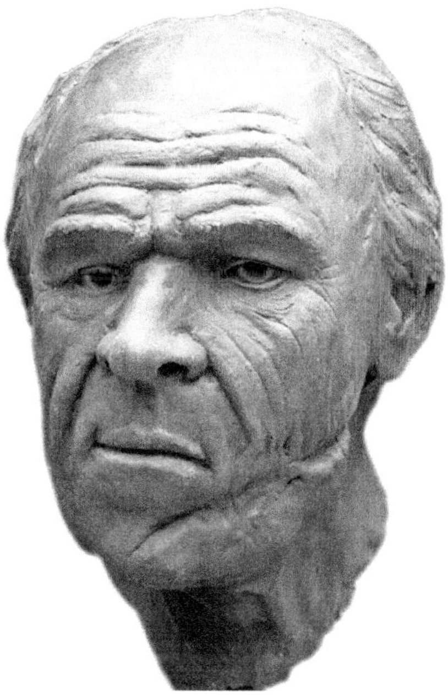

Figure 1.8. Facial reconstruction of Towton 16, with scarring of the mandibular wound and loss of muscle tone and retraction at the left corner of the mouth. Facial depiction courtesy of Professor Caroline Wilkinson and the University of Manchester.

**27** Trevor Huff, Luke J Weisbrod, and Daniel T. Daly, "Neuroanatomy, Cranial Nerve 5 (Trigeminal)," *StatPearls [Internet]* (2024): 1–9.

**28** Caroline Wilkinson and Richard Neave, "The Reconstruction of a Face showing a Healed Wound," *Journal of Archaeological Science* 30, no. 10 (October 2003): 1343–48.

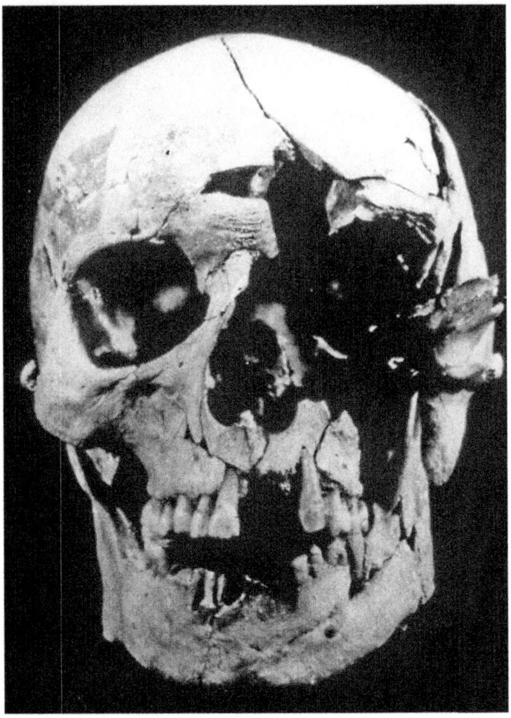

Figure 1.9. The extent of Towton 16's perimortem injuries after cranial reconstruction from fragments, with comminution (crushing) of the left side of the face. The mandibular injury in Figure 1.7 can also be seen to the lower right-hand side (left-side mandibular corpus) of this image. © BARC (Biological Anthropological Research Centre), University of Bradford, UK. Used with permission.

Moreover, his body was buried in the midst of the mass grave, face-down, with limbs splayed, a disposition that contrasts with the more commonly encountered practice of supine position with the upper limbs crossed at the pelvis or at the chest, or extended and aligned along the torso, with the lower limbs adducted (aligned with the mid-line of the body) and extended, the commonplace position during the late medieval period. In the high and late medieval periods burials are typically found within or near a church, with the body in an east to west alignment, head to the west.[29] Towton 16's burial position—prone and with limbs outstretched and head to the east[30]—contrasts with the more commonplace and highly regularized, symbolic orientations thought to aid resurrection. The lack of these features shows lack of care and, potentially, abnegation. Towton 16's injuries were so extensive—crushing (comminution of) the left side of the face—that they would have made his body difficult to identify (figure 1.9). He was one of the oldest (forty-six to fifty years of age at death) and one of the most

29 Gillian Stroud and Richard L. Kemp, *Cemeteries of St. Andrew, Fishergate*, vol. 12.2 of *The Archaeology of York: Medieval Cemeteries* (York: Council for British Archaeology, 1993); Christopher Daniell, *Death and Burial in Medieval England, 1066–1550* (London: Routledge, 1997), 118.

30 Tim Sutherland, "Recording the Grave," in *Blood Red Roses*, 36–44.

strongly lateralized individuals in the grave, with the left elbow being more robustly built than the right, and an avulsion of the left medial epicondyle of the humerus showing signs of the remodelling of healing.[31] These skeletal changes resulted from prolonged training for and performance of two-handed activities since right shoulder developmental asymmetry suggests that he was right-handed. The avulsion injury would have occurred when he was a juvenile, prior to fusion of the medial epicondylar growth centre at fourteen to sixteen years of age, in males.[32]

In the late medieval period, this type of orthopaedic injury associates him with a group of individuals in burial contexts of high social status and/or martial pursuits related to training for weapon use in the adolescent years.[33] Perhaps surprisingly, although gravely impaired at least for a time, neither of these injuries was sufficient to disable him for combat, to which he returned and during which he eventually perished. In this case, disability includes wounds and injuries received as result of both training for and participation in warfare.

## Antemortem (Healed) Weapon Injuries in Medieval Burial Population Samples

At the early (eleventh century) and high medieval (thirteenth-fourteenth centuries) Fishergate site, York, UK, fifteen and thirty-two individuals, respectively, survived infra-cranial trauma (Table 1.1). All cranial trauma, however, seems to have been fatal, with no signs of healing. This site contrasts with the fifteenth-century Towton site. While twenty-seven of twenty-eight crania, some 96 percent, exhibit perimortem injuries, Novak also notes that nine (32 percent) individuals from the Towton mass grave exhibit antemortem, healed cranial injuries. These attest to injuries received in previous aggressive encounters and participation in armed aggression, much of which may have been incurred in battle but could also have been sustained in aggression not linked directly to the field of battle but from inter-personal

---

**31** Knüsel, "Activity-related Changes in Casualties from the Medieval Battle of Towton," 103–18.

**32** J. Louise Scheuer and Sue M. Black, *Developmental Juvenile Osteology* (San Diego: Academic, 2000), 285, figure 8.9.

**33** Christopher J. Knüsel, "Men Take Up Arms for War: Sex and Status Distinctions of Humeral Medial Epicondylar Avulsion Fractures in the Archaeological Record," in *Breathing New Life into the Evidence of Death: Contemporary Approaches to Bioarchaeology*, eds. Aubrey Baadsgaard et al. (Santa Fe: School for Advanced Research, 2011), 221–50.

Table 1.1. Number of individuals with perimortem wounds and number of individuals with antemortem (healed) cranial wounds (Fishergate, parish cemetery; Fishergate, monastic cemetery; Battle of Towton; Battle of Good Friday, Uppsala).

| **Site** | | | |
|---|---|---|---|
| Fishergate, parish cemetery | Fishergate, monastic cemetery | Battle of Towton | Battle of Good Friday, Uppsala |
| **Date** | | | |
| 11th century | Late 13th to mid-14th centuries | March 29, 1461 | April 6, 1520 |
| **Number of individuals with perimortem wounds (Total number of wounds)** | | | |
| 21 (152) | 10 (58) | 38 (156) | 54 (103) |
| **Number of individuals with antemortem (healed) cranial wounds (Total number of healed wounds)** | | | |
| 0 | 2 (2) | 9 (16) | 3 (6) |
| **Comments** | | | |
| 15 infracranial healed injuries | 32 infracranial healed injuries | 16 wounds, five wounds in Towton 41 (maximum) alone—blunt and sharp force injuries | 15 bones show evidence of healed trauma, including four depressed fractures on two crania, A4:12 and A4:26, and two superficial linear fractures and one penetrating wound, all healed, in the single individual, A4:26 |
| **Source** | | | |
| Stroud and Kempe (1993): 225–31 | Stroud and Kempe (1993): 225–31 | Novak (2000): 94–95 | Kjellström (2005): 36–37 |

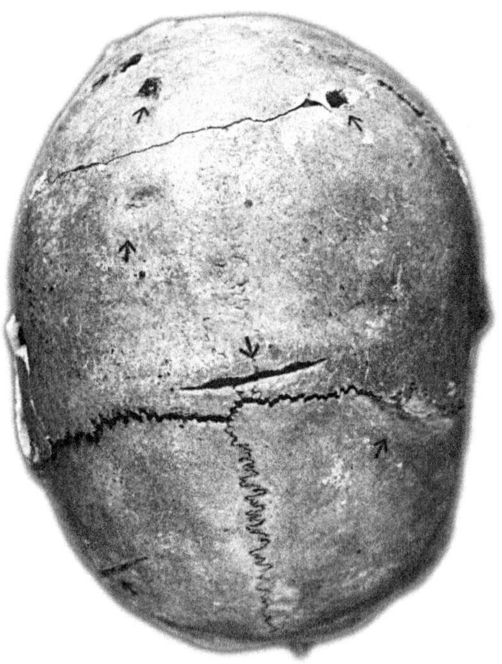

Figure 1.10. Superior view of the cranium of Towton 41, a male of twenty-six to thirty-five years of age at death, who had sustained five previous antemortem cranial injuries, a sharp-force antemortem wound affecting the top of the cranium seen here in the centre of the image and a depressed fracture of the right parietal, arrowed lower wound on the top left of the image. There are also three arrowed penetrating wounds on the posterior of the cranium, to the extreme left of the image, and two perimortem sharp force injuries: one to the frontal bone, lower right of the image (arrowed), and another, deeper, although not penetrating the vault, affecting the coronal suture in the central part of the image (arrowed). © BARC (Biological Anthropological Research Centre), University of Bradford, UK. Used with permission.

aggression involving weapons in other encounters. Of these injuries, six are due to healed blunt-force trauma, while ten are of a sharp-force origin, with three individuals being especially noteworthy: Towton 16 (two related mandibular injuries, one blunt-force, one sharp-force trauma), Towton 40 (two antemortem blunt-force injuries of the cranium and mandible), while Towton 41, a male of twenty-six to thirty-five years of age at death, sustained five previous antemortem cranial injuries, two of which were sharp-force wounds affecting the top of the cranium (head), with two others affecting the face, one on the right frontal, and a depressed fracture of the left frontal just above the orbit, with yet another affecting the right parietal, just off the sagittal suture (figure 1.10). He had additionally sustained three perimortem penetrating wounds of the posterior parietal bones, which match the cross-section of the top-spike of a poleaxe, in addition to nine perimortem infra-cranial wounds affecting the neck and the right and left upper limbs, specifically the right hand and shoulder.[34] While he had survived five cranial injuries of both sharp and blunt-force variety, likely because these injuries were superficial ones that did not penetrate deeply into the endocranial cavity and were therefore remedially treatable without the need to apply extensive procedures, he seems to have been hacked to death by multiple blows to the body and head subsequently at Towton. This individual bearing multiple wounds, some well-healed, from at least two aggressive encounters matches the profile of an injury recidivist,[35] as indeed do Towton 16 and 40 (described above). These were individuals inured to the mass violence of warfare, having participated in it on at least two occasions.

Based on the healed nature of their wounds, it seems they may have had access to remedial medical treatment. This access may have increased from the early and high medieval periods to the late medieval period, based on the increase in survival in the latter period, but this hypothesis warrants further assessment due to the restricted samples analyzed to date. One is left to wonder at the mental state of these men after having survived these injuries, and these can be perceived only through later accounts of similar injuries and their effects (see below).

---

**34** Novak, "Case Studies."

**35** Margaret A. Judd, "Ancient Injury Recidivism: An Example from the Kerma Period of Ancient Nubia," *International Journal of Osteoarchaeology* 12, no. 2 (March 2002): 89–106; Margaret A. Judd, "Injury Recidivism Revisited: Clinical Research and Limitation," in *Broken Bones, Broken Bodies: Bioarchaeological and Forensic Approaches for Accumulative Trauma and Violence*, eds. Caryn Tegtmeyer and Debra Martin (Lanham: Lexington Books, 2017), 1–24.

Similarly, at sixteenth-century Uppsala, three individuals had sustained six cranial wounds, comprising four depressed fractures on two crania, A4:12 and A4:26. A single individual, A4:26, had sustained two antemortem superficial linear fractures as well as one penetrating wound.[36] These two can also be identified as recidivists, having sustained wounds that had healed and also those that were perimortem (and thus without signs of healing), which resulted from death in violent circumstances.

Contrasting experience of trauma and the presence of recidivists for traumatic injuries likely reflects the historical circumstances of these conflicts, with the thirteenth-fourteenth century occurrences from York relating to unknown, but recurrent brushes with violence. Perimortem fatal injuries appear to relate to the different origins of combatants that pitted experienced combatants against more poorly trained and less experienced civilian feudal levies,[37] perhaps like those from Fishergate, York. The greater preponderance of both unhealed and healed injuries at Towton derives from successive confrontations and what appears to have been, in some cases, running battles that characterized the Wars of the Roses' Battle of Towton, a critical encounter that confirmed the Yorkist Edward, Earl of March, to the throne as King Edward IV. Rather than being a single day-long encounter, the battle seems to have taken place over a period of days.[38] The Wars of the Roses were at once a series of aristocratic feuds (see Tirosh, in this volume, on this type of sustained and highly personalized vengeance-fuelled confrontation in medieval Iceland) between the powerful northern scion Percy and Neville families. It was a double dynastic revolt in that both sides, Lancastrians and Yorkists, considered the other to be traitors to one of the two crowned monarchs, Henry VI of the House of Lancaster and Edward IV of the House of York. It was a civil war affecting much of the populace, the entire kingdom, and its resources, stretching over the years 1455 to 1487. With both royal treasuries exhausted, seized lands and goods acted as payments to victorious nobles of both houses, a situation which led to acts of attainder (a declaration of ignoble (bad) aristocratic blood) and summary executions in the aftermath of military

**36** Anna Kjellström, "A Sixteenth-Century Warrior Grave from Uppsala, Sweden: The Battle of Good Friday," *International Journal of Osteoarchaeology* 15 (September 2005): 23–50.

**37** Knüsel, "Courteous Knights and Cruel Avengers."

**38** Tim Sutherland, "Killing Time: Challenging the Common Perceptions of Three Medieval Conflicts—Ferrybridge, Dintingdale and Towton—'The Largest Battle on British Soil,'" *Journal of Conflict Archaeology* 5, no. 1 (June 2009): 1–26.

encounters that denied inheritance, which acts of attainder nullified.[39] These circumstances may explain the number and extent of injuries; these men were fighting as much for their livelihoods and social status as for their lives, with much to gain from removing foes. Although noble fatalities were recovered from the field of battle for interment elsewhere, the retainers of non-noble status were usually interred on the field of battle or near where they fell in unmarked graves at Towton. For instance, the Lancastrian noble adherent Lord Randolph Dacre of Gilsland (today, part of Cumbria, UK) was buried in the churchyard of nearby Saxton, West Yorkshire, where his tomb can still be seen, and Henry Percy, Lord Poynings and 3rd Earl of Northumberland, was interred at the parish church of Saint Denys in York. The relocation of elites bodies in this manner similarly occurred after earlier confrontations—such as that at Agincourt in October 1415—and later conflicts.[40]

The social ramifications of injuries are difficult to obtain from skeletal remains, although some general aspects of survival can be ascertained from burial contexts,[41] while some of the outcomes can be gleaned from more recent cases of combatant head trauma. The latter type of source is highly informative, but even then, most patients were discharged and the subsequent lives over the longer term remain unknown (see also Verreycken and Depreter in this volume). How such individuals survived and what care was required in later years is lost today. Essentially, we lack sufficiently detailed follow-up medical records to provide all but anecdotal examples. Yet, even so, some insights can be gained.

**39** On these executions, see John Gillingham, *The Wars of the Roses: Peace and Conflict in 15th Century England* (London: Weidenfeld, 1990); Anthony Goodman, *The Wars of the Roses: Military Activity and English Society* (London: Routledge, 1981). As summarized in "The Human Remains in their Medieval Context," in *Blood Red Roses*, 169–88.

**40** Knüsel, "Courteous Knights and Cruel Avengers"; Catherine Rigeade, "Approche archéoanthropologique des inhumations militaires," *Socio-anthropologie* 22 (2008): 93–105; Malin R. Holst and Tim L. Sutherland, "Towton Revisited: Analysis of the Human Remains from the Battle of Towton 1461," *Forschungen zur Archäologie im Land Brandenburg* 15 (2014): 97–129.

**41** Christopher J. Knüsel, "Orthopaedic Disability: Some Hard Evidence," in "Disability and Archaeology," ed. Nyree Finlay, special issue, *Archaeological Review from Cambridge* 15, no. 2 (January 1999): 31–53.

### Treatment of the Wounded

Access to skilled practitioners as part of aristocratic and ecclesiastical households was a likely inducement to fight in aristocratic retinues. For example, in the fourteenth century, Guy de Chauliac was the personal physician of the Avignon popes, while later, in the sixteenth century, Ambroise Paré was a servant of the French Crown. This situation arose because those skilled in maintaining health and treating conditions were often tied through patronage to entitled aristocrats and ecclesiastics, becoming members of their retinues.

The organization of skilled medical aid was variable and may not have existed at all for many outside the entourage of aristocrats and monarchs. From the fifth to the eleventh century, Mounier-Kuhn could count only nineteen textual references to *medici* (roughly equivalent to doctor-surgeons) present on battlefields, which the author sees as a conservative estimate.[42] These battlefield medics commonly attended a named person, often an aristocrat, who may also have, in turn, been attended by multiple doctors and surgeons in the course of consultation and treatment, the two occupations being separate and at times at odds with one another for much of the High and Late Middle Ages.[43]

By the High and Late Middle Ages, this situation had changed considerably, however, and there are many more references to, variably, doctors, surgeons, barber-surgeons, and apothecaries who are named as present in medieval retinues of kings and aristocrats. Mounier-Kuhn counts some 228 surgeons present in Western European armies in the fourteenth to fifteenth centuries, with the grand majority being present in the armies of the French and English kings and the dukes of Burgundy or in the employ of the towns of Flanders.[44] The English king Edward I, who bore the epithet "Hammer of the Scots," a reflection of his bellicose tendencies, had in his retinue what Mounier-Kuhn describes as a veritable military medical service ("un véritable service de santé militaire")[45] during his early thirteenth-century campaigns in Scotland. These medical practitioners' associations with other wounded more generally can only be conjectured, but those accompanying

**42** Mounier-Kuhn, *Chirurgie de la guerre*, 105.

**43** Roy Porter, *The Greatest Benefit of Mankind: A Medical History of Humanity from Antiquity to the Present* (London: HarperCollins, 1997), 119–20.

**44** This probably mirrors the origins of the sources he accessed. Mounier-Kuhn, *Chirurgie de la guerre*, 122.

**45** Mounier-Kuhn, *Chirurgie de la guerre*, 115.

Edward I were under contract to attend to *all* of the wounded.[46] Even in those aggressive encounters where all casualties were stipulated to be treated, hierarchy, as well as wealth and status played a prominent role in prioritizing those who received treatment and the speed with which it could be administered.

Mounier-Kuhn notes a fundamental change at the end of the thirteenth and beginning of the fourteenth century when university-trained surgeons, such as the literate Henri de Mondeville, personal surgeon of Philippe le Bel, King of France, and Guy de Chauliac were progressively replaced by a new group of practitioners, the barber-surgeons.[47] Although less well-grounded than these university-trained practitioners, by the fifteenth century, based on their daily civilian practices, they began to appear more regularly on the battlefield to develop experience of trauma and its treatment, benefitting as did later military surgeons from the extreme circumstances of their situations to develop innovative therapeutic surgical procedures, treatments, and instruments in the absence of the more constrained atmosphere of the daily civilian sphere. They were often offering last-ditch treatments *in extremis*, so had the opportunity to take chances and apply experimental procedures to save those who otherwise had little hope of survival.

The number and extent of those offering treatment and their proximity to the battlefield improved over the course of the Middle Ages according to the text-based analysis of Mounier-Kuhn.[48] This did not categorically exclude the lowly-born from surgical treatment, but aristocrats and those of high rank were favoured in this triage by status, and those of lower rank were treated if higher-ranking casualties had already been treated. Based on feudal obligation and individual aristocratic preferences and resources, practices varied greatly from one territory to another, from one battle to another and from one practitioner to another, and by the later Middle Ages, with increasing numbers of those offering treatment, this applied more "democratically" to all wounded, more often removed from the dangers of the field of battle to be treated elsewhere.[49] In the best circumstances, instruments and *materia medica* were prepared in advance to aid both treatments and healing.

---

**46** Mounier-Kuhn, *Chirurgie de la guerre*, 117.

**47** Mounier-Kuhn, *Chirurgie de la guerre*, 283–84.

**48** Mounier-Kuhn, *Chirurgie de la guerre*, 173. Mounier-Kuhn's account is heavily reliant upon—and made more detailed as a result—sources documenting France, England, and Burgundy.

**49** Mounier-Kuhn, *Chirurgie de la guerre*, 172–73.

Treatment administered on the field of battle and rapid evacuation from the field of battle were major innovations in military medicine, and these practices appear to have been much more piece-meal even in the late medieval period compared with subsequent developments. This may also explain why animal scavenging has been found among the remains, at Uppsala's Battle of Good Friday, where bodies of the Swedish rebels were intentionally left on the field of battle without burial to eventually freeze in the cold of spring, April 6, 1520, only to be buried later.[50]

## Texts, Conflicts, the Wounded, and Casualties

It is undeniable that textual references likely underplay the number of people who practised curing and healing during the late medieval period.[51] In this light, the evidence from human remains plays an important complementary role to augment the number and details of treatments. However, the circumstances of these treatments are often only revealed through their association with a known or archaeologically attested building, settlement, or location, but they are rarely associated with a named individual. In short, we know neither the names of those bearing injuries, nor those bearing signs of treatment, nor those offering such treatments. Reference to the specific treatments of battle casualties—and those who performed such treatments and where they performed them—are difficult to study from written sources alone and, prior to the late medieval period and the appearance of the first literate military barber-surgeons, are few, hindered by vagaries of source and quality of content. In the modern era—from the nineteenth century—these medical practitioners treated wounded on the battlefield prior to evacuating individuals to another location, often as in the case of the wounded soldiers alluded to below, by train to more distant hospitals. In the absence of these institutions in their modern curative guise, treatment and transport were much more variable, sometimes systematically organized, and often restricted to high-ranking individuals or only that offered by comrades in arms on an ad-hoc basis.

Although medical treatments existed in written form, it is often unclear if the writer had first-hand experience, or if they relied on previous compilations of known and unknown sources. Some of the best evidence of war-related trauma and treatments comes from the study of human remains. Although occurring in unnamed individuals and unrecorded by history, they

---

**50** Kjellström, "Sixteenth-century Warrior Grave from Uppsala, Sweden," 44–46.

**51** Knüsel, "The Unwritten History of Medical Treatment," 206–16.

provide insights that complement, but also greatly extend textual sources. Human remains often provide the most unequivocal evidence for violence and, when repeated and sustained for a period of time, to warfare,[52] but the context of these wounded individuals also adds much fundamentally informative evidence which can confirm a variety of behavioural aspects surrounding conflict and its aftermath, as well as their historical development.

Even if the violent circumstances surrounding injuries are reasonably well-attested, the specifics leading to injury of individuals are often omitted or unclear, inadequately described, or in a manner that does not easily equate to more recent terminology and understandings of weapon trauma (see Depreter in this volume). In many cases, there were no surviving witnesses, in others no literate witnesses and, in many, no motivation to document not only the deaths, except in some well-known cases, but also the survivors, or minimally survivors whose rank made them "worthy of mention."

The development of remedial medical treatment of injuries sustained in conflict can be appreciated from surviving textual sources, but their relative incompleteness and scarcity or complete absence for certain places and times limits their usefulness. In this case, as in consideration of peri-mortem weapon trauma the *sine non qua* for armed aggression, the evidence for treatments leaving tell-tale osseous signs is critical in any assessment of treatment and survivorship, their frequency reflecting, at once, on the skills of those undertaking such actions, as well as their efficacy for preserving human lives.

In his survey covering the thousand years of the Middle Ages, Mounier-Kuhn characterizes developments in the following way: "While their [the wounded] situation appears relatively better from the twelfth century onwards, at least for those on the victorious side, it is difficult to determine the situation in earlier centuries. This is not because there is evidence of deliberate refusal of care, but simply because sources are too scarce to allow a broad enough assessment of what happened to the wounded."[53] Therefore,

---

**52** Philip L. Walker, "A Bioarchaeological Perspective on the History of Violence," *Annual Review of Anthropology* 30 (2001): 573–96; Clark Spencer Larsen, *Bioarchaeology: Interpreting Human Behavior from the Human Skeleton* (Cambridge: Cambridge University Press, 1997); Clark Spencer Larsen, "Bioarchaeology: The Lives and Lifestyles of Past People," *Journal of Archaeological Research* 10, no. 2 (June 2002): 119–66; Knüsel, "The Physical Evidence of Warfare."

**53** "Autant leur [the wounded wariors'] situation apparaît relativement meilleure à partir du xii$^{e}$ siècle, du moins pour ceux du camp vainqueur, autant elle est difficile à cerner pour les siècles antérieurs, non pas que des preuves existent d'un refus délibéré de soins, mais simplement les sources trop rares ne permettent

analyses of well-contextualized late medieval human remains revealing healed and healing injuries are key indicators of not only the occurrence of traumatic injuries but also treatment and survival. Given the proportion of healed and healing weapon-related injuries, efficacy can be assessed through continued subsequent participation in armed conflict, which would require a certain level of physical, if not mental, fitness. The relatively meagre findings of this study based on physical remains of combatants seem to confirm this longer-term perspective. By the late medieval period, there seems to be greater evidence for survival from even quite severe injuries.

The study of traumatic injuries inflicted in aggressive encounters can be viewed in two ways: as a complement to historical treatments, or as a type of unwritten history documenting violent acts in the past that are otherwise undocumented. In short, such studies address the following questions: What are the personal consequences of participation in medieval warfare, and how can these incidents contribute to the historical record? This type of endeavour can also provide insight into the motivations for participation in hostilities that centre around social advancement, access to resources, better positioning for social alliances and coalitions, and improved healthcare and well-being. Usually the effects of warfare are measured with respect to its demographic effects on a population level, or with regard to destruction of material and infrastructure, but the injuries received, both physical and especially mental (see Turner, in this volume, on "mania or melancholia," medieval terms for mental illness, the formulaic "having lost his senses" or "madness" being the description used for Burgundian cases (Depreter in this volume) and Aleksandra Pfau, in this volume, for the mental affliction of French king Charles VI), are less easily perceived because they are experienced on an individual level, but what is the effect of participation in warfare on the human body?

What seems clear is that impairment did not necessarily equate to incapacity or disability: rather it signalled and symbolized in visible healed lesions the reverse: previous experience of arms, survival, and perhaps associated sagacity (cf. Giulia Morosini, pers. comm., contribution on Renaissance-period Italy, as part of the oral presentations for this volume). This sentiment is reflected in Stephan Crane's fictional unnamed young American Civil War soldier's experience: "At times he regarded wounded soldiers in an envious way. He perceived persons with torn bodies to be peculiarly

pas d'apprécier avec une perspective assez large, ce que devenaient les blessés." Mounier-Kuhn, *Chirurgie de la guerre*, 74 ; translation by the author.

happy. He wished that he, too, had a wound, a red badge of courage."[54] The youthful soldier considers himself a "man of experience" after his survival of injury.[55] As has been previously established by contributors to this volume (see also Verreycken and Tirosh in this volume), rather than individuals being seen as handicapped in the sense of an inability to participate in armed conflict, previous scars from battle wounds enhanced an individual's reputation and social identity as a warrior combatant, producing what the novelist Stephen Crane referred to as the "red badge of courage," a wound and scar that served as a physical sign of bravery to dispel any suspicion of cowardice and also indicative of active participation as well as a testament of survival.

## Antemortem, Perimortem, and Mortal Injuries

At Towton, roughly a quarter, nine of thirty-eight, of individuals who died from head injuries had previously survived head injuries, with the majority, twenty-nine of thirty-eight, three-quarters, dying after receiving head injuries for the first time. Some had survived more than one injury, with Towton 41, unusually for the samples reviewed here, having survived five such injuries (see Table 1). The effects of such trauma on behaviour and the extent of impairment and incapacity can be better perceived in later accounts that can then be retrodicted into the late medieval period, where such detailed accounts are absent. The longer-term effects, though, are difficult to surmise even in these accounts due to a paucity of information.

## Head Injuries and Their Sequelae: Concluding Remarks and More Recent Historical Sources

In Barnes's late nineteenth-century account head injuries were often fatal, or assumed to be fatal, as in the case of Private Thomas Dillon, twenty-seven years of age, wounded at the Battle of Chancellorsville (Virginia), May 31, 1863, by a musket ball, which had entered the brain after striking the superior angle of the occipital bone. There was no comminution, fissuring, or depression of bone around the wound entrance, nor herniation of brain tissue through the wound. The wound was not immediately dressed, "probably because of the natural supposition that the case would prove speedily fatal...The patient received little attention, the case being regarded as

54 Stephen Crane, *The Red Badge of Courage* (s.l.: Mockingbird, 2015), 54.

55 Crane, *The Red Badge of Courage*, 87.

hopeless."[56] Delirium set in and the patient was restrained on a mattress on the floor of his tent. He experienced no sensation of pain. Despite lack of subsequent treatment to remove the missile, other than shaving the head and removing some bone fragments (cf. Towton 16, above, as described by Hans von Gersdorff, see Frohne in this volume) and then dressing the wound, his strength had returned by the first week of June, the wound had closed, and all his functions returned, except his memory of the incident and he did not recognize intimate relations. On June 13, 1863, he was transferred to Philadelphia, at which time he was well enough recovered to be able to walk to the station, a distance of nearly half a mile (over 800 metres). "In April, 1864, he was returned to his regiment in the field, perfectly well physically, but with an intellect somewhat impaired." His mental impairment was not sufficient to prevent him from active service, and he was not deemed to be disabled, followed by the comment that "he is not a pensioner." Here, mental impairment was not sufficient reason to exclude this young soldier from active duty.

In others, injuries prevented them from working, as in the case of Private Garrett Rozell, sixteenth New York Battery. Aged thirty-six years of age, he was wounded in an engagement at Chapin's Farm, Virginia, September 29, 1864, by a piece of shell, which tore away the eyebrow, eyelid, and part of the temporal and malar bones of the left side, completely extirpating the left eye, and opening a wound into the nasal bone one-fourth by one-eighth of an inch (3.18 to 3.65mm) in extent, leaving the loose appendages turned inward and hanging over the cheek as low as the middle of the nose. In his report of 1867 the attending examiner, John G. Orton, MD, described his face as "so badly disfigured that he will ever be an object of pity, and unable to gain a living, except in seclusion from society."[57] It seems he was expected to face a life of potential poverty and social exclusion. If, indeed, he did so, the sources do not inform us. This type of detailed information on the longer-term effects of injury is also missing from other more personalized medieval accounts (see Depreter in this volume), like that of the Swiss combatant Heinrich Schönbrunner (1489–1537) from canton Zug in central Switzerland, who received a serious head wound, possibly blinding him in one eye, but as Bianca Frohne notes in her contribution to this volume, "he was not interested in relaying his pain in detail or in expanding on the emotional experience related to his injury." Schönbrunner went on to fight in other campaigns, became

**56** Barnes, *The Medical and Surgical History of the War of the Rebellion*, 190–91.

**57** Barnes, *The Medical and Surgical History of the War of the Rebellion*, 368.

a councilman, held important offices, and served as a military captain. It seems whatever the lasting effects of his injury, they did not bar him from professional pursuits, some of them of a military nature. The fate of those suffering facial disfigurement from their injuries seems to bode poorly for those afflicted, a sentiment shared through very similar statements concerning the facial disfigurement of Jehan de Savoye, a squire, who was said to have been marred for life, as described in Michael Depreter's chapter in this volume for this late fifteenth-century medieval Burgundian combatant.

In other cases of head injury, there was no attempt to remove the missile and some returned to fighting still retaining missiles in their heads, some of whom were described as "not a pensioner," many were discharged, as in the case of Private John Wolstenholm, twenty-five years of age, having received a penetrating wound of the right mastoid process of the temporal bone from a musket ball that had entered the brain. He is described as being "entirely deaf in the right ear, the right eye irritable and injected [i.e., blood-shot], with constant pain in the right side of the head, impairment of the mental faculties, tendency to vertigo upon slight exertion."[58] His disability was rated as "total and permanent"; the missile had not yet been removed on later examination by the pension officer, and he was discharged from the service on July 24, 1865. The use of "total" in the classification of the Pension Bureau, implied incapacity to earn a livelihood by either physical or mental exertion. Specific causes of this classification include: "Vision...[being] destroyed in two instances, and more or less impaired in seven others. Complete deafness resulted in one case; hemiplegia in one case, paraplegia in another, and local paralysis in three others; and nearly all of the patients suffered from vertigo, headache, defective memory, and various forms of impairment of the mental faculties."[59] The longer-term impact of these brain lesions could not be reported due to a lack of sufficient detail in the reports, according to practitioners. This absence of long-term follow-up remains a hindrance to disability research (also Verreycken for a lack of elaboration on the longer-term consequences of battle injuries in medieval French petitions for pardon and Depreter, this volume, for medieval Burgundy, which are similarly affected by absent information).

With regard to incised (i.e., linear) fractures of the cranium, more similar to late medieval sharp-force trauma from a heavy-bladed weapon, Barnes makes the following observation:

---

**58** Barnes, *The Medical and Surgical History of the War of the Rebellion*, 194.

**59** Barnes, *The Medical and Surgical History of the War of the Rebellion*, 209.

> Of the ten patients who were discharged for disabilities resulting from sabre fractures of the skull, one became insane, one lost vision in an eye, three suffered from attacks of vertigo or dizziness, and, in two of these, the mental faculties were impaired, loss of memory being particularly noticeable. A sixth patient was hemiplegic, and his mind was much deteriorated. The other four men discharged, and the four paroled men, suffered only from occasional headaches or from slight disabilities. In eleven of the forty-nine patients, fragments of bone were removed by the forceps, elevator, Hey's saw [a type of incising saw used to cut through the cranial vault], or trephine [a drill for performing craniotomies to release the pressure of the accumulated blood of haematoma]. But one of these eleven cases terminated fatally. In thirty-seven cases, the site of fracture is definitely described. The frontal bone was principally involved in seven cases. Two of these terminated fatally; from tetanus [muscle spasms of the jaws and, progressively, other muscles], in one instance; in the other, with fracture of the outer table only, secondary encephalitis and abscess of the brain supervened. There were two fractures of the temporal region, which recovered. In twenty-two cases, one or both parietals were fractured, and six of these cases resulted fatally. Of six patients with incised fractures in the occipital region, three recovered and three died. These statistics corroborate the observation of Hennen[60] and others, that sabre wounds on the top of the head are not, by any means, so dangerous as those of the sides.[61]

So, head wounds to the superior cranial vault did not systematically kill but led to impairment and substantial disability as indeed may have been the case of Towton 41's linear wound to the top of the head (figure 1.10), being left with serious impairment, both physical, in some cases, mental, or both. In the nineteenth century, disability was judged on the basis of associated poverty and economic hardship, focusing on the ability or inability to perform wage-labour. This is the part of the story that is most difficult to perceive in the late medieval past at present due to difficulties in determining the relative timing of bone changes in different parts of the body. By historical physical analogy, it seems highly likely that the cranial injury survivors described above experienced similar longer-term mental effects far more long-lasting than their physical injuries. This challenge is one of the chief concerns addressed in the following contributions to this volume.

**60** John Hennen, *Principles of Military Surgery, Comprising Observations on the Arrangement, Police, and Practice of Hospitals, and on the History, Treatment, and Anomalies of Variola and Syphilis*, 3rd ed. (London: John Wilson, 1829), 286 (cited in Barnes, *The Medical and Surgical History of the War of the Rebellion*, 23).

**61** Barnes, *The Medical and Surgical History of the War of the Rebellion*, 23.

Chapter 2

# DISABILITY AND TRAUMA IN BATTLE IN THE MEDIEVAL ICELANDIC SAGAS

YOAV TIROSH

IN AN EPISODE of *Mad Men*'s third season, "Guy Walks Into an Advertising Agency," we encounter the show's most gory scene. Guy is the newest member to join the Madison Avenue ad men, an account manager belonging to the British company that had recently bought their agency. In a night of merriment and alcohol, a secretary drives a small John Deere tractor over Guy's foot, shredding it off in a very gut-wrenching scene, uncharacteristic of what was usually an aesthetically pleasing show representing men in suits and women in dresses, always looking "sharp." Later, when an ad agent meets the company's British owners to discuss Guy's situation, the boss has this to say:

> "It's a terrible tragedy. One that surely could have been avoided, although, Mrs. Harris, thank you for your quick thinking. You may have saved his life. *Such as it is.* He was a great account man. A prodigy. He could talk a Scotsman out of a penny. Now that's all over. *The man is missing a foot. How is he going to work? He can't walk. The doctor said he'll never golf again.*"[1]

This is an almost on-the-nose example of how society disables people based on their embodied difference. But another interesting point in this conversation is the American characters' reaction to it. The Americans are visibly perplexed by their British boss's connection between one's ability

1 My emphasis. Lesli Linka Glatter, dir., "Guy Walks Into an Advertising Agency," *Mad Men*, season 3, episode 6, September 20, 2009, AMC.

**YOAV TIROSH** is based in Scandinavian Studies and Experience Economy, Aarhus University, and Center for Disability Studies at the School of Social Sciences, University of Iceland. His first monograph, *How Genre Governs Creation in the Medieval Icelandic Sagas* (2025), offers a new analytical perspective on saga literature. Yoav Tirosh's research was also supported by Marie Skłodowska-Curie Actions grant agreement no. 101064468 and by a Rannsóknasjóður grant from the University of Iceland 1010-1013145.

to be an advertising agent, and their ability to walk. By emphasizing a supposed inability to play golf, the British man exhibits a systemic lack of imagination: business can only be done one way (and golf can only be played one way, at that!). Here the show illustrates clear cultural differences between the 1960s US and UK. If during the same period, two societies speaking more or less the same language could still have such vastly different understandings of disability, can we ever truly understand what disability was in the Middle Ages?[2]

When I was invited to write this chapter by editors Ninon Dubourg and Christophe Masson, my first reaction was to write them saying that there are no wars in the Icelandic sagas. This was, on second thought, wildly inaccurate. There were a few large-scale battles in Iceland's thirteenth-century civil unrest, as well as an abundance of battles in the various sagas' descriptions of the Viking Age and in the sagas chronicling Norwegian kings. However, when thinking about the *Íslendingasögur*, the sagas of early Icelanders, small (yet violent) skirmishes between farmers rather than large-scale martial encounters come to mind. The famous summary of these texts, "bændur fljúgast á" ("farmers fight each other"), remains quite accurate.[3] The lion's share of these sagas describes what could be called small scuffles, with few deaths and a fair number of injured parties. Furthermore, as noted in this book's introduction, warfare can be described as "organized and sustained violence." As a consequence, medieval Iceland is lucky enough to receive a chapter dedicated to its people's battle-related trials and tribulations.

High and late medieval Icelanders' culture produced texts that were often preoccupied with the measure of a *man*.[4] The sagas feature constant comparisons between individuals, with less regard to wealth and more to

**2** Acknowledging that this is a fictional representation of such differences. The difficulty of determining instances of historical violence has also been pointed out (Christopher J. Knüsel and Bonnie Glencross, "Çatalhöyük, Archaeology, Violence," *Contagion: Journal of Violence, Mimesis, and Culture* 24, no. 1 (2017): 23–36. https://doi.org/10.14321/contagion.24.1.0023), much of it due to "how notoriously resistant it has proven to formal definition." Oren Falk, *Violence and Risk in Medieval Iceland: This Spattered Isle* (Oxford: Oxford University Press, 2021), 25.

**3** Jón Ólafsson úr Grunnavík, *Safn til íslenskrar bókmenntasögu*, eds. Guðrún Ingólfsdóttir and Þórunn Sigurðardóttir (Reykjavík: Stofnun Árna Magnússonar í íslenskum fræðum, 2018), 7.

**4** Note, e.g., Edna Edith Sayers's comment about the sagas being written by and about men. (Edna Edith Sayers (published as Lois Bragg), *Oedipus Borealis: The Aberrant Body in Old Icelandic Myth and Saga* (Madison: Fairleigh Dickinson University Press, 2004), 12.

how many supporters and how much political influence a person had. By way of evidence, one of the most famous northeastern Icelanders, Bjarni Brodd-Helgason, ended his life in relative poverty, despite being considered one of the Eastfjord's region's most powerful people. Indeed, to this day we read stories about this man, proving that he did well to preserve his legacy. On the other hand, one of the famously richest chieftains of the medieval Icelandic North, Guðmundr inn ríki Eyjólfsson, was the constant target of humiliating quips and attacks due to his perceived cowardice and unmanliness. Despite his prestige, his shame is remembered to this day in sagas, articles, and Instagram webcomics. The importance of honour was inherent to Icelandic politics, and feud was its means of expression.[5] When discussing martiality in medieval Iceland, it is more common than not to address it through the viewpoint of feud. Indeed, the language of vengeance and the societal concern with litigation lends very much to thinking in that vein.

Most recently, however, it was my privilege to read a doctoral thesis chapter draft written by Michael Hansen, who researches martiality in high and late medieval Iceland. One of his more fascinating observations was that more than kinship ties or coercive obligation, the participants of battles were in it to be on, simply put, the winning side. There was more prestige in following a respected leader than a disgraced one, and there was much glory to be gained in fighting for a great man or a great family, even at the cost of life or limb. Hansen's model suggests that positive prestige rather than negative coercive considerations explains the enthusiastic battle participation that we see in the sagas. While it is not a catch-all solution, it does help to explain why people in general would risk so much to participate in the dangerous political struggles of the rich and famous.

In the saga dealing with events contemporary to its writing, the *Sturlunga saga*, one can find the named victim Þórðr daufi (the deaf) among the list of dead in the (in)famous Battle of Örlygsstaðir.[6] While Þórðr is not otherwise mentioned in the text, his presence in the battle means that he was trusted to fight.[7] *Sturlunga saga*, despite being written with a literary and

5 On the dynamics of medieval Icelandic feud, see, e.g., Falk, *Violence and Risk*; William Ian Miller, *Bloodtaking and Peacemaking: Feud, Law, and Society in Saga Iceland* (Chicago: University of Chicago Press, 1990); and Jesse L. Byock, *Feud in the Icelandic Saga* (Berkeley: University of California Press, 1993). For a different emphasis regarding honour, see Viðar Pálsson, *Language of Power: Feasting and Gift-Giving in Medieval Iceland and Its Sagas* (Ithaca: Cornell University Press, 2016).

6 *Sturlunga saga*, ed. Örnólfur Thorsson (Reykjavík: Svart á hvítu, 2010), 1:424.

7 This scene was pointed out to me by Michael Hansen.

political agenda,[8] describes events that happened relatively close to the time of composition. As Meulengracht Sørensen has argued, this closeness to events makes it difficult to veer too much from facts: a person's children or grandkids might be reading or listening, so you had better get things right.[9] That being said, sometimes it is the truth itself that is perceived as shaming. Even if Þórðr was a historically real person, it is currently impossible to ascertain what degree of deafness was enough to justify a nickname such as *daufi*: you need to hear to be given orders aurally (the option of lip reading is a possibility, of course), but you do not need to hear to swing a sword.[10] Þórðr shows us that mental, physical, and sensory differences make an appearance in the sagas. But sometimes one needs to look hard to find them.

A larger point must also be made: Old Norse did not, in fact, have a clear word for "disability" or "embodied difference."[11] The closest that comes to that is *ómagi*, which might be translated as "dependent."[12] *Ómagi* is incongruous with embodied difference or disability. *Ómagi* is simultaneously apt

---

**8** W. P. Ker, *Epic and Romance, Essays on Medieval Literature* (New York: Dover, 1957 [1908]); Stephen Norman Tranter, *Sturlunga Saga: The Rôle of the Creative Compiler* (Frankfurt am Main: Lang, 1987); Úlfar Bragason, *Ætt og saga: Um frásagnarfræði Sturlungu eða Íslendinga Sögu hinnar miklu* (Reykjavík: Háskólaútgáfan, 2010).

**9** Preben Meulengracht Sørensen, *Unmanly Man: Concepts of Sexual Defamation in Early Northern Society*, trans. Joan Turville-Petre (Odense: Odense University Press, 1983), 80–81.

**10** Archaeological evidence shows that the phenomenon of deafness must have existed in medieval at least to some extent (Cecilia Collins, "The Palaeopathology of Maxillary Sinusitis, Otitis Media and Mastoiditis in Medieval Iceland," PhD diss., University of Reading, 2019), though deafness as a socio-linguistic identity marker did not appear on the island until much later. Kristín Lena Thorvaldsdóttir and Valgerður Stefánsdóttir, "Icelandic Sign Language," in *Sign Languages of the World: A Comparative Handbook*, eds. Julie Bakken et al. (Berlin: de Gruyter, 2015), 409–29, at 410–11; see also Stefan C. Hardonk and Yoav Tirosh, "'Svá daufr orðinn, at hann mátti eigi heyra': A Critical Exploration of Depictions of Deaf and Non-Speaking Characters in Medieval Icelandic Literature," *The Journal of Deaf Studies and Deaf Education* 30, no. 3 (2025): 384–395.

**11** Ármann Jakobsson, Anna Katharina Heiniger, Christopher Crocker, and Hanna Björg Sigurjónsdóttir, "Disability Before Disability: Mapping the Uncharted in the Medieval Sagas," *Scandinavian Studies* 92, no. 4 (2020): 440–60; Christopher Crocker, Yoav Tirosh, and Ármann Jakobsson, "Disability in Medieval Iceland: Some Methodological Concerns," in *Understanding Disability Throughout History: Interdisciplinary Perspectives in Iceland from Settlement to 1936*, eds. Hanna Björg Sigurjónsdóttir and James G. Rice (New York: Routledge, 2022), 12–28, at 14–17.

**12** On this see Ryder Patzuk-Russell and Yoav Tirosh, "Icelandic Hospitals, Clergy, and Disability in the *Saga of Bishop Lárentíus*," *Mirator* 24, no. 1 (2024): 1–17.

and highly inapt for describing disability. A disabled person could certainly be dependent on someone's financial and practical assistance. But not all medieval disabled people were dependents. And, furthermore, *ómagi* can and does often refer to a widow, a poor person, or an underage child. *Ómagi* emphasizes the intersectional element that is inherent to disability. A man could remain independent if he becomes blind,[13] while a non-disabled widow who remains unmarried and cannot maintain her household alone could be rendered a dependent. As such, this chapter does not attempt to do injustice to the past by applying anachronistic categories to its denizens (though some of these will, inevitably, make an appearance), but will instead try to focus on the uses of the human body and embodied difference.[14]

This chapter will cover two aspects of disability and battles: participation in battle by individuals with embodied difference, and trauma and disability resulting from battles. These aspects reflect the book's theme of becoming, surviving, and managing. One acquires embodied difference, becoming disabled, and acquires the status of fighter as well, becoming a soldier, warrior, or henchman. Surviving battle-related injuries is not so much an event as it is a process. One that often involves trauma, and the development of chronic medical issues. Finally, this chapter also discusses ways by which such battle related disability and trauma are mitigated, or managed. The signs of battle inscribed on the body become symbolic of a person's participation in violent activities, both for matters of prestige, as well as for matters of infamy.

Many of its cases are found in the texts commonly referred to as the *Íslendingasögur*, or sagas of early Icelanders, which I have recently defined thus:

> The *Íslendingasögur* are a group of prose or prosimetric texts that concern the medieval Norse world, usually taking place in the period between the end of the ninth and the mid-eleventh centuries, and usually focusing on Iceland. Their structure usually revolves around a feud or feuds, usually with at least one family of elite farmers or landowners. Common themes include

13 See, e.g., Christopher Crocker, "Narrating Blindness and Seeing Ocularcentrism in *Þorsteins saga hvíta*," *Gripla* 31 (2020): 267–92; Crocker, Tirosh, and Ármann Jakobsson, "Disability in Medieval Iceland," 19.

14 See discussions in Bianca Frohne, "Heutige Modelle von Dis/Ability—tauglich für die Vormoderne?: The Cultural Model," in *Dis/Ability History der Vormoderne: Ein Handbuch* = Premodern Dis/Ability History: A Companion, eds. Cordula Nolte et al. (Affalterbach: Didymos, 2017), 61–63; Wendy J. Turner, "Models of Disability: Connecting the Past to the Present," *Zeitschrift für Disability Studies* 1 (February 2022): 1–18.

> interactions with the paranormal, violent competition over matrimony and status, regional politics, and travel. Stylistically, they are terse, concretely grounded in time and space, and give an illusion of objectivity. They reflect an oral tradition stemming from the Viking Age, written down between the thirteenth and fifteenth centuries, and are earliest preserved in manuscripts dated to the late medieval and early modern periods. While their intended audience is a general Icelandic one, they mesh well with the sentiments of an independent and Christian-minded medieval farmer.[15]

While this chapter concerns mostly characters in literary texts that deal with Viking Age (i.e., eighth to eleventh century) Iceland and Scandinavia, the focus is rather on the period in which these texts were written, the thirteenth to fifteenth century. While the degree to which the sagas were seen as historical evidence chronicling true events is an ever-challenged debate that currently lacks resolution,[16] I generally adopt the approach of collective memory that frames medieval representations of the past as revealing the concerns of the authorial present.[17]

## Weaponizing the Body

Before speaking about how people could experience disability following battle, or whether or not people with physical, mental, or sensual difference were permitted to participate in battle in medieval Iceland, it would benefit us to first address how embodied difference was not always a disadvantage in battle. In fact, the sagas' characters occasionally would and did use their embodied difference to their advantage in battle. This is not to say that the experience was necessarily an empowering one, but it was surely not a black and white matter of equating embodied difference with persistent disadvantage in battle.

---

**15** Tirosh, *How Genre Governs Creation in the Medieval Icelandic Sagas*, xxii.

**16** A good summary of the topic could be found in Ralph O'Connor, "History or Fiction? Truth-claims and Defensive Narrators in Icelandic Romance-Sagas," *Mediaeval Scandinavia* 15 (2005): 101–69. See also Ármann Jakobsson, "History of the Trolls? *Bárðar saga* as an Historical Narrative," *Saga-book of the Viking Society* 25 (1998): 53–71.

**17** See for example the introductory articles: Pernille Hermann and Stephen A. Mitchell, "Constructing the Past: Introductory Remarks," *Scandinavian Studies* 85, no. 3 (2013): 261–66; and Simon Nygaard and Yoav Tirosh, "Old Norse Studies and Collective Memory: An Introduction," in "Old Norse Studies and Collective Memory," eds. Yoav Tirosh and Simon Nygaard, special issue, *Scandinavian–Canadian Studies* 28 (2021): 24–35.

In *Ragnars saga loðbrókar*, which takes place in legendary times but does concern individuals to whom Icelanders would often trace their lineage, Viking leader Ragnarr Lóðbrók has a son dubbed Ívarr *hinn beinlausi* (the bone-less) due to a condition where his bones are replaced with connective tissue.[18] Interestingly, in the show *Vikings* Ívarr is stereotypically portrayed as an evil and bitter man with a despotic nature, but in the medieval saga he is the wisest of Ragnarr's sons, who travels by having attendants carry him around. When fighting the Swedish cow-god Síbilja, Ívarr has his men catapult him at the cow, killing her on impact with no injury to himself due to his lack of bones. In the romance *Sigrgarðs saga frækna*, a character named Hörðr smashes his hunched back into enemies in battle. Later it is disclosed that Hörðr's hunched back is, in fact, bags of iron held together using dwarfish technology.[19] In *Svarfdæla saga*, the belligerent character Klaufi takes fighting with embodied difference to the extreme; after the man is decapitated by his enemies, he returns as an animated corpse and assists his kinsmen in a battle by smacking people with his disembodied head. Lucia Simova points at a connection between Klaufi and the cephalophores, beheaded martyrs who carry their own decapitated heads. Simova hints at the warrior as a kind of inverted saint, staying loyal to his family and fighting alongside them as compared with the martyr who keeps his Christian faith.[20]

In *Grettis saga*, we learn about the late ninth-century Önundr Ófeigsson, who is called *tréfótr*—Wooden-Leg—following the loss of his leg in a battle against the up and coming Norwegian king Haraldr hárfagri.[21] As has been pointed out, this byname *tréfótr* becomes a marker of his identity, preserved in the very name of his gravemound, *tréfótshaugr*.[22] But while Önundr frames his limb loss as tragic, the saga itself does not necessarily share the sentiment.

---

**18** *Völsunga saga ok Ragnars saga loðbrókar*, ed. Magnus Olsen (Copenhagen: S. L. Møllers, 1906–1908), 129.

**19** See also Gagné in this volume for a discussion of the use of iron hands in premodern settings. See Frohne in this volume for a discussion of Gottfried (Götz) von Berlichingen's use of a prosthetic hand and his emotional reaction to this necessity. See also Crocker, Tirosh, and Ármann Jakobsson, "Disability in Medieval Iceland," 17–20.

**20** Lucia Simova, *The Dead Deserve Rest Too: The Treatment and Perception of Corpses in Medieval Icelandic Literature* (Master's thesis, University of Iceland, 2022), 65.

**21** *Grettis Saga Ásmundarsonar, Bandamanna Saga, Odds þáttr Ófeigssonar*, ed. Guðni Jónsson (Reykjavík: Hið íslenzka fornritafélag, 1936), 3–25; Gareth Lloyd Evans, *Men and Masculinities in the Sagas of Icelanders* (Oxford: Oxford University Press, 2019), 87–92; Sayers, *Oedipus Borealis*, 240–45.

**22** John P. Sexton, "Difference and Disability: On the Logic of Naming in the Icelandic

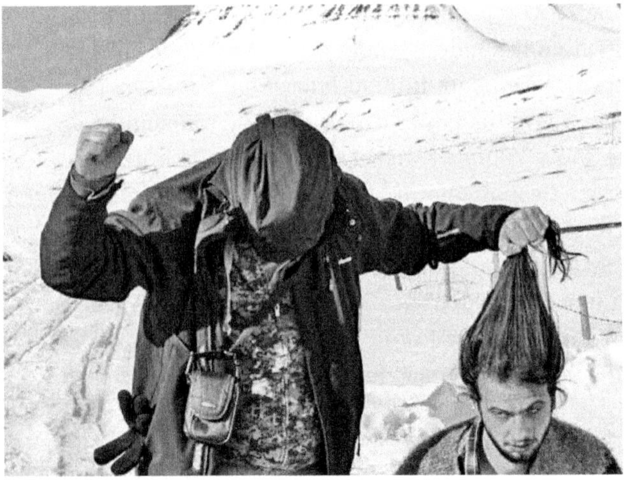

Figure 2.1. Recreating Klaufi's weaponized-head scene in the Svarfdaela saga set in the snowy landscape of Svarfaðardalur in North Iceland, April 2013. Pierre de Lépinay features as Klaufi's severed head and an unidentified person (Yoav Tirosh?) as the decapitated Klaufi. Photograph by author.

If before a certain battle an enemy Viking Vígbjóðr mocks Önundr's embodied difference, it is Önundr who laughs last, when the man swings his sword at Önundr and it gets lodged in his wooden leg prosthesis, allowing Önundr to swiftly cut off his hand, rendering Vígbjóðr *óvígr* (not in fighting form). This suggests that the "author" (a term I am using quite irresponsibly in the context of the medieval sagas) was able to capture both the mental effects of limb loss, as well as an awareness of the complexity of the experience of being a warrior with embodied difference. While most of these accounts are fantastical, they indicate that it was not beyond probability to imagine how embodied difference could be weaponized to someone's advantage in battle.

Another example to the opposite would be when someone's own physical difference is weaponized against their own person. *Vápnfirðinga saga*, a text that is highly concerned with embodied difference,[23] describes the feud between the Northeastern Icelandic cousins Þorkell Geitisson and Bjarni Brodd-Helgason. Throughout the saga, Þorkell's attempts at taking Bjarni's life are frustrated by manifestations of the would-be killer's embodied difference. They show that while in some cases embodied difference does not

Sagas," in *Disability in the Middle Ages: Reconsiderations and Reverberations*, ed. Joshua R. Eyler (London: Ashgate, 2010), 149–63, at 151–57.

**23** Christopher Crocker and Yoav Tirosh, "Health, Healing, and the Social Body in Medieval Iceland," in *Understanding Disability Throughout History: Interdisciplinary Perspectives in Iceland from Settlement to 1936*, eds. Hanna Björg Sigurjónsdóttir and James G. Rice (New York: Routledge, 2021), 113–27; and Yoav Tirosh, "Is There a Doctor on Vopnafjord? Disability, Health, and Embodied Difference in *Vápnfirðinga saga*," *Scandinavian-Canadian Studies*, forthcoming.

hinder a person from participation in battles, it often does put a barrier between a person and access to violence. One clear example of this can be found when Bjarni travels over a certain heath in the district. When Þorkell and a force of men suddenly appear before him and close in on him, Bjarni quickly thinks of a clever ruse. He has a chopping block dressed like him and fitted on a horse, and while his two companions ride with it as if it were Bjarni, he runs away into the woods to hide. The success of this plan lies in Þorkell's ocular abilities; during this episode the narrator informs us that "Þorkell was not a far-sighted man."[24] Þorkell suspects that it is not Bjarni who is riding with his companions and wishes to seek him elsewhere, but he must rely on the reports of his far-sighted men, who confidently ablesplain (in the spirit of "mansplain") him that the person riding the horse is his enemy Bjarni. By the time the ploy is revealed, Bjarni has escaped to safety.[25]

Overall, what these episodes point to is a kind of supercrip narrative construction. José Alaniz suggests that comic-book superpowers "'overcompensate' for a perceived physical defect, difference, or outright disability. Often, the super-power will erase the disability, banishing it to the realm of the invisible, replacing it with raw power and heroic acts of derring-do in a hypermasculine fashion."[26] While there is a large gap in time between the medieval sagas and modern comic-books, here Wendy J. Turner's useful term "parallel diagnosis" can assist. Applied in cases where similar embodied phenomena can be found in medieval and modern circumstances, Turner highlights that cross-cultural and cross-temporal comparisons can be fruitful if done in a thoughtful manner.[27] Along the same lines, when discussing the phenomenon of the supercrip, it is possible to observe elements that are shared between the cultures, despite the vast ocean separating them. As mentioned with the example of Klaufi, his use of his own head to bludgeon people certainly counts

---

**24** My translation. "Þorkell var maðr eigi skyggn"; *Austfirðinga sögur*, ed. Jón Jóhannesson (Reykjavík: Hið íslenzka fornritafélag, 1950), 56.

**25** On the morality of such unchivalric tactics such as trickery in the battlefield, see James Titterton, *Deception in Medieval Warfare. Trickery and Cunning in the Central Middle Ages* (Woodbridge: Boydell, 2022), 171–201.

**26** José Alaniz, "Supercrip: Disability and the Silver Age Superhero," *International Journal of Comic Art* 6, no. 2 (2004): 304–24, at 307; quoted in Sami Schalk, "Reevaluating the Supercrip," *Journal of Literary & Cultural Disability Studies* 10, no. 1 (2016): 71–86, at 81.

**27** Wendy J. Turner, "Medieval English Understanding of Mental Illness and Parallel Diagnosis to Contemporary Neuroscience," in *Cognitive Sciences and Medieval Studies: An Introduction*, eds. Juliana Dresvina and Victoria Blud (Cardiff: University of Wales Press, 2020), 97–112.

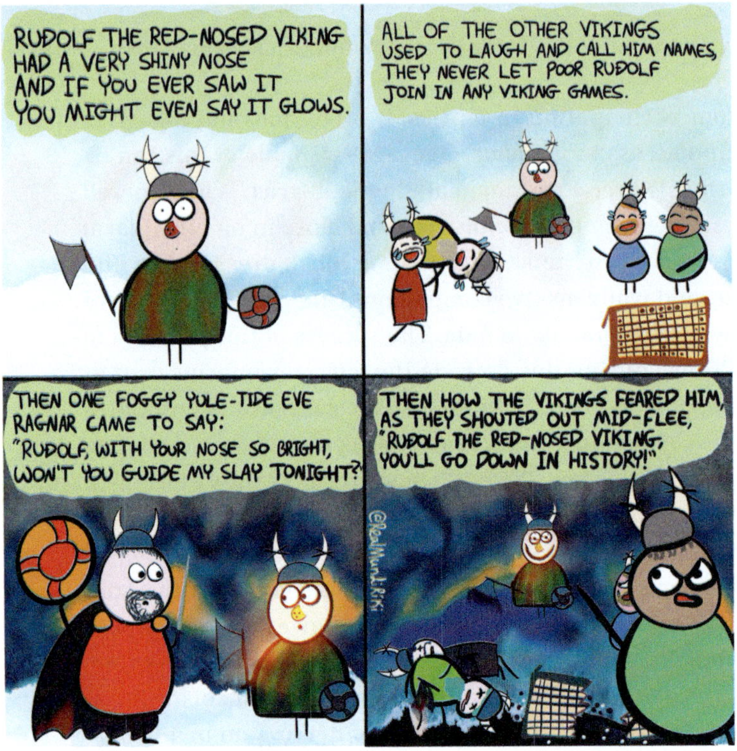


Figure 2.2. Yoav Tirosh (@RealMundiRiki), "Ruðolf the Red-Nosed-Viking." Drawn by author with Procreate on iPad Pro. Four-panel webcomic.

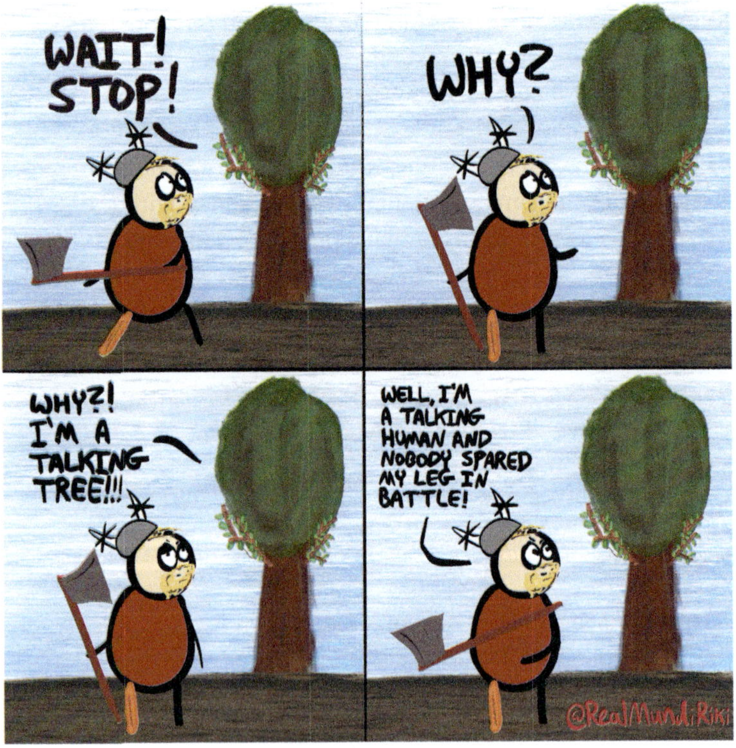


Figure 2.3. Yoav Tirosh (@RealMundiRiki), "A Talking Human." Drawn by author with Procreate on iPad Pro. Four-panel webcomic.

as a certain "super power," while the possible connection to Christian saints enhances the perception of Klaufi's loyalty to his kinsmen. As noted by William Sayers, homological patterning was at play in Old Norse narratives: one lack could be compensated for by a corresponding ability. In *Brennu-Njáls* saga, "absence of facial hair is compensated for by the seer's power, seated in the mind; the mark of masculinity active in the present is suppressed in favour of knowledge of the future outcomes of such male activity."[28] While the concepts of homology and supercrip are not identical phenomena, they point to similar ways of thinking about and describing disability.[29]

## Physical Injury Sustained in Battle

In terms of people who acquire permanent physical difference as a result of battle, there are limitless examples to be drawn from a literature as focused on fighting as the Icelandic sagas and Old Norse literature in general. Some specific considerations related to battle-related permanent physical difference can be fruitful for further debate and research. Sean Lawing has framed compensation for lost limbs and other battle-related disfigurement "as a form of medical disability payment."[30] In his research of mutilation, Lawing touches upon Old Norse approaches to limb loss as "'a fate worse than death.'" He argues that:

> At stake seems to be a quality of life issue. The phrase in Gulaþingslög "worse off living than dead" is a value statement to be situated along a continuum of dismemberment and choice. The implication according to the passage is that, in the balance, missing either both hands or both feet is still better than being dead. But, when faced with the option of losing both feet and hands, death is to be preferred.[31]

---

**28** William Sayers, "Njáll's Beard, Hallgerðr's Hair and Gunnarr's Hay: Homological Patterning in Njáls Saga," *TijdSchrift voor Skandinavistiek* 15 (1994): 5–31, at 12.

**29** See also the idea of "narrative prosthesis" as described in David T. Mitchell and Sharon L. Snyder, *Narrative Prosthesis: Disability and the Dependencies of Discourse* (Ann Arbor: University of Michigan Press, 2000). See also the criticism of the concept in Michael Bérubé, *The Secret Life of Stories: From Don Quixote to Harry Potter, How Understanding Intellectual Disability Transforms the Way We Read* (New York: New York University Press, 2016), 41–53.

**30** Sean Lawing, "Perspectives on Disfigurement in Medieval Iceland: A Cultural Study Based on Old Norse Laws and Icelandic Sagas," (PhD diss., University of Iceland, 2016), 144.

**31** Lawing, "Perspectives on Disfigurement," 144.

We find here echoes of the *Mad Men* scene discussed at the beginning of this chapter, where the benefit of living with permanent physical difference is questioned. In the Old Norse corpus, this notion is not limited to the lawbooks. For example, in *Vápnfirðinga saga*, when describing the list of a battle's casualties, we find this sentence: "Eilífr was also felled by Hallbjörn, and went on living, so to speak."[32] Despite this attitude, we can see medieval Scandinavian law providing legal accommodations for physical and sensory differences that originated from acts of violence. For example, the Norwegian Frostaþing lawbook provides special instructions for a man whose tongue is cut out by another, with an emphasis on his ability to identify the person who did the act to him; "He shall then point at that man [who did the deed] with the handle of his axe, and then he shall become an outlaw. But if he [the perpetrator] is not at the assembly, then he shall inscribe his name if he knows runes, but if he does not then he shall make those gestures so that a person can know the truth most accurately."[33] These kinds of provisions are not only a sign of social responsibility, but also a matter of liability and caregiving, as pointed out in Lawing's research. By enforcing the culpability of the man who did a certain injury, he becomes legally obligated to pay compensation, therefore limiting the need for social intervention in maintaining the person. People had enough on their plate as it is, figuratively—though often not literally—speaking. Anna Katharina Heiniger also argues that the legal settlement plays the role of a "narrative prosthesis," providing closure to the legal case and an endpoint in the event's telling. As is often the case, a silence is present when discussing a person who was impaired in battle with regard to their past injury; compensation has been paid, it is a done deal.[34]

Access to legal recourse and agency over one's own fate was a right mainly available to free men. In case of battle-related injuries, women would usually have to rely on their husbands or male kin to pursue their case by law or by sword. In *Eyrbyggja saga*, for example, Auðr and other women try to quell a violent skirmish between her husband Þórarinn's men and their

**32** My translation. "Eilífr fell ok fyrir Hallbirni, ok lifði hann þá at kalla," *Austfirðinga sögur*, 62.

**33** My translation. "Þá skal hann stinga á þann mann øxarskafti sínu, þá skal sá vera útlagr. En ef hann er eigi á þingi, þá skal hann rista nafn hans ef hann kann rúnar, en ef hann kann eigi þá bendi hann þeim bendingum er mann viti hvat sannast sé." *Norges gamle love indtil 1387*, eds. Rudolf Keyser and Peter Andreas Munch (Christiania: Gröndahl, 1846), 1:171.

**34** Anna Katharina Heiniger, "The Silenced Trauma in the *Íslendingasögur*," *Gripla* 31 (2020): 233–65.

enemies. As a result, Auðr's hand gets hacked off. Rather than seeking vengeance or compensation, she tries to hide the injury from her husband for as long as possible (perhaps to delay "hot blooded" vengeance), and does not state explicitly who cut off her hand. The otherwise peaceful man seeks his enemies out and overhears them say that it was Þórarinn himself who amputated his own wife's hand, a statement which they pay for in blood. After this new act of violence Þórarinn flees the island, and his wife is no longer mentioned. Auðr is robbed of her agency throughout her appearance. First, she tries to bring peace by intervening in the fighting, but the battle-eager men end up cutting off her hand. Then, she wishes to delay the revelation of her limb loss so that violent vengeance would not be sought, but this plan too is foiled. We never hear Auðr directly name the culprit whose actions cost her her hand, but rather her mother-in-law alleges to speak in her name, possibly using her silence as an opportunity to deflect her own son's blame for his wife's amputation.[35] She does nudge her husband out of the house during his outlawry, perhaps concerned about paying a further price for the district's political wranglings. Finally, her husband seems to leave her, provided for financially by his kinsmen, presumably, with no mention of her fate.[36]

## Battle Scars

The following two scenes from *Heiðarvíga saga* reveal a complex attitude to battle scars. The first describes a skirmish between the confusingly named Þorgísl and Þorgísl, and the second between Eyjólfr and Oddr:

> Thorgisl struck a blow which hit him on the brow toward his nose, and said, "Now you have been well marked, as you deserve; more of you should get such treatment." Thorgisl then said, "Not a fair mark, but more's the hope that I'll bear it bravely. You've little cause to be proud of yourself yet," and

**35** It is also possibly her way to settle an old score in the dispute between the district's two witches. On this fascinating case see further Ármann Jakobsson, "Two Wise Women and Their Young Apprentice: A Miscarried Magic Class," *Arkiv for nordisk filologi* 122 (2007): 43–57.

**36** *Eyrbyggja saga*, ed. Einar Ólafur Sveinsson (Reykjavík: Hið íslenzka fornritafélag, 1935), 33–60. See Heiniger, "Silenced Trauma"; Sean Lawing, "Re-membering Auðr's Hand in *Eyrbyggja Saga*," International Medieval Congress: The Literature of Medieval Scandinavia, III: Political, Cultural, and Mythological Empires, Leeds, July 7, 2014 [accessible online: https://www.academia.edu/13176735/Re_membering_Au%C3%B0r_s_Hand_in_Eyrbyggja_saga]; Crocker, Tirosh, and Ármann Jakobsson, "Disability in Medieval Iceland."

> struck him a blow which put him out of action. There followed a pause in the fighting, while men bound up their wounds.[37]

> Eyjolf turned to [Oddr] and the two of them fought together, both courageous men. Eyjolf struck [Oddr] a blow which landed on his cheek and cut into the side of his mouth, causing a gaping wound. Eyjolf then said, "Your widow may well find your face the worse for the kissing." [Oddr] answered, "It may not have been much good for some time, but now it's been really spoiled. You may not, however, get the chance to tell your girlfriend of this," and dealt him a blow which caused him a great wound.[38]

These scars are simultaneously treated as a source of wound and pride. In the first case, Þorgísl both states that the wound is not "fair," but also that it should be bravely borne, presumably as a battle scar. The comments in the second scene treat Eyjólfr's injury as something that reduces his physical attractiveness, or possibly as reducing its functionality in intimate settings.

*Svarfdæla saga* describes an ongoing feud in which a man named Skíði receives a scar from his enemies' mistreatment. Later on, when Skíði wishes to win the hand of Yngvildr, she states that she will only marry him if his scar is healed, meaning that his honour is reclaimed. Skíði then avenges his earlier injury by killing the powerful Karl the Red. This results in Yngvildr stating that Skíði's scar was healed. Some years later, Karl the Red's son, also named Karl, disturbingly tortures Yngvildr until she admits that Skíði's scar did, in fact, not heal. While it becomes a metonym for the ex-husband, the scar also takes on its own separate identity. His scar takes on a life of its own, disconnected from the body and face it occupies, representing rather the violence that Yngvildr demanded to accept Skíði's hand. The scar's disappearance was a sign of honour; its reappearance, a sign of shame.

---

**37** "The Saga of the Slayings on the Heath," in *The Complete Sagas of Icelanders, Including 49 Tales*, trans. Keneva Kunz, eds. Viðar Hreinsson et al. (Reykjavík: Leifur Eiríksson, 1997), 4:67–129, at 118. "Þorgísl ræzk honum í móti, bróðir Þórodds, ok eigusk við lengi, ok eigi skortir harðfengi hvárntveggja; ok eitt hǫgg høggr Þorgísl til hans ór brúnunum ofan nefit ok mælti: 'Nú fekk þú gott mark ok þér hœfiligt; slíkt skyldu þér fleiri hafa.' Þá mælti Þorgísl: 'Eigi er markit gott, en meiri ván, at þora ek at bera hreystiliga, ok lítt þurfi þér enn at hœlask,' og høggr til hans, svá at hann fellr ok er óvígr." *Borgfirðinga sögur*, eds. Sigurður Nordal and Guðni Jónsson (Reykjavík: Hið íslenzka fornritafélag, 1938), 306.

**38** "Saga of the Slayings," 118. "Eyjólfr gengr í móti Oddi, ok berjask þeir, ok er þar hvárrtveggi inn bezti drengr; ok nú høggr Eyjólfr til Odds, ok kemr á kinnina ok í hváptinn, ok verðr þat mikit sár. Þá mælti Eyjólfr: 'Vera kann, at ekkjunni þykki versna at kyssa þik.' Hann segir: 'Lengi hefir eigi gott verit, en þó mun nú mikit um hafa spillzk, ok þó kann vera, at eigi segir þú þetta þinni vinkonu,' ok høggr til hans, svá at hann fekk mikit sár." *Borgfirðinga sögur*, eds. Nordal and Jónsson, 306.

Elsewhere in the corpus, battle scars are seen rather as a sign of honour, as indication of a willingness to put oneself in harm's way and expose oneself to risk.[39] In that sense, it is almost the opposite of the *Svarfdæla saga* scar-as-shame. In the knightly tale *Ásmundar saga kappabana*, the protagonist's hands scarred from battle give him an edge as a suitor for the hand of a vengeance-minded princess.[40] This is interesting when compared with Önundr tréfótr (wooden-leg) discussed above. While Önundr did bemoan his limb loss and the saga does reveal some societal apprehension in relation to this injury, it is also a mark of honour, the prosthesis by-name a constant reminder of the price he paid for his bravery at battle.

What is the difference between the body scarred in battle and the face scarred in battle? Honestly, I am not sure, but I suspect it could connect to physiognomy, the notion that one's face indicates one's nature. As Cock and Skinner state in relation to the face, "The vulnerability of the face to change and non-normativity exposed the vulnerability of the self to alteration, including non-human identification."[41] Icelandic society clearly had awareness of humourism and its physiognomical applications,[42] a worldview in which a person's appearance reflected their specific character traits, influenced by the concentration of liquids (humours) in their bodily system. While the connection between one's character and battle scars might not

**39** See Knüsel's discussion of scars as a "red badge of courage" in this volume. See also Stephen Crane, *The Red Badge of Courage* (s.l.: Mockingbird, 2015).

**40** Sarah Künzler, *Flesh and Word: Reading Bodies in Old Norse: Icelandic and Early Irish Literature* (Berlin: de Gruyter, 2016), 259–65; Crocker, Tirosh, and Ármann Jakobsson, "Disability in Medieval Iceland," 21.

**41** Emily Cock and Patricia Skinner, "(Dis)functional Faces: Signs of the Monstrous?" in *Monstrosity, Disability, and the Posthuman in the Medieval and Early Modern World*, eds. Richard H. Godden and Asa Simon Mittman (London: Palgrave, 2019), 85–105, at 87–88. See Bianca Frohne, "Object Lesson: St. Roch," *Manual* 17 (2022) [Last modified April 03, 2024. Accessed December 28, 2024.] https://risdmuseum.org/issue-17-variance/object-lesson-st-roch, for an accessible entry point on bodies and aesthetics in medieval Europe.

**42** On humoral theory in the Icelandic context see Brynja Þorgeirsdóttir, "Humoral Theory in the Medieval North: An Old Norse Translation of *Epistula Vindiciani* in Hauksbók," *Gripla* 29 (2018): 35–66. For a study of humoral theory's manifestations in saga literature, see Lars Lönnroth, "Kroppen som själens spegel—ett motiv i de isländska sagorna," *Lychnos* 4 (1963–1964): 24–61. See also Christopher Crocker, "Emotions," in *The Routledge Research Companion to the Medieval Icelandic Sagas*, eds. Armann Jakobsson and Sverrir Jakobsson (New York: Routledge, 2017), 240–52, at 242–3; and Yoav Tirosh, "Milk, Masculinity, and Humor-Less Vikings – Gender in the Old Norse Polysystem," in "Constructing Masculinity in Old Norse Culture," ed. Cord. Remigiusz Gogosz, special issue, *Limes* 13 (2020): 136–50, at 143–46.

be intuitively understood, it is worth considering that in the worldview of the romance—which had its influences on medieval Iceland and certainly on the greater Scandinavia[43]—one's facial features would often be perceived as a consequence of one's actions, rather than as indicating inherent features fated by birth.[44] The above-mentioned Haraldr hárfagri, enemy of *Grettis saga*'s Önundr tréfótr, exemplifies the importance of appearance in the context of battle as well. Haraldr's by-name *hárfagri* could be translated as "fair-hair." But he only acquires this name after he manages to unite all of Norway under his reign; before this he is in fact called *lúfa*, which means "tangled hair," a reference to his vow to avoid cutting his hair or combing it before achieving his grand goals. Haraldr's getting rid of his tangled hair is here seen as a sign of an oath kept, of his honour standing. Önundr and his nemesis Haraldr reveal that bodies were open to interpretation: there remains a fine line between reading embodied difference as a (potentially instrumentalizing) metaphor, and using embodied difference as a helpful metonym.[45] Yet one would be hard pressed to fully understand disability without understanding performance, and reading disability performance requires reading bodies.[46] The fighting ethos itself is also intertwined with injury and the consequences of embodied difference.[47] To what extent facial disfigurement should be considered a disability is also up for debate,[48] but like much other embodied difference, is dependent on factors like time, place, gender, or class.[49]

---

**43** See Sif Rikhardsdottir, *Medieval Translations and Cultural Discourse, the Movement of Texts in England, France and Scandinavia* (Cambridge: Brewer, 2012); and Sif Rikhardsdottir, *Emotion in Old Norse Literature: Translations, Voices, Contexts* (Cambridge: Brewer, 2017).

**44** For an example of such discussion see Bonnie Millar, "Dis/enabling Courtesy and Chivalry in the Middle English and Early Modern Gawain Romances and Ballads," in *Approaching Facial Difference: Past and Present*, eds. Patricia Skinner and Emily Cock (London: Bloomsbury Academic, 2018), 11–25, esp. 17–22, which touches on the mirroring of facial difference resulting from violence with that resulting from corruption.

**45** Sexton, "Atypical Bodies," 31; Michael Bérubé, "Disability and Narrative," *PMLA* 120, no. 2 (2005): 568–576.

**46** On reading bodies in the Old Norse and Early Irish literatures, see Künzler, *Flesh and Word.*

**47** See Hildebrand in this volume.

**48** Emily Cock and Patricia Skinner, "Introduction: Situating the Different Face," in *Approaching Facial Difference*, 1–8, at 1–3.

**49** See, for example, in this volume: Verreycken "A Vulnerable Military Masculinity: Soldiers and Disability in Late Medieval Pardon Letters (France, England, and the

## Battle Trauma

In a 2023 editorial credited to the *Washington Post* editorial board, it was opined that

> If we owe our veterans every support, we also owe them a measure of fiscal responsibility. Today, we offer suggestions about how to carefully prune the department's kudzu-like spending growth...Payments rise, on a scale of 1 to 100, from minor injuries to complete impairment. The ratings were established in 1945 and in many cases have not changed in decades. That means payments are generally based on the ability to perform work most needed generations ago, or what the Congressional Budget Office described as "manual or physical labor." The skill sets needed and jobs available today—in an information and service economy—are in many cases different from those needed in the months and years after World War II.[50]

The *Washington Post* here offers a reform to VA disability compensation, which functions as a series of cutbacks. Why this matters in the present context is that the *Washington Post* does so by redefining what qualifies as a disability, and who is qualified to receive money from the government. The editorial board is doing nothing new here. In fact, as Peter Levenda has noted—in his characteristic conspiratorial yet compelling habit—the very definition of Post Traumatic Stress Disorder (PTSD) originated in the United States military's need for categorizing battle-related physical and mental injuries, partially in order to determine compensation.[51] While arguing that certain periods are more or less traumatic could be controversial, it is quite clear that manifestations of what we would today call trauma were present in medieval Iceland, and more specifically medieval Icelandic literature.[52] Anna

---

Low Countries)," and Pfau "Traumatic Repercussions: Warfare and Disability in the French Countryside."

**50** Editorial Board, "Veterans Deserve Support. But One Benefit Program Deserves Scrutiny," *Washington Post*, April 3, 2023; https://www.washingtonpost.com/opinions/2023/04/03/veterans-affairs-disability-payments-overdue-update/, accessed January 7, 2024. See Depreter in this volume for a discussion of a medieval form of veteran benefits.

**51** Peter Levenda, *Sinister Forces: A Grimoire of American Political Witchcraft. Book Three: The Manson Secret* (Walterville: TrineDay, 2011), 6–8. For a less explicitly sinister take on the military's involvement, see Allan V. Horwitz, *DSM: A History of Psychiatry's Bible* (Baltimore: Johns Hopkins University Press, 2021), 21–27.

**52** Torfi H. Tulinius, "I: 17 Trauma Studies," in *Handbook of Pre-Modern Nordic Memory Studies: Interdisciplinary Approaches*, eds. Jürg Glauser et al. (Berlin: de Gruyter, 2018), 250–55; and Torfi H. Tulinius, "II: 15 Trauma," in *Handbook of Pre-Modern Nordic Memory Studies*, 495–501.

Katharina Heiniger has explored the silence regarding battle-related physical difference as the manifestation of trauma. [53] Often such injuries would remain infused in a person's identity through their by-names, such as the case of Ófeigr tréfót (wooden-leg) discussed above.[54] Yet, as Heiniger shows, these will usually remain unaddressed by the characters. While trauma is not limited to the realm of battle,[55] it certainly invites events that stay ever-present in people's psyche after the fact. *Svarfdæla saga*'s tortured Yngvildr has already been mentioned, and it is worth considering that despite not participating in the battlefield, Yngvildr's trauma and possible subsequent suicide is certainly violence-related.[56] Violence and trauma, thus, do not skip non-combatants. In a late medieval Icelandic letter of protest written by Hólar bishop Jón Vilhjámsson Craxton, the following scene is described:

> you took and imprisoned like a picaroon our kinswoman Ragnfríður Gautadóttir when she was home in Hólar, and shut her and her twelve year old son in [a shed?] without clothes in the biting frost and cold. And when they came out men saw that she was both blue and bloody. And then you took from her her property without legal warrant, and uncourteously those goods that belonged to the Holy Church of Hólar. And she was cut by your knife that you have in your possession. And you wanted her to be distressed, as she often attests.[57]

---

**53** Heiniger, "Silenced Trauma."

**54** See Sexton, "Difference and Disability" and Sexton, "Atypical Bodies," 29–32.

**55** See, for example, Pernille Hermann's discussion of the Norse settlement of Vínland—modern day Canada—which admittedly did involve much violence, but also the exploration of a brave new world. Pernille Hermann, "The Horror of Vínland: Topographies and Otherness in the Vínland sagas," *Scandinavian Studies* 93, no. 1 (2021): 1–22.

**56** See also Marion Poilvez, "A Troll Did It? Trauma as a Paranormal State in the *Íslendingasögur*," in *Paranormal Encounters in Iceland 1150–1400*, eds. Ármann Jakobsson and Mariusz Mayburd (Berlin: de Gruyter, 2020), 71–88, at 74.

**57** My translation, with help from Þórdís Edda Jóhannesdóttir. "þu tok(t) oc fangader sæm ræningia ragnfridæ gautadottur uora frendkona heima a holum oc brygder hana med sinom syni tolf vetra gomblum bædi saman mestu klædlaus j miklu frostæ oc kulda oc þa þau komu vt sa mænn hana bædi blaa oc bloduga oc þar med tokt þu vpp hennar godz an doms oc laga oc æi sidr þat godz sem reiknadh uar heilagre hola kirkiu oc hon skæindizst af þinom knifæ sem þu hafder a þær j ykaræ samæighn oc þu vilder henne þrugat hafua sæm hon hefuer fram boret firir oss optliga." *Diplomatarium Islandicum: Íslenzkt fornbréfasafn sem hefir inni að halda bréf og gjörninga, dóma og máldaga, og aðrar skrár er snerta Ísland eða íslenzka menn*, eds. Jón Sigurðsson et al. (Copenhagen: Hið íslenzka bókmenntafjelag, 1857–1972), 4:528.

Ragnfríður's repeated provocations of the bishop smack of trauma. Once again, Turner's notion of parallel diagnoses alerts us to the advantages and disadvantages of taking what is good about retrospective diagnosis without committing full-heartedly to our results. It nevertheless seems that whatever happened to her and her son in that shed seems to have shaken her to her core, remaining with her since.[58]

Expressions of trauma are often characterized by a belated response to a violent event. An occurrence might not be perceived as traumatic at the time, but it will eventually manifest in one's dreams, flashbacks, thoughts, or behaviours.[59] Trauma sends us on an awkward trajectory that does not mesh well with what we might think of as the heteronormative experience of time. Here the concept of crip time, an offshoot of queer time, is relevant. These two concepts suggest that both queer and crip people experience time differently than non-disabled and heteronormative trajectories.[60] Disability involves planning and time management that non-disabled people often do not experience. Chronic pain, medical interventions, planning out accessible travel routes: all of these impact one's sense of time and interactions with it.[61] This, both on a mental level as well as practical. On the mental side, it is

---

**58** Vilborg Davíðsdóttir's historical novel on the Icelandic fifteenth century, *Galdur: Skáldsaga* (Reykjavík: Mál og menning, 2002), is based on the description of this very item in the bishop's letter, showing its piercing potency and potential.

**59** The classic texts dealing with the expression of trauma in literature are Cathy Caruth, *Unclaimed Experience: Trauma, Narrative, and History* (Baltimore: Johns Hopkins University Press, 1996), and Shoshana Felman and Dori Laub, *Testimony: Crises of Witnessing in Literature Psychoanalysis and History* (London: Routledge, 1992). Since then, much criticism has been shared on this theoretical application as appropriating the term from actual trauma survivors (Wulf Kansteiner and Harald Weilnböck, "Against the Concept of Cultural Trauma or How I Learned to Love the Suffering of Others without the Help of Psychotherapy," in *Cultural Memory Studies: An International and Interdisciplinary Handbook*, eds. Astrid Erll and Ansgar Nuenning (Berlin: de Gruyter, 2008), 229–40), or even at the very highlighting of a traumatic "event" as Western-minded (Stef Craps, "Beyond Eurocentrism: Trauma Theory in the Global Age," in *The Future of Trauma Theory: Contemporary Literature and Cultural Criticism*, eds. Gert Buelens et al. (London: Routledge, 2013), 45–61). See also Robert Eaglestone, "Knowledge, 'Afterwardsness' and the Future of Trauma Theory," in *The Future of Trauma Theory: Contemporary Literature and Cultural Criticism*, eds. Gert Buelens et al. (London: Routledge, 2013), 11–21, at 13–14.

**60** J. Halberstam, *In a Queer Time and Place: Transgender Bodies, Subcultural Lives* (New York: New York University Press, 2005); Alison Kafer, *Feminist, Queer, Crip* (Bloomington: Indiana University Press, 2013), 25–46.

**61** Emma Sheppard, *Chronic Pain, BDSM and Crip Time* (New York: Routledge, 2023), 65–83.

hard to say that one lives a linear existence when one is often abruptly transported into the past. A certain scent, word, or emotion triggers a return to a moment or moments that distressed your psyche. A person experiencing trauma is thus somewhat outside of time, living an existence that is unique in its temporal interactions. As mentioned at the beginning of this chapter, in *Ljósvetninga saga*, the protagonist Guðmundr inn ríki invades the home of his enemy Þorkell hákr to avenge insults against his masculinity. Þorkell refuses to go down without a fight, and he reaches the point where he fights Guðmundr and his men with his guts sticking out. Furthermore, in the process of the battle, not only does Guðmundr fail to show impressive military prowess, he also falls into a vat of white liquid milk, thus perpetuating the very rumours regarding his masculinity that he fought so fiercely to quell. Even worse, Guðmundr's spy Rindill is killed as vengeance for the deed, an act that infuriates *Ljósvetninga saga*'s protagonist to the brink of a murderous rampage.[62] The whole experience, you see, is visceral, humiliating, and altogether traumatizing.

Following this killing and its violent aftermath, Guðmundr inn ríki experiences recurring dreams of Þorkell hákr's bloody head. Seeking solace, Guðmundr visits his victim's brother, Drauma-Finni the dream interpreter, and gets him to explain the vision's meaning. By soliciting Drauma-Finni's services and reminding him of his brother's unavenged state, one could hardly be blamed for thinking that Guðmundr is in fact enacting a death-wish. If this is the case, it succeeds, as a few scenes later, Drauma-Finni brings about Guðmundr's death by paranormal means.[63] The dream and the urgent need to rid himself of it give the reader the feeling that this particular saga character is struggling with symptoms of battle-related post trauma. On a practical level, experiencing trauma can also take a toll on an individual's interactions with time itself: *Grettis saga*'s protagonist Grettir finds himself in quite a pickle. Following his battle with the undead Glámr, Grettir becomes afraid of the dark, having trouble sleeping alone. The harrowing ghostbusting stays with Grettir: When he closes his eyes, he can see Glámr's eyes shining from the moonlight.[64] This battle related trauma affects Grettir's decision making

---

**62** Yoav Tirosh, "*Argr* Management: Vilifying Guðmundr inn ríki in *Ljósvetninga saga*," in *Bad Boys and Wicked Women: Antagonists and Troublemakers in Old Norse Literature*, eds. Daniela Hahn and Andreas Schmidt (Munich: Utz, 2016), 240–72.

**63** *Ljósvetnínga saga: Eptir gömlum hdr. útg. at tilhlutun hins konúngliga Norræna fornfræða félags*, eds. Þorgeir Guðmundsson and Þorsteinn Helgason (Copenhagen: Möller, 1830), 67–70.

**64** Poilvez, "A Troll Did It?" 75–77.

and eventually leads to his (and his brother's) death: Later in the saga Grettir is outlawed, and since he cannot be by himself at night, he finds himself seeking out the company of others, despite the associated dangers.[65]

## Conclusion

> Difference, if it is to yield insight into any mind-set but our own, must be examined as a function and outcome of context.[66]

As mentioned above, it is very difficult to discuss disability in medieval Iceland when the concept of *ómagi*—dependent—covers an entirely different category of class, gender, and embodied difference that more often than not does not correlate with our modern understandings of the concept. Add to that the difficulty in determining in what cases embodied difference would be treated as disability, and whether any consistent attitude towards this could even be found, and you get a very distant and very constructed past to contend with. While in Old Norse literature war, feud, and violence tend to target men, this is generally the case, but not always the case. A woman could lose a limb or suffer trauma. Disability in battle likewise transcends class. Þórðr daufi from the Örlygsstaðir battle has no other clear identity markers, implying that he did not come from an elite progeny. Countless slaves are injured in battle, fighting somebody else's fight. Disability and trauma are at once loose categories, but also with very real-life implications. Those who experience mental, physical, and sensory difference resulting from battle go through something that is very real and must be addressed. When discussing the past, we cannot ignore these people's fates simply because they might not have had a word to describe their situation. In a society so culturally focused on violence as the medieval Icelandic one, it should not surprise us that its literature would feature so many examples of disability and trauma.

If in the imagined 1960s UK of Mad Men a person missing a foot cannot be employed as an advertising agent, and in the reality of 2020s USA some *Washington Post* editors might not consider battle-related physical

---

**65** See also, in this volume, chapters by Hildebrand, "Hungry for Love: Disabling the Knightly Body and Mind through Starvation in Sir Thomas Malory's *Le Morte Darthur*," Pfau, "Traumatic Repercussions: Warfare and Disability in the French Countryside," and Turner, "Investigating the Lifecycle of the Medieval English Soldier: Disability, Mental Trauma, and Medicine in Connection with War in Late Medieval English Records."

**66** Sexton, "Atypical Bodies," 24.

difference as a disability per se, it is clear that disability is a fluid concept. It is worth studying the very different past because its people deserve to be studied in and of themselves. But we also gain an understanding of the complexities of our own post-modern situation through the process of research. In a thirteenth- to fourteenth-century Icelandic saga, when a Viking loses his foot in battle, he might be cranky about it, but nonetheless continues to live and fight. In an American 2010s television drama, when a small John Deere runs over the foot of a British ads man, his life is no longer worth living.

Chapter 3

# HUNGRY FOR LOVE

## DISABLING THE KNIGHTLY BODY AND MIND THROUGH STARVATION IN SIR THOMAS MALORY'S *LE MORTE DARTHUR*

KRISTINA HILDEBRAND

INJURY AND DISABILITY are natural results of war, for obvious reasons, and knightly romances deal with this kind of temporary or permanent disability. In this chapter I will discuss love-madness as a disability, its aggravation by starvation, and the parallels between physical disability through wounding with mental disability through love-madness, in Sir Thomas Malory's *Le Morte Darthur*.

### Malory, the Text, and War

In the ninth year of the reign of Edward IV—1469 or 1470—Sir Thomas Malory wrote his *Le Morte Darthur*.[1] This is a compilation, translation, and rewriting of various prose and poetry romances in French and English, some of which are identifiable and some not. Regardless of the sources to which Malory constantly refers, this is no mere copy, but a unique text. Where we have the sources, we can see that Malory rewrites them, including deleting parts, and adding new ones; it is reasonable to assume that he does so also where we do not know the source—and also to consider the possibility that those parts might be original writing.

The manuscript also has a complex history. It was printed by Caxton in 1485, and this was the only extant version until, in 1934, a manuscript

1 Sir Thomas Malory, *Le Morte Darthur*, ed. P. J. C. Field, 2 vols. (Cambridge: Brewer, 2013). Further references will be in the text as (page number. line number), this being the standard quotation format for this text.

**KRISTINA HILDEBRAND** is Lecturer in English at Dalarna University, Sweden, and an Associate Member of the Centre for Arthurian Studies at Bangor University, Wales. Her work on gender, sexuality, and disability, especially in medieval and modern Arthurian texts, has appeared in *Arthuriana* and in various anthologies.

containing a different, and longer, version of it was discovered at Winchester College. The relationship between the Winchester manuscript and Caxton's printed version is not clear, although markings on the Winchester manuscript show that it has been at Caxton's printing press.

While the scholarly community has spent some time arguing about who Sir Thomas Malory was, there is largely a scholarly consensus agreeing with P. J. C. Field's *The Life and Times of Sir Thomas Malory*,[2] which identifies him as a knight from Newbold Revel, who fought in the War of the Roses under the earl of Warwick. Due to a rather extensive career in crime—robbery, extortion, rape, and attempted murder—as well as following Warwick to the then losing Lancastrian side in the war, he spent a lot of time imprisoned. It was presumably during one of these stints in prison that he wrote his book, as the text repeatedly refers to its author being a prisoner.

A significant part of Malory's life and work is his experience of battle. While many romances had been written in various monasteries, this text was created by someone who had undoubtedly seen fighting. Malory was also possibly present, or knew those who were, at the Battle of Towton in 1461.[3] Christopher Knüsel's text in this volume, with its examples of the extensive, not to say excessive, injuries to the bodies indicates the violence of that battle.[4] The text is by no means a depiction of contemporary warfare; wars are fought as series of individual combats, with rarely an archer in sight. Nevertheless, almost all fighting appearing in the text, whether it takes place in wars or as individual combat, is set in a "context of organized and sustained violence involving structured groups of individuals."[5] The knights at Arthur's court, and in particular the Round Table knights, constitute a

---

**2** P. J. C. Field, *The Life and Times of Sir Thomas Malory* (Cambridge: Brewer, 1993).

**3** Field discusses the possibility that Malory was at Towton, based on both his active participation in the War of the Roses and on his description of a horrific final battle at Camlann. He states that "the year of [Malory's] apparent release [1460–1461] was the most active and bloody of the War of the Roses...Since one of the warring parties had repeatedly tried to free him, and the other had shown itself determined to keep him in prison, Malory had reason to be in the thick of things. If he was, however, there is no reliable evidence of it." Malory's addition to his sources when describing Arthur's final battle, with the wounded being killed by pillagers for their armour and valuables, reminiscent of Towton, "could have been prompted by a different battle or by Malory's imagination alone." Field, *Life and Times*, 126.

**4** In this volume, Christopher Knüsel, "The Recidivists: Healed Cranial Trauma from Conflicts in the Late Medieval Period."

**5** Ninon Dubourg and Christophe Masson, "Disability and War: Becoming, Surviving, Managing," in this volume.

battle force participating in wars, judicial combat, and general policing of the realm, with no real distinction made between those functions. In Malory's text, despite the absence of contemporary warfare, the depiction of injuries, disability, and scarring, as well as of people plundering the bodies on the battlefield (924.16–20), testify to a profound familiarity with battle and its effects, including temporary or permanent disability.

## Knightly Disability

In medieval romances, knights and disability are inextricably intertwined. In these, disability—explicit or as the absence of ability—unavoidably features as a major part of knightly life. While, as Pearman points out, Malory's *Morte Darthur* "on the surface...figures ability as the normative centre of the chivalric code,"[6] physical injury is integral to knighthood, being an unavoidable consequence of combat. Shichtman and Finke point out that "violence provides the foundation for an elaborate structure of exchange which determines hierarchies among men."[7] Injury, including temporary or permanent disability, is a consistent fact of life—indeed, without the wounding there is no knighthood. The wounding does, in fact, prove the knighthood: when people "saw so many wounds on [Sir Launcelot] they judged that he had been a man of honour" (648.21–22).[8] The scars testify to the ability of the knight. Furthermore, as Hodges points out, "the injuries sustained give weight and worth to the abstract issues being fought about."[9] Pearman points out that "the division between knighthood and disability is not so unambiguous: instead, a knight must perpetually oscillate between disability and ability in order to maintain his status, making (dis)ability central to knighthood."[10] Like physical injuries, the mental ones can be temporary or

---

**6** Tory V. Pearman, *Disability and Knighthood in Malory's Morte Darthur* (London: Routledge, 2019), 7.

**7** Laurie R. Finke and Marty Schichtman, "No Pain, No Gain: Violence as Symbolic Capital in Malory's *Morte d'Arthur*," *Arthuriana* 8, no. 2 (Summer 1998): 115–34.

**8** "sawe so many woundys uppon [Sir Launcelot] they demed that he had bene a man of worshyp." Translations of Malory's text are my own, and intended to facilitate the reading for non-experts, not as the final word on the exact meaning of the text. The original text will be provided in the footnotes, and I refer the reader to that as the basis for my analysis.

**9** Kenneth Hodges, "Wounded Masculinity: Injury and Gender in Sir Thomas Malory's *Le Morte Darthur*," *Studies in Philology* 106, no. 1 (Winter 2009): 14–31, at 16.

**10** Pearman, *Disability and Knighthood*, 1.

permanent: Wendy J. Turner and Aleksandra Pfau's articles in this volume both point out that mental disability was seen as possible to recover from.[11] In Malory, knights become mentally disabled from love, generally survive the experience, but mostly do not manage the disability: instead they are cured by various means. While it lasts, the mental disability is generally all-encompassing, to the extent that knights lose their identity. Nevertheless, it is not permanent—unless the madness leads to suicide—and thus little long-term management is required.

There is much excellent work on disability in the Middle Ages, by scholars such as Irina Metzler and Henri-Jacques Stiker,[12] as well as work on disability in fiction by for example Ato Quayson, David T. Mitchell, and Sharon L. Snyder.[13] Work on disability in medieval romance is rarer, but some excellent scholarship in this field is emerging. Among this we see Tory V. Pearman's work on disability in medieval literature, Jonathan Hsy's work on disability in the global Middle Ages, their *A Cultural History of Disability in the Middle Ages*, and articles like Christine Marie Neufield's "A Dwarf in King Arthur's Court: Perceiving Disability in Arthurian Romance."[14] This is an expanding and highly active field, covering both history and literature, and the intersections between them.

However, physical injury is only one form of disability threatening the knights. Other writers in this volume, specifically Pfau and Turner, discuss mental trauma and disability, as does Tirosh. While their discussions have

---

**11** See, in this volume, Wendy J. Turner, "Investigating the Lifecycle of the Medieval English Soldier: Disability, Mental Trauma, and Medicine in Connection with War in Late Medieval English Records"; and Aleksandra Pfau, "Traumatic Repercussions: Warfare and Disability in the French Countryside."

**12** Irina Metzler, *Disability in Medieval Europe: Thinking about Physical Impairment during the High Middle Ages, c. 1100–1400* (London: Routledge, 2006); *A Social History of Disability in the Middle Ages: Cultural Consideration of Physical Impairment* (New York: Routledge, 2013); Henri-Jacques Stiker, *A History of Disability*, trans. William Sayers (Ann Arbor: University of Michigan Press, 1999).

**13** Ato Quayson, *Aesthetic Nervousness: Disability and the Crisis of Representation* (New York: Columbia University Press, 2007); David T. Mitchell and Sharon L. Snyder, *Narrative Prosthesis: Disability and the Dependencies of Discourse* (Ann Arbor: University of Michigan Press, 2000).

**14** Tory V. Pearman, *Women and Disability in Medieval Literature* (New York: Palgrave, 2010); "Disability, Blood, and Liminality in Malory's 'Tale of the Sankgreal,'" *Journal of Literary & Cultural Disability Studies* 10, no. 3 (2016): 271–86; Jonathan Hsy et al., eds., *A Cultural History of Disability in the Middle Ages* (London: Bloomsbury, 2020); Christine Marie Neufield, "A Dwarf in King Arthur's Court: Perceiving Disability in Arthurian Romance," *Arthuriana* 25, no. 4 (Winter 2015): 25–35.

added much to my understanding of war and disability, they focus on the perceived mental disability of historical figures, even when presented in semi-fictional form. In Pfau and Turner, the sources show how the mental disabilities had real-world consequences for the sufferers and their immediate surroundings, and in the case of Charles VI, for the realm. In the Icelandic sagas, as Tirosh points out, the writing refers to historical figures who lived recently enough that their "children or grandkids might be reading or listening, so you had better get things right."[15] This relationship to historical fact is largely absent from Malory's text—regardless of the readers' belief, or lack thereof, in Arthur as a historical king. The knights' disabilities, thus, do not need to adhere to anybody's lived experience, but are—as everything about them tends to be—larger than life. This is not mere fictional exaggeration, but a fundamental aspect of the text, depicting as it does, the "flower of knighthood": a brief moment of near-perfection not of individuals but of a community. Disability is an integral, although complicated and ambiguous, part of this perfect community.

I will here focus on the mental disability caused by love-madness, and especially its connection to starvation. Pearman defines love-sickness as "a disabling chronic illness" and differentiates love-madness as involving a "complete loss of sanity."[16] As the love-madness might appear even in mutual love relationships, due to misunderstandings or physical separation, this mental disability is a constant possible consequence of love—which is itself also unavoidable for the knights. Malory comments that "there was never an honourable man nor an honourable woman that didn't love someone better than any other, and honour in arms can never be thwarted" (841.24–26).[17] Malory's knights are defined by combat and love, and both these things frequently result in disability.

Love-madness also carries a risk of starvation. Love-sickness might result in loss of appetite, as it does with Sir Gareth; however, love-madness not only causes the knight to lose interest in eating, but also removes him from one of the central focuses of the chivalric society, courtly communal dining. Even were he willing to eat, he lacks the social context, and the serving of food, that the court he has left provides. Consequently, this lack of food increases the disabling and dysfunction of the knightly body in romance texts.

**15** Yoav Tirosh, "Disability and Trauma in Battle in the Medieval Icelandic Sagas," in this volume.

**16** Pearman, *Disability and Knighthood*, 47

**17** "there was never worshypfull man nor worshypfull woman but they loved one bettir than anothir, and worshyp in armys may never be foyled."

## Love Madness

It is of course *de rigueur* for knights disappointed in love to run mad through the forest. This can be seen in Chrétien de Troyes's Yvain, who becomes mad after failing to return to his lady and thus being rejected by her. Already in this text we see the association of madness and inability to acquire the right kind of food: Yvain is forced to eat raw meat.[18] The great lovers of the stories, Launcelot and Tristram, but also minor characters, display this excess of distress caused by unrequited love, their lover rebuking them, or the belief that their lady loves another. The madness is sometimes fleeting and passes quickly, in other cases lasts for years. As Pearman points out, "[love-mad] knights experience full removal from the courtly realm, often disappearing into the wilderness for weeks or years."[19] This retreat to a world outside the civilization of the court is a consequence of madness, but also a symptom: Jean-Marie Fritz notes that "the mad person is a being from outside, out of all civilized or socialized space, out of himself, out of his senses, and thus some of the expressions which habitually designate the frenetic in our romances are those such as *hors du sen*, *hors de son mimoire*, *issir del sen*, and not *fol*."[20] Mental disability places the sufferer outside normal human interaction. Yet despite this, in Malory's text mental disability, compared to physical disabilities, is not as subject to slippage and invisibility. In Malory, the permanently physically disabled knights move from a liminal position to extensive marginalization, with names, plotlines, and thematic functions shifting between characters and occasionally disappearing entirely.[21] This is not the case with mental disability due to love-madness. Furthermore, while the narrative breaks down at the points where it concerns physical disability, it remains largely stable and coherent on this mental disability.

The expression of the mental disability of love-sickness and love-madness is markedly gendered. The most common format is a man driven to mental distress and disability by the beauty of a woman he loves, from Uther's love for Igraine to Launcelot's love for Guinevere, which Pearman

---

**18** Chrétien de Troyes, *Le Chevalier au lion*, ed. Corinne Pierreville (Paris: Champion, 2016), 2827–28.

**19** Pearman, *Disability and Knighthood*, 47.

**20** Jean-Marie Fritz, *Le discours du fou au Moyen Âge* (Paris: Presses universitaires de France, 1992), 16, quoted and translated in Aleksandra Pfau, "Mental Health Issues: Folly, Frenzy, and the Family," in *A Cultural History of Disability*, eds. Hsy et al., 157–73, at 160.

**21** Kristina Hildebrand, "Sitting on the Sidelines: Malory and Disability," *Arthuriana* 27, no. 3 (Fall 2017): 66–81.

argues bookend *Le Morte Darthur*. Pearman also notes that women act as "instruments of (dis)ability" who might not even be aware of the love-sickness they cause in men.[22] However, women, too, suffer from madness due to excessive love: as Pearman also notes, Ettard and Elaine of Astolat are examples of this.[23] This takes a gendered form of expression, as the women suffering from it do not have the knightly option of physically removing themselves from the courtly context: love-madness disables women—and sometimes leads to death from the illness or from suicide—but they rarely, if ever, run wild through the forest.

The expression of love-madness is, as noted, gendered, but whether it leads to gender-transgressing behaviour in the knights is more complex. Knightly masculinity in Malory focuses on prowess and courtly love rather than rationality and logic. Pearman argues that disability, including mental disability due to love-madness, feminizes the knights: they lose rational thought, and exhibit behaviours that are traditionally coded feminine.[24] Yet we should note that they retain their martial abilities, even if practising them irrationally. As long as they retain their prowess, despite their loss of rational thought they have not been fully feminized. Disability is a complex matter that can be read both as causing feminization and as proof of masculine valour, and mental disability, like physical, sits uneasily between forms of gendering, causing both feminine irrationality and hypermasculine physical action.

The love-madness that drives the knight into the forest is an uncanny parallel to the knightly adventures. The wilderness is a necessary arena for knightly endeavour: it holds adventures and wonders, and disappearing from court into the forest is a regular occurrence in knightly life. From this wilderness, the knights then return to court to tell of their experiences and have their successes celebrated. The mad knight, then, is following procedure in entering the wilderness; the divergence from normality comes from the state in which he does so. The mad knight often enters the forest without armour, or on foot, and in all cases unable to avail himself of the guidance offered by the miscellaneous damsels, hermits, and other advisors normally encountered in the wilderness. Sir Tristram, made desperate by the belief that Isoud loves another, "fell down off his horse in a faint,"

22 Pearman, *Disability and Knighthood*, 24–25, at 21.

23 Pearman, *Disability and Knighthood*, 27.

24 Pearman, *Disability and Knighthood*, 49.

and will not eat or drink (388.35–398.1, 389.17).[25] Sir Launcelot, doubly distressed by Elaine's repeated rape of him and Guinevere's belief he has consented, runs off as "an unarmoured man in his shirt with a sword in his hand" (635.35).[26] Palomides, crazed with envy of Sir Tristram for his winning tournaments—but also jealous of his relationship with Isoud, whom Palomides also loves—"made many strange signs and token, and so due to his bitterness he threw his sword in that fountain" only to go into the fountain to recover it (416.17–19, 20–21).[27] The entrance into the wild world outside court thus happens without the deliberation and control normally present, and differs in fundamental ways from the standard adventuring. The mad knight is also unable to re-enter the court, or any court, and is cut off, by his madness, from the community which normally fulfils both his physical and social needs.

## Courtly Dining

Among the knights' needs is food, which has both a physical and social function. Eating together is a significant part of courtly life: Arthurian romance, after all, is largely defined by its dining table. The dinners at Arthur's court involve a certain amount of ritual, such as waiting for a "wonder" before sitting down to dine, and they are often interrupted by the arrival of petitioners asking assistance from the knights. Courtly dining, thus, manifests both the unity of Arthur's court, and the primary function of the knights—to uphold the king's authority by risking their bodies in combat. The entire "Tale of Sir Gareth," in *Le Morte Darthur*, depicts a young knight's way from kitchen boy to respected landed lord, all of it presenting increasingly sophisticated and communal eating. The dining is not restricted to knights, but also offers a display of courtly manners in front of women. In speaking of his brother Sir Launcelot's perfection as a knight, Sir Ector praises him as "the meekest man and the gentlest that ever ate in a hall among ladies" (939.20–21).[28] Even though the knights leave the court to go adventuring, they are still part of this community, even when they dine alone: as they fulfil the function of knighthood, they still constitute a communal court. While love-mad knights retain their martial ability, they exercise it randomly and incoherently, rather than

**25** "felle downe of hys horse in a sowne."

**26** "a naked man in his shurte wyth a swerde in hys honde."

**27** "made many straunge sygnes and tokyns, and so thorow the rageynge he threw hys swerde in that fountayne."

**28** "the mekest man and the jentyllest that ever ete in hall emonge ladyes."

as knights of King Arthur. Their fights do not carry any authority and do not promote Arthur's court as containing the flower of chivalry.

As I have argued elsewhere, physically disabled knights lack access to this community of diners, and the restoration of ability restores that access, too.[29] The mentally disabled knights removing themselves from court to run off into the wilderness, might then be read not only as having their madness removing them from civilized company, but as mental disability, like physical, being utterly incompatible with presence at court. Love-mad knights are occasionally cared for in various manors and castles, after being found by the inhabitants, but they are not normally included in communal courtly life.

Knights disabled by love-madness suffer hunger, partly because they refuse to eat, but partly also because, unable to function as part of the court, they are deprived of proper knightly food in sufficient amounts. This hunger, in its turn, results in further disabling. Lack of proper food is tied to both bodily and mental decline, sometimes to the extent that the knights become unrecognizable even to their family and friends. However, this seems rarely to affect their martial ability, which they retain despite madness and starvation. Obviously, knights errant do otherwise spend time in the forest, fed by hermits who are often also nursing them back to health from whatever injuries they have suffered. This food does not seem to cause them mental or physical disability. However, the love-mad knights suffer long periods of no access to courtly context, as they cannot dine with noblemen and ladies whose castles they encounter while adventuring: mostly, they are entirely cut off from courtly life.

## Starvation

There is a sliding scale from pangs of love confusing the knight and making him unable to eat, and the serious despair that results in long-lasting mental disability. Gareth, on not being allowed to meet his lady, "rode now here, now there, he knew not whither" (255.31) and "had no rest, but wallowed and writhed for the love of the lady of that castle" (255.34–35).[30] On meeting her again he "so . . .burned in love that he went far from his reason and might not eat, for his love was so hot that he did not know where he was"

**29** Hildebrand, "Sitting on the Sidelines."

**30** "rode now here, now there, he wyste nat whother"; "had no reste, but walowed and wrythed for the love of the lady of that castell."

(259.17–20).[31] As Gareth is soon preparing to marry the lady, he recovers and "was much inclined to eat, and fully knightly and eagerly he ate his food... and some said they never saw a more courteous man nor one eating so well" (279.23–25).[32] This reads as a brief episode of love pangs and inability to eat, quickly resolved by marriage.

The knights who cannot achieve such success, most commonly because the lady already loves someone else, suffer more severe episodes of love-madness and starvation, becoming unrecognizable to others but also to themselves. Palomides, being in the company of Isoud but unable to get her love, "weakened and mourned, that all men marvelled why he faded away so" (614.17–18),[33] and finally sees himself:

> in the water he saw his own face, how he was discoloured and faded away, nothing like how he used to be. "Lord Jesus, what might this mean?" said Sir Palomides. And thus he said to himself: "Ah, Palomides, Palomides! Why are you thus faded away, that was always likely to be called one of the fairest knights of the world? Indeed, I will no longer live this life, for I love what I will never have or achieve." (614.21–28)[34]

The most extreme change is Launcelot's, after the death of Guinevere: "he ever after ate but a little food, nor drank, until he died, for he became more and more ill, and dried and wasted away...he was grown a cubit shorter than he used to be, so that people did not recognize him" (937.6–8, 9–10).[35] However, Launcelot's decline is a more complex situation than sheer love-sickness and will be dealt with below.

---

**31** "so...brenned in love that he passed hymself farre in his reson"; "myght nat ete, for his love was so hoote he wyst nat where he was."

**32** "lyste well to ete, and full knyghtly he ete his mete and egirly...and som seyde they nevir sawe a goodlyer man nother so well of etynge."

**33** "faded and mourned, that all men had merveyle wherefore he faded so away."

**34** "in the watir he sawe his owne vysayge, how he was discolowred and defaded, a-nothynge lyke as he was. 'Lorde Jesu, what may this meane?' seyde Sir Palomydes. And thus he seyde to hymselff: 'A, Palomydes, Palomydes! Why arte thou thus defaded, and ever was wonte to be called one of the fayrest knyghtes of the worlde? Forsothe, I woll no more lyve this lyff, for I love that I may never gete nor recover.'"

**35** "never after ete but lytel mete, nor dranke, tyl he was dede, for than he seekened more and more, and dryed and dwyned awaye...that he was waxen by a kybbet shorter than he was, that the peple coude not knowe hym."

## Launcelot and Tristram

The two major examples of mental distress on loss of love, followed by disabling starvation, are Tristram and Launcelot. As they are the two greatest lovers of the cycle, it seems fitting they should also be the most distressed by the loss—real or imagined—of their love.

Malory's Tristram finds a letter his lover Isoud has written to another man, out of pity for his hopeless love for her. Predictably, he takes it amiss, and rides off into the forest where, after fighting a few knights, he "sighs and makes great sorrow" (388.32) and "was so sorrowful he fell down off his horse in a faint, and this sorrow lasted three days and three nights" (388.35–389.1).[36] Here, clearly, the sorrow brought on by the (imagined) infidelity of Isoud is such that Tristram cannot stay on his horse. This recalls knights being unhorsed in battle, and indicates that Tristram is vanquished by his distress.

Throughout his love-madness, Tristram has a problem finding and/or consuming food, which leads to starvation. This runs consistently through the narrative, in a pattern of avoidance and inability. Initially, a damsel who knows him attempts to feed him: "then she brought him food and drink, but he would have none" (389.16–17). Tristram, however, not only refuses food but avoids any contact with the helpful damsel: he "escaped away from the damsel" (389.18)[37] as if threatened by the offer of food. The damsel recruits a lady to help her, and she states that "he will have food and drink of the best" and that she will also bring him a harp (389.29–30). Nevertheless, "this lady and the damsel brought him food and drink, but he ate little of it" (389.32–33).[38] During this time his love-madness worsens, as he "put his horse away and unlaced his armour, and so he went to the wilderness and broke trees and boughs" (389.33–35).[39] This follows immediately upon his refusing food, and marks a loss of identity: he loses his armour and horse, markers of knighthood, and attacks the trees instead of other knights. Despite his loss of identity, he plays the harp the lady has given him, and she

36 "'syeth and makith grete dole'"; "made such sorow that he felle downe of hys horse in a sowne, and in such sorow he was inne thre dayes and thre nyghtes."

37 "than she broughte hym mete and drynke, but he wolde none"; "ascaped away frome the damesell."

38 "he shall have mete and drynke of the beste"; "thys lady and damesell brought hym mete and drynke, but he ete lityll thereoff"

39 "put hys horse frome hym and unlaced hys armour, and so he yeode unto the wyldirnes and braste downe treys and bowis."

learns to attract him by playing herself: "then she would sit down and play the harp, and at once Sir Tristram would come to the harp" (390.3–5).[40] The harping attracts Tristram, but the offers of food are refused or even escaped physically. The music constitutes a link to Tristram's past, as he is known to be a good harper, and a connection to his former self. The food, however, is unacceptable outside the social structure which supports knightly eating.

Predictably, Tristram suffers some physical effects of his starving: "then he was unarmoured, and became lean and poor in flesh" (390.9). The madness also leads to his joining some shepherds, who "would daily...give him some of their food and drink," although they also beat him (390.10–12).[41] He seems not to refuse this food, in spite of having turned down the food from the damsel and the lady. It would appear that the basic food of the common people can still be eaten, as it is not part of the courtly connection for which he is currently not eligible.

Tristram is explicitly removed from the courtly and civilized environment: "Sir Tristram endured there for half a year without armour and would never come into town" (390.24–25).[42] Tristram retains—as knights often do—his martial ability, but seems at this point not to know who he is. Nevertheless, wearing no armour, he kills a squire after getting his hands on Sir Dagonet's sword (392.2), and later kills a giant (393.35–394.1). While it may be argued that he demonstrates some adherence to the chivalric code in protecting the herdsmen who have provided for him,[43] his actions—taking up the cause of the herdsmen who have also mistreated him, against the squires—simultaneously indicate his inability to interact with a courtly context and its inhabitants.

After this encounter with Sir Dagonet, Tristram is briefly fed by a hermit:

> So meanwhile Sir Tristram ran unarmoured in the forest with the sword in his hand, and so he came to a hermitage, and there he lay himself down and slept. And in the meanwhile the hermit stole away the sword and lay food down by him. Thus was he kept there for a tenday, and at the end he departed and came to the herdsmen again. (393.6–11)[44]

---

**40** "than wolde she set hir down and play uppon the harpe, and anone Sir Trystamys wolde com to the harpe."

**41** "than was he naked, and waxed leane and poore of fleyshe"; "dayly...wolde gyff hym som of theire mete and drynke."

**42** "Sir Trystram endured there an halff-yere naked, and wolde never com in towne."

**43** As Pearman points out, *Disability and Knighthood*, 53.

**44** "So thys mean whyle ran Sir Tristram naked in the foreyste with the swerde in hys honde, and so he cam to an ermytayge, and there he layde hym downe and slepte.

This initially reads as a straightforward narrative: finding a man with a sword asleep outside his home, the hermit very sensibly takes the sword away before attempting to feed him. However, the removal of the sword again reduces Tristram to a non-knight, lacking the accoutrements of knighthood. Leaving the hermit, he returns to the shepherds. It is interesting to consider if the sword, and the retaining of martial ability, could have sped Tristram's return to mental health.

The restoration of Tristram from madness comes when he is returned to a courtly setting. King Mark's knights, finding him asleep, take him to Tintagel "safely and kindly" where "they bathed him and washed him, and gave him hot broth, until they had brought back his memory of himself" (394.20–23).[45] Tristram's knowledge of this identity is restored through this courtly attendance, and food served in the castle rather than in the forest. The loss of identity, however, is twofold: not only have his madness and the starvation connected to it meant the loss of his sense of self—"hys remembraunce"—it has also made him unrecognizable to others. When he is found by King Mark, who is his uncle and knows him well, neither Mark nor his court is able to recognize him: "all this time there was no one who recognized Sir Tristram nor what kind of man he was" (394.23–25).[46] He has been rendered unrecognizable both as an individual and as a member of the knightly community. Even Isoud is unable to place him: "so when the queen looked upon Sir Tristram she did not remember him, but all the time she said to Dame Brangwayne, 'It seems to me I must have seen this man here before in many places'"(394.34–395.2).[47] While he looks familiar to her, which is more than he does to the rest of the court, Isoud cannot recognize him. He is finally identified, significantly, by his dog which "felt the scent of Sir Tristram" and then leaps at him, smells him all over, and thus identifies him (395.10–13).[48] Tristram's own restoration of his mental health is thus followed

---

And in the meane whyle the ermyte stale away the swerde and layde mete downe by hym. Thus was he kepte there a ten dayes, and at the laste he departed and com to the herdemen ayen."

**45** "savely and fayre"; "they bathed hym and wayched hym, and gaff hym hote suppyngis, tylle they had brought hym well to hys remembraunce."

**46** "all thys whyle there was no creature that knew Sir Trystamys nothir what maner man he was."

**47** "So whan the quene loked uppon Sir Trystamys she was nat remembird of hym, but ever she seyde unto Dame Brangwayne, 'Mesemys I shulde have sene thys man here before in many placis.'"

**48** "felte a savoure of Sir Trystram."

by recognition, even though he is still clearly visually unrecognizable. At this point, he temporarily rejects Isoud and rides off to Arthur's court, returning to the primary courtly context in the Arthurian world.

The other great lover of the Arthurian world, Launcelot, is driven mad by having been sexually assaulted by Elaine of Corbenic, and being then rejected by Queen Guinevere, who is unaware that the sexual encounter was non-consensual. His madness is similar to, but considerably more serious than Tristram's. Like Tristram, "he fell down to the floor in a faint" (633.17), and then

> leapt out of a bay window into a garden, and there he was all badly scratched by thorns on his face and his body, and so he ran forth he knew not whither, and was as wildly insane as anyone ever was. And so he ran two years, and never anyone had the grace to recognize him. (633.19–24)[49]

There are several similarities to Tristram's love-madness; Launcelot is also "naked," as in without armour, yet still retains his ability to fight. He defeats a fully armoured knight in battle (644.25–31); defeats two brothers while not only unarmed but injured (646.8–21); kills a wild boar with a sword stroke (647.7–15); and reacts to harassment by town youngsters by breaking their arms and legs (648.15–17). Indeed, Launcelot seems to have lost none of the skills that make him the best knight in the world. However, Launcelot, unlike Tristram, has little access to any food except that foraged in the forest. He suffers "cold hunger and thirst" (636.26); and "lived on fruits and such as he might get, and drank water for two years" (643.32–33).[50] It is not clear whether he would have avoided food, like Tristram does, as it is not at this point offered.

Launcelot is eventually found by a knight's dwarf and tentatively identified: "'it seems to me,' said the dwarf, 'the he looks much like Sir Launcelot'" (645.10–11).[51] He is brought to a castle, in a process also very similar to Tristram's: carried, still sleeping, on a feather bed on a horse litter, and given "good food and drink" (645.22–25, 26). The food and drink "brought

---

**49** "fell downe to the floure in a sowne"; "lepte oute at a bay wyndow into a gardyne, and there wyth thornys he was all to-cracched of his vysage and hys body, and so he ranne furth he knew nat whothir, and was as wylde woode as ever was man. And so he ran too yere, and never man had grace to know hym."

**50** "colde hungir and thyrste"; "lyved by fruyte and suche as he myght gete, and dranke watir too yere."

**51** "'mesemmyth,' seyde the dwarff, 'that he resembelyth much unto Sir Launcelot.'"

him back to his strength and fairness" (645.26–27).[52] However, unlike Tristram, this does not cure his mind: "they could not bring him back to his wits, nor to know himself" (645.27–28).[53] In this castle, he spends a year and a half, "decently clothed and kindly dealt with" (645.29–30) but still kept in chains (646.9–10).[54] After Launcelot rescues the owner of the castle and his brother from two other knights, breaking his chains in the process, the owner regrets chaining him and releases him (646.27-28). In his breaking of the chains, Launcelot injures his hands: Pearman points out that "the subsequent injury to his hands—two tools necessary to successful knights—demonstrates that the possession of both a lack of reason and a surplus of physical capability is inconsistent and untenable."[55] However, I would like to note the parallel to Launcelot's injured hands at Meleagant's castle, where he breaks the bars keeping him out of Guinevere's room and injures himself in the process (852.14–18). The injury to his hands here foreshadows the injury his love for Guinevere causes him, and marks him as a good man of his hands, as knights are so often termed in Malory's text. Here, Launcelot occupies a liminal space: chained like a madman yet partly treated as the knight they know he is.

On leaving the castle after impulsively joining a boar hunt, Launcelot again suffers starvation. While he stays with a hermit for the wound inflicted by the boar, the hermit "could not find him sustenance, and so he weakened and grew feeble both of body and of his wit: for lack of sustenance he grew more insane than he was before" (648.5–8).[56] It is unclear here whether the hermit simply cannot feed him sufficient food, or if the food available is not nourishing enough. I would argue that the "sustenaunce" Launcelot requires cannot, again, be found outside a courtly context, and thus he declines in health. It is significant that even though good food and drink have previously made him healthy physically but not mentally, lack of the right food not only fails to sustain him physically but worsens his mental state. On finding himself yet again at a castle, Launcelot is recognized as having been "a man of honour" (648.22), While he is disabled by his madness, he cannot be

---

**52** "good metys and good drynkys"; "brought hym agayne to hys strengthe and hys fayreness."

**53** "in hys wytte they cowde nat brynge hym agayne, nother to know hymselff."

**54** "honestly arayed and fayre faryn wythall."

**55** Pearman, *Disability and Knighthood*, 57.

**56** "myght nat fynde hym his sustenaunce, and so he empeyred and wexed fyeble bothe of body and of hys wytte: for defaute of sustenaunce he waxed more wooder than he was aforetyme."

part of courtly life: instead, he is given "clothes for his body, and straw and rushes to lie on under the gate of the castle" (648.23–24). He is fed, but not waited on: "every day they would throw him food and set down drink, but there were only a few who would bring him food to his hands" (648.24–26); he is given clothes but not admitted to the communal environment of the castle.[57] His food is thrown to him and he is living at the castle gate—neither in nor out of the castle—much like a dangerous watchdog. He seems here to be included in a court context, despite being mentally disabled still, and to accept food.

Launcelot is finally recognized by Elaine, who on finding him in her garden "came to remember him and recognized him truly as Sir Launcelot" (649.10–11).[58] While Launcelot, unlike Tristram, is to some extent recognizable to others even in his starved state, he is considerably more mentally disabled. It is implied that Launcelot's disabling madness is a permanent state, as one character states "I saw and heard by his behaviour that he is insane forever" repeating that "he is marred forever" and Queen Guinevere says that "we have lost him forever" (633.29–30, 634.9–10, 14).[59] While Sir Launcelot is finally cured of his madness, it is achieved by the Grail and termed a "myracle"(650.6). The implication is clearly that the disability would have been permanent without divine intervention. His miraculous return to mental health results in his being provided with a castle of his own, complete with ten knights and "twenty of the fairest young ladies that are in this country" (651.19–20),[60] emphasizing again the need for a court with its community of courtiers for proper knightly life.

The miraculous cure by Grail that Launcelot receives is one of the few places in Malory's text where a religious aspect of disability might be present. The medieval views of this aspect are complex and varied: as Metzler points out, disability could be seen as requiring physical healing, as punishment for sin, or as a way to spiritual improvement.[61] These different views overlapped and co-existed. Malory's text shares in this complex relationship between religion and disability. However, it can be noted that of the

**57** "clothis to hys body, and straw and lytter undir the gate of the castell to lye in"; "every day they wolde throw hym mete and set hym drynke, but there was but feaw that wolde brynge hym mete to hys hondis."

**58** "felle in remembraunce of hym and knew hym veryly for Sir Launcelot."

**59** "I saw and harde by his countenance that he ys madde for ever"; "he ys marred for ever"; "we have lost hym for ever."

**60** "twenty of the fayryste yonge ladyes that bene in thys contrey."

**61** Metzler, *Disability*, 46–47, 187.

two lovers suffering from madness and starvation, Tristram dies without the benefit of clergy, murdered by King Mark, and Isoud dies of grief on his grave (865.6–9, 14–15; 881.12–15), whereas both Launcelot and Guinevere die in holy orders, and in Launcelot's case a holy death. A bishop dreams that he sees "angels bring Sir Launcelot to heaven, and the gates of heaven opened for him"(938.11–12).[62] Their shared suffering from love madness seems to have had no shared outcome at their deaths: the complexity of mental disability in Malory as punishment for sin, a way to spiritual improvement, or both, deserves a study of its own.

The origin of Launcelot's love-madness—as opposed to Tristram's—is never explicitly addressed in Malory's text. Elaine blames Guinevere, Sir Bors blames both of them (633.28–30; 634.24–25). Arthur suggests it is due to Launcelot's (non-existent) love for Elaine (657.15–17), and the text states that "Sir Launcelot's kinsmen knew for whom he went out of his mind" (657.22–23).[63] Nevertheless, the text makes it clear that Launcelot is not only suffering from love-madness, but from a posttraumatic reaction to having been twice sexually assaulted, drugged and tricked into sexual contact with Elaine. I have shown elsewhere that this coerced sexual contact impacts Launcelot's sense of identity, to the point that even when he recovers from his madness, he chooses not to use his name.[64] Launcelot's having suffered rape should be considered a significant feature aggravating his attack of insanity.

Pearman argues that Launcelot's final days are marked by a last return of his love-sickness: "after Guinevere's death removes the possibility of a future reunion, Lancelot experiences his final symptoms of love-madness; he swoons, falls into a deep depression, experiences insomnia, and is unable to eat or drink for six weeks, after which he becomes bedridden until his death."[65] However, this final illness is complicated by several aspects, and not least by Launcelot's own words on the subject. When previously admonished, during the Grail quest, for his love of Guinevere, Launcelot weeps and admits to its being excessive and sinful (696.11–24), and the text refers to it as such (790.10–15). While characters in Malory may be incorrect on facts, their

**62** "angellys heve up Syr Launcelot unto heven, and the yates of heven opened ayenst hym."

**63** "Sir Launcelottys kynnesmen knew for whom he wente oute of hys mynde."

**64** Kristina Hildebrand, "'I love nat to be constreyned to love': Launcelot and Coerced Sex," *Arthurian Literature* 37 (2022): 175–92.

**65** Pearman, *Disability and Knighthood,* 62.

statements—especially Launcelot's—on the state of their feelings should be treated as valid. Launcelot is firm and explicit on his sexual coercion by Elaine, and he is equally so on the causes of his final illness. Being reprimanded by a hermit for his sorrow over Guinevere, Launcelot responds:

> Truly, I trust I do not displease God, for He knows my intention, for my sorrow was not, and is not, for any enjoyment of sin. But my sorrow can never end, for when I remember their beauty and their nobility, which was both with her king and her, so when I saw his body and her body so lie together, truly my heart could not sustain my sorrowful body. And also when I remembered how by my fault and my arrogance and my pride that they were both stricken, that were peerless among all Christians ever living, know you . . . this remembered, of their affection and my lack of it, went so to my heart that I could not support myself. (936.29–937.5)[66]

Launcelot nowhere here refers to his courtly love for Guinevere, rejecting it instead outright as a source for his sorrow ("not for ony rejoysyng of synne"). Instead, he focuses on the perfection of Arthur and Guinevere and on his own guilt over the fall of the Round Table and of Arthur. The separation between Launcelot and Guinevere has already been achieved by both of them entering holy orders, and the grief that finally kills Launcelot is over the whole court and its unique quality, rather than the loss of Guinevere.

## Conclusion

The knights who suffer mental disabling from love, if serious, are unable to attend court. The milder forms are cured either by reconciliation with the lady or by their resigning themselves to being true lovers without recompense. The greatest lovers of the story, Tristram and Launcelot, suffer more serious mental disabling, presumably due to their stronger love.

This love madness leads to starvation for a number of reasons: unwillingness to eat; inability to access sufficient or high-quality food; and absence of a courtly community with which to eat. This refusal/inability to eat like

---

**66** "'Truly...I trust I do not displease God, for he knoweth my entente, for my sorow was not, nor is not, for ony rejoysyng of synne. But my sorow may never have ende, for whan I remembre of hir beaulté and of hir noblesse, that was bothe wyth hyr kyng and wyth hyr, so whan I sawe his corps and hir corps so lye togyders, trule myn herte wold not serve to systeyne my careful body. Also whan I remembre me how by my defaute and myn orgule and my pryde that they were bothe layed ful lowe, that were pereles that ever was lyven of Cristen people, wyt you wel...this remembred, of their kyndenes and myn unkyndenes, sanke so to myn herte that I myght not susteyne myself.'"

knights brings them further physical and mental injury. In Tristram's case, bathing and hot broth return him to his senses, though not before he has suffered disfiguring starvation; in Launcelot's, even that cannot bring him to mental health, but a miracle is required. It is unclear whether reconciliation with Isoud and Guinevere, respectively, would have cured them, as those reconciliations happen after their recoveries. On recovering, they are again reabsorbed into the courtly life of proper knightly food eaten communally, and presumably return also to their looks and physical health.

The starvation caused by love-madness is complex and does not follow a simple pattern; it functions both as cause and effect. The love-madness causes loss of appetite, resulting in starvation: yet the removal from court and its communal eating is also a cause of the starvation. Simultaneously, the starvation causes further mental injury, including the loss of looks and even identity that means the knight is not recognized even by those closest to him—which, in itself, increases the risk of starvation as the knight cannot draw on the support of his fellow knights and other members of the court. Starvation thus places itself as both cause and effect of mental disability.

The representation of mental disability brought on by love rests in its relationship to the two main signifiers of knighthood: prowess in battle and courtly love. The knights suffering madness are all of them still fearsome fighters, often able to vanquish their opponents despite disadvantages such as lack of armour or even proper weapons. Indeed, the disability seems not to affect their martial ability at all. As noted above, this martial ability is closely connected to the risk of injury and the inevitability of at least temporary disability. Just as physical injuries prove not only the skill and valour of a knight, they also prove the importance of the matter for which they fight. Winning unscathed cannot prove this commitment, but the injury and possible disability can. As Hodges argues,

> A victorious knight...proves his commitment to other causes—honour, justice, a claim to a given piece of land, an assertion that one woman is the most beautiful—not by injury to the loser but by injury on his side: to his own body or to those who matter to him.[67]

Similarly, the risk of love-madness and starvation proves the commitment to love and the worth of that love. Even when the sufferers do not know who they are or are unable to remember their ladies, their love-sickness is a direct effect of their knightly love; that it drives them insane supports rather than contradicts the strength and purity of their love. Pearman also comments

**67** Hodges, "Wounded Masculinity," 16.

on the parallel between the "implied ability/disability system" that runs through both the knights' martial activities and their love for a lady.[68] As with physical disability, "a knight must perpetually oscillate between disability and ability"[69] in his love-sickness or love-madness. I would therefore argue that the mental disability brought about by love-madness and the resulting starvation is not entirely negatively constructed. While the love-madness does remove the knights from the society which provides for their physical needs and recognition both of them as individuals and of their value as knights, it also seems an unavoidable consequence of one of the characteristics that construct said value: their ability to love faithfully. The disfigurement and increased disability brought on by starvation further prove the importance of the love for which they suffer. The knights must love, successfully or not, as "there was never an honourable man nor an honourable woman that didn't love someone better than any other" (841.24–26),[70] and thus must risk love-madness. In the cases of Tristram and Launcelot, the love-madness and starvation disable them, but that very disability also establishes the strength and knightliness of their love, placing them even more firmly as the best knights of the world.

**68** Pearman, *Disability and Knighthood*, 62.

**69** Pearman, *Disability and Knighthood*, 1.

**70** "there was never worshypfull man nor worshypfull woman but they loved one bettir than anothir."

Chapter 4

# A VULNERABLE MILITARY MASCULINITY

## SOLDIERS AND DISABILITY IN LATE MEDIEVAL PARDON LETTERS (FRANCE, ENGLAND, AND THE LOW COUNTRIES)

QUENTIN VERREYCKEN

IN APRIL 1446, a soldier named Jehan Chauvet was granted an abolition letter by Charles VII, which pardoned him the pillaging and robberies he had repeatedly committed against the subjects of the king of France over the past few years. The lieutenant of the captain of the abbey of Charroux in Poitou, Jehan Chauvet was a seasoned combatant of the Hundred Years' War, as exposed in his letter. At the age of 16 or 18, he had become the servant of Guillaume d'Albret, lord of Orval, following him at war as soon as he "was strong enough to bear armor."[1] After his master died at the Battle of Rouvray in 1429, Jehan continued to serve in the king's armies under the command of Jehan Foucault, lord of Saint-Germain-Beaupré, and Charles II d'Albret, Count of Dreux and Guillaume's eldest brother. After a decade of military service, he sustained a severe spear wound while taking part in the siege of the castle of Mareuil in Guyenne in February 1438. Consequently, he was brought to the castle of Courbefy in Limousin to be treated, where he remained ill for a long period of time. After partially recovering from his injury, Jehan found himself without any money. Prompted by the soldiers of the garrison of Courbefy, he decided to remain in the Limousin region to pillage and plunder the coun-

1 Paris, Archives Nationales (hereafter AN) JJ 177, fols. 125v–126r, no. 184, published in Paul Guérin and Leonce Celier, eds., *Recueil des documents concernant le Poitou contenus dans les registres de la Chancellerie de France* (Poitiers: Société des archives historiques du Poitou, 1898), 8:266–70: "quant fut puissant pour porter harnoiz."

**QUENTIN VERREYCKEN** is a Permanent Researcher of the Fund for Scientific Research-FNRS at UCLouvain Saint-Louis Brussels. His research revolves around the exercise, perception, and regulation of violence at war in late medieval and early modern Western Europe. His second book, *Crimes et gens de guerre au Moyen Âge*, was published by the Presses universitaires de France in 2023.

tryside for the next two years. Even after he was summoned again to join the king's service, he pursued the same habit, pillaging, robbing, and ransoming the French population to compensate for the lack of regular pay in the armies. At one point, he even briefly joined the company of Jehan de la Roche, the notorious former *écorcheur* captain who participated in the revolt of the French nobility known as the *Praguerie* in 1440—although Jehan Chauvet claimed that he did not take part in this rising.[2]

In fact, Jehan's crimes were so numerous that "he could not describe them all"[3] and so he knew that he risked finding himself in serious trouble for his actions, as royal legislation punished pillaging, plundering, robbing, and ransoming the king's subjects by death.[4] So, in 1445, when Charles VII made a royal proclamation in which he promised to grant an abolition letter to pardon and erase any crime committed by his soldiers during the war against the English, Jehan quickly took his chance and petitioned for such pardon, which he received in April 1446.[5]

Over the course of the next few years, dozens of soldiers received an abolition letter similar to Jehan Chauvet's, describing comparable scenes of violence and abuses committed against the French population. This could make Jehan's story seem rather unoriginal—after all, he claimed in his petition that he had acted "as men of war are accustomed to do"[6]—if the soldier

---

**2** Gustave Clément-Simon, "Un capitaine de routiers sous Charles VII, Jean de La Roche," *Revue des questions historiques, nouvelle série* 14 (1895): 41–65.

**3** AN, JJ 177, fols. 125v–126r, no. 184: "il ne pourroit bonnement dire ne exprimer."

**4** Valérie Bessey, ed., *Construire l'armée française: Textes fondateurs des institutions militaires* (Turnhout: Brepols, 2006), 1:88–101; Quentin Verreycken, *Crimes et gens de guerre au Moyen Âge: Angleterre, France et principautés bourguignonnes au xv^e siècle* (Paris: Presses universitaires de France, 2023), 42.

**5** For the context of this *abolition générale*, see Loïc Cazaux, *Les capitaines dans le royaume de France: Guerre, pouvoir et justice au bas Moyen Âge* (Paris: Champion, 2022), 648–56; Christophe Furon, *Les écorcheurs: Violence et pillage au Moyen Âge, 1435–1445* (Paris: Arkhê, 2023), 196–201; Claude Gauvard, "Pardonner et oublier après la guerre de Cent Ans: Le rôle des lettres d'abolition de la chancellerie royale française," in *Pardonner et oublier? Les discours sur le passé après l'occupation, la guerre civile et la révolution*, eds. Reiner Marcowitz and Werner Paravicini (Munich: Oldenbourg Wissenschaftsverlag, 2009), 27–55, at 38–40; Valérie Toureille, *Robert de Sarrebrück ou l'honneur d'un écorcheur (v. 1400–v. 1462)* (Rennes: Presses universitaires de Rennes, 2014), 140–51; Quentin Verreycken, "Mercy at War: Military Violence and the Politics of Royal Pardon in Fifteenth-Century France," *French Historical Studies* 47, no. 2 (2024): 187–218, at 205–6.

**6** AN, JJ 177, fols. 125v–126r, no. 184: "ainsi que gens de guerre avoient accoustumé de faire."

had not provided a fascinating explanation of the circumstances that drove him to become such a prolific military offender. According to the narrative account of his abolition letter, which was largely based on Jehan Chauvet's initial petition for pardon, it was only after he had been severely injured during the siege of Mareuil, underwent a long convalescence, and was left out of money that he resorted to plundering to survive. The soldiers of the Courbefy garrison also appear to have played a significant role in this affair, encouraging Jehan Chauvet to loot the region as they themselves were used to do—perhaps urging him to demonstrate that he was still physically capable of bearing arms. The abolition letter does not clarify if, after his recovery, Jehan Chauvet was permanently impaired, although it gives us an interesting clue. Indeed, the letter indicates that Jehan Chauvet's nickname was *Piedebeuf* ("beef foot"), a sobriquet suggesting that the soldier may have suffered from some sort of foot defect that could be congenital (like clubfoot) or caused by a war injury, like the one inflicted at Mareuil. Permanent or not, his impairment had dramatic consequences for Jehan Chauvet, turning him into a persistent pillager and plunderer, because of which he eventually sought royal pardon.

This contribution examines the pardon letters and petitions for pardon of impaired soldiers like Jehan Chauvet, from fifteenth-century France, England, and the Burgundian Low Countries. The three main belligerents of the Hundred Years' War, the kings of France and England as well as the duke of Burgundy were particularly generous towards their soldiers, pardoning them their crimes and allowing them to remain in the army while escaping the rigor of ordinary and military justice. Although combatants made up only a minority of those granted royal or princely mercy—since any subject could request a pardon after committing a crime—they represented a *significant* minority, accounting for between 1% and 18% of pardon recipients depending on the region and the period. These letters reveal the extreme violence soldiers could exhibit outside the battlefield, plundering, ransoming, and raping—which was considered criminal committed in allied territories. Yet, as with the rest of the population, the most frequently pardoned crime among soldiers in the fifteenth century was homicide resulting from a spontaneous dispute that escalated into a deadly brawl, such as a drunken altercation in a tavern or a quarrel between two soldiers over lodging arrangements.[7]

7 Verreycken, *Crimes et gens de guerre*, esp. 50–54, 85–105 and 199–241.

Despite this particular attention of the French, English, and Burgundian monarchs towards those who served them at war, finding disabled soldiers among the recipients of pardons is often like searching for a needle in a haystack—only a few dozen cases can be found among the several thousand letters recorded in fifteenth-century chancery records. Using this limited sample, this article explores how maimed combatants accounted for their injuries and disability while seeking mercy, questioning how these disclosures of physical impairment affected soldiers' self-representations of masculinity. When discussing "physical impairment," I adopt the typology developed by disability historian Irina Metzler, which categorizes somatic and sensory impairments as: 1) "extreme deformations or monstrosities"; 2) " impairments which notably restrict normal functions"; 3) "little or no restriction of normal function," such as deficit of toes or fingers.[8] Moreover, since no instances of extreme deformation appear in the pardon letters reviewed, this study focuses exclusively on Metzler's second and third categories.

Since the late 1980s, there has been an extensive body of literature on the value of pardon letters and their interest in the history of violence[9]. French and Burgundian pardon letters (called *lettres de rémission* and *lettres d'abolition*), in particular, are well-known for their rich narrative content. The first part of each letter is a slight adaptation of the initial petition for pardon or *supplique* submitted by the supplicants, in which they extensively describe the circumstances of their crimes.[10] Comparatively, English pardon letters are briefer and more formulaic, as they rarely include a narrative account of the pardoned crime. Fortunately, about 600 original petitions for pardon have been preserved in the archives for the late medieval period, including a few dozen from soldiers. These petitions, although often

**8** Irina Metzler, *Disability in Medieval Europe: Thinking about Physical Impairment during the High Middle Ages, c. 1100–1400* (London: Routledge, 2006), 5.

**9** For a historiographical survey, see Quentin Verreycken, "The Power to Pardon in Late Medieval and Early Modern Europe: New Perspectives in the History of Crime and Criminal Justice," *History Compass* 17, no. 6 (2019), https://doi.org/10.1111/hic3.12575.

**10** Peter Arnade and Walter Prevenier, *Honor, Vengeance, and Social Trouble: Pardon Letters in the Burgundian Low Countries* (Ithaca: Cornell University Press, 2015); Rudi Beaulant, *Les pratiques de la grâce des ducs et duchesses de Bourgogne à la fin du Moyen Âge* (Paris: Classiques Garnier, 2024); Natalie Zemon Davis, *Fiction in the Archives: Pardon Tales and Their Tellers in Sixteenth-Century France* (Stanford: Stanford University Press, 1987); Claude Gauvard, *"De grace especial": Crime, état et société en France à la fin du Moyen Âge* (Paris: Publications de la Sorbonne, 1991).

less detailed than the French and Burgundian remission letters, enrich our understanding of the identity and crimes of English petitioners.[11] However, thanks to the seminal work of Natalie Zemon Davis, historians have been aware of the particular biases present in late medieval pardon letters and petitions for pardon.[12] Written in collaboration between petitioners and professional scribes or clerks, these letters are "narratives, artfully constructed legal texts"[13] subjects to the rules of chancery and pardon procedure. To make their case eligible for a pardon, petitioners must insist on the positive circumstances of the crime (such as killing in self-defence, by accident, or anger, rather than by premeditation) as well as demonstrate that they were good and loyal subjects. However, because their declarations were subject to rigorous scrutiny during the pardon process—first when the petition was reviewed by the royal or ducal council, then when the pardon letter was ratified by a local court—petitioners had to shape a story that was both credible and verifiable through witness testimony. This explains the presence of literary artifices alongside legal arguments in pardon letters. The result of these efforts was rich but scripted testimonies, using self-narrations and self-descriptions tailored to meet the expectations of both royal or ducal counsellor as well as local justices.[14] "Neither biography nor autobiography, pardon letters are carefully constructed feats of self-presentation, guided by a notary's hand, that perform multiple rhetorical acts: defence of reputation, assertion of honour, denunciation of an adversary."[15]

Interestingly, similar observations have been made regarding other forms of petitioning in the late medieval and early modern periods, including

---

**11** Helen Lacey, "Petitioners for Royal Pardon in Fourteenth-Century England," in *Petitions and Strategies of Persuasion in the Middle Ages: The English Crown and the Church*, eds. Thomas W. Smith and Helen Killick (York: York Medieval Press, 2018), 40–63; Verreycken, *Crimes et gens de guerre*, 151.

**12** Davis, *Fiction in the Archives*.

**13** Arnade and Prevenier, *Honor, Vengeance, and Social Trouble*, 13.

**14** Luke Giraudet, "Witnesses, Witnessing and the Crafting of Pardon Letters: The Case of the Habsburg Privy Council of the Spanish Netherlands (1540–1633)," in *"Voor Ons Sijn Verscheenen" (Oog)Getuigen En Hun Verklaringen in de Vroegmoderne Periode*, eds. Dries Raeymaekers and Gerrit Verhoeven (Leuven: Leuven University Press, 2024), 41–65; Quentin Verreycken, "'En nous humblement requerant': Crime Narrations and Rhetorical Strategies in Late Medieval Pardon Letters," *Open Library of Humanities* 5, no. 1 (2019): 1–31.

**15** Peter Arnade and Elizabeth Colwill, "Crime and Testimony: Life Narratives, Pardon Letters, and Microhistory," *Journal of Medieval and Early Modern Studies* 47, no. 1 (2017): 147–66, at 148.

within the field of disability history. In a recent article, Lloyd Bowen shows how petitions for pension from maimed veterans of the English Civil War were shaped by the generic conventions employed by the scribes responsible for drafting these requests, discussing to what extent these rhetorical artifices prevent the reader from accessing the petitioners' "authentic" experiences of war and disability.[16] Similarly, Ninon Dubourg's groundbreaking monograph on petitions submitted by disabled clerics to the Papal Chancery in the Late Middle Ages offers valuable insights into how petitioners' disclosure of their impairment was a means "to receive formal recognition of their disability," which ultimately "enacted a shift in supplicants' own sense of identity, and fundamentally transformed their relationship with the ecclesiastical institution."[17]

These considerations of authorship, identity, and the public recognition of physical disability are central to this article. The ambivalence of medieval society toward disabled people—articulating charity and piety with social exclusion and mockery—prompts us to ask why soldiers would disclose their impairments when petitioning for pardon.[18] As the embodiment of a virile masculinity rooted in strength and martial prowess,[19] the figure of the late medieval combatant seems at first glance challenged by the descriptions of the weakened bodies of military petitioners who laid their

**16** Lloyd Bowen, "Genre, Authorship and Authenticity in the Petitions of Civil War Veterans and Widows from North Wales and the Marches," in *The Power of Petitioning in Early Modern Britain*, eds. Brodie Waddell and Jason Peacey (London: University College London Press, 2024), 33–60; Geoffrey L. Hudson, "Arguing Disability: Ex-Servicemen's Own Stories in Early Modern England, 1590–1790," in *Medicine, Madness and Social History*, eds. Roberta Bivins and John V. Pickstone (London: Palgrave, 2007), 105–17.

**17** Ninon Dubourg, *Disabled Clerics in the Late Middle Ages: Un/Suitable for Divine Service?* (Amsterdam: Amsterdam University Press, 2023), 276.

**18** Ninon Dubourg, "European Medieval Disability History: An Overview," in *Handbook of Disability*, eds. Marcia H. Rioux et al. (Singapore: Springer, 2022), 1–18, at 9–11.

**19** Matthew Bennett, "Military Masculinity in England and Northern France *c.* 1050–*c.* 1225," in *Masculinity in Medieval Europe*, ed. Dawn Hadley (London: Longman, 1999), 71–88; Hervé Drévillon, "Du guerrier au militaire," in *Histoire de la virilité*, ed. Georges Vigarello (Paris: Seuil, 2011), 1:289–321; Ruth Mazo Karras, *From Boys to Men: Formations of Masculinity in Late Medieval Europe* (Philadelphia: University of Pennsylvania Press, 2003), 21–66; Craig Taylor, *Chivalry and the Ideals of Knighthood in France during the Hundred Years War* (Cambridge: Cambridge University Press, 2013), 91–98.

physical vulnerabilities bare for all to see.[20] Building on the consideration that *impairment* and *disability* are both the products of social activities,[21] this article argues that by situating their wounded body at the core of their narrative, soldiers transformed their condition into legal and moral argument for pardon. In so doing, they framed their physical impairment as a mark of pride rather than shame, attesting to their past military services. From these petitions therefore emerges a portrayal of a vulnerable military masculinity that contrasts with the chivalric ideal of physical prowess. Although their wounds and scars testified to honourable wartime service, they also left soldiers exposed to poverty and social exclusion—an injustice that could only be addressed through the mercy of their sovereigns.

## Describing War Disabilities in Pardon Letters

The study of disability through pardon letters has been the subject of a number of recent studies, focusing more specifically on mental disability.[22] Aleksandra Pfau, in particular, in her contribution to this collective volume as well as in her past work, has shown how fourteenth- and fifteenth-century remission letters provide instances of mental disturbances caused by war—although these letters mainly concern peasants who suffered from the destructions and brutalities caused by the Hundred Years' War, rather than soldiers experiencing some sort of post-traumatic stress disorder acquired in battle.[23] In contrast, there has been—to my knowledge—little or no his-

---

**20** Cathy McClive, "Masculinity on Trial: Penises, Hermaphrodites and the Uncertain Male Body in Early Modern France," *History Workshop Journal* 68, no. 1 (2009): 45–68.

**21** Bianca Frohne, "The Cultural Model," in *Dis/Ability History Der Vormoderne: Ein Handbuch = Premodern Dis/Ability History: A Companion*, eds. Bianca Frohne et al. (Affalterbach: Didymos, 2017), 61–63. See also Wendy J. Turner, "Models of Disability: Connecting the Past to the Present," *Zeitschrift für Disability Studies* 1 (February 2022): 1–18.

**22** Aleksandra Pfau, *Medieval Communities and the Mad: Narratives of Crime and Mental Illness in Late Medieval France* (Amsterdam: Amsterdam University Press, 2021), esp. 34–45; Maud Ternon, *Juger les fous au Moyen Âge: Dans les tribunaux royaux en France* XIV$^{e}$–XV$^{e}$ *siècles* (Paris: Presses universitaires de France, 2018), esp. 15–16.

**23** See Aleksandra Pfau, "Warfare, Trauma, and Madness in French Remission Letters of the Hundred Years War," in *The Hundred Years War (Part III): Further Considerations*, eds. L. J. Andrew Villalon and Donald J. Kagay (Leiden: Brill, 2013), 437–54, and *Medieval Communities and the Mad*, 169–75, as well as her chapter in the present volume.

torical research on physical disability based on pardon letters, despite the valuable information they provide.[24]

Take, for instance, the French remission letter granted to eighteen-year-old Jehan Dorin, who had become hunchbacked in one shoulder after falling from a bed in his early childhood.[25] Although this case does not concern a soldier, it remarkably highlights the social exclusion and mistreatment experienced by disabled individuals in the Late Middle Ages, while also demonstrating how these experiences could be integrated into the petitioner's narrative as an argument to be pardoned. The letter recounts how, in June 1453, a heated argument erupted between Jehan Dorin and a servant named Jehanne Loye, who mocked him, threw him to the ground, and beat him, as Jehan "did not have the strength to resist her because she was a strong woman."[26] Crafting this image of vulnerability and inferior status, the narrative of the remission letter strategically contrasts Jehan's frailty, a young man with a hunched back and a fragile constitution, with the physical strength of Jehanne Loye, portrayed as a "plump, fat woman aged 25 or 30, and quite tall"[27] and prompt to resort to violence—traits typically attributed to men in criminal records.[28] It is this difference in physical strength that justifies why, in an attempt to protect himself, the young man drew a knife and stabbed the woman twice.

In the case of soldiers, the type of handicap suffered by Jehan Dorin, whether congenital or acquired in infancy, seems incompatible with the physical condition required for the profession of arms. While it is beyond

**24** Symptomatically, Irina Metzler, *A Social History of Disability in the Middle Ages: Cultural Considerations of Physical Impairment* (New York: Routledge, 2013), 147, 278 briefly quotes a fourteenth-century French remission letter concerning the case of an old man suffering from dementia who had killed his wife, but she ignores the letters describing physical impairment.

**25** AN, JJ 182, fols. 74v–75r, no. 136, published in Guérin and Celier, eds., *Recueil des documents*, 9:344–49: "se foula telement qu'il en devint bossu d'une espaule et a ceste occasion a esté et encores est faible et de petite stature et n'est pas bien sain." A more in-depth analysis of this compelling case will be the subject of a future publication.

**26** AN, JJ 182, fols. 74v–75r, no. 136: "il n'avoit pas la force de resister contre elle qui estoit forte femme."

**27** AN, JJ 182, fols. 74v–75r, no. 136: "grosse femme replette, de l'aage de XXV. à trente ans ou environ et bien grande."

**28** Beaulant, *Les pratiques de la grâce*, 344–49; Gauvard, "*De grace especial*," 307–16; Diane Roussel, "La description des violences féminines dans les archives criminelles au XVIe siècle," *Tracés: Revue de sciences humaines* 10, no. 19 (2010): 65–81.

the scope of this contribution to discuss the complexities of late medieval military structures and recruitment systems, it is worth noting that French, English, and Burgundian armies encompassed a broad spectrum of socio-professional profiles—from peasants temporarily enlisted through feudal levies to noble military careerists. This complexity is further obscured by the generic terminology often employed in pardon letters, such as "man of war" (*homme de guerre*), "companion in war" (*compaignon de guerre*), or "soldier" (*soldeour*), to describe these individuals.[29] Although not all those performing military service viewed themselves as professional soldiers or received advanced training, a basic proficiency in handling weapons was typically required. This is well-illustrated by the 1469 feudal levy in Burgundy, commissioned by Duke Charles the Bold, which categorized male adult residents of the duchy into eight categories, from those described as "strong and swift" (*forts et vifs*) to those labelled as "feeble and old" (*débiles et âgés*) and therefore unsuitable for service.[30] Likewise, fifteenth- and sixteenth-century military memorialists often highlight how aging and accumulated war injuries gradually forced them to end their career. The physical decline resulting from these wounds often became a source of frustration and even shame for these veterans, who found themselves unable to continue the armed service to which they had devoted a significant portion of their lives.[31]

Nevertheless, chancery records occasionally reveal signs of physical impairment among military offenders who applied for a pardon. A first indication can be observed in how soldiers introduced themselves as petitioners. Alongside their name, profession, military rank, or marital status, late medieval petitioners frequently mentioned a nickname, which often referenced their regional origin (such as André Belleau, known as *le Liégeois*)[32] or a physical trait (like Jehan le Roy, called *le Roux*).[33] In at least one instance, the case of Jehan Chauvet, known as *Piedebeuf*, such nickname probably alluded to a form of impairment of the petitioner. Moreover, the remission letter granted in 1474 to the man-at-arms Jehan de Dorguir, who recounts having

**29** Verreycken, *Crimes et gens de guerre*, 21–25, 50–61.

**30** Jules de La Chauvelays. "Mémoires sur la composition des armées de Charles le Téméraire dans les deux Bourgognes," *Mémoires de l'Académie des sciences, arts et belles-lettres de Dijon* 5 (1878–1879): 138–369, at 150.

**31** Quentin Verreycken, "Une noblesse à l'épreuve de la guerre: *L'Aventurier rendu a dangier* ou les mémoires d'un soldat-brigand au début du XVI$^{e}$ siècle," *Revue historique* 712, no. 4 (2024): 567–609, at 600–602.

**32** AN, JJ 207, fol. 80v, no. 173.

**33** Lille, Archives départementales du Nord (hereafter ADN), B 1695, fols. 46v–47r.

killed another soldier named Jehan de Fillebert, also called *le Borgne* ("the one-eyed"), shows that the victim of a pardoned crime could receive similar nickname.[34] As John P. Sexton observes, nicknames in medieval Europe frequently "served as a record of salient features that might enter into public record"[35] to differentiate one person from another, while also reflecting individual reputation as well as the significance of the visible wounded body in society.

Even more revealing are the pardon letters in which petitioners explicitly described the severe injuries they sustained during military service, even when such injuries were directly related to the crime for which they sought forgiveness. For instance, in his petition seeking pardon for a homicide committed while attempting to stop a riot in the village of Hanslope in Buckinghamshire, Roger Skrowe emphasizes his long-standing service to King Edward IV, insisting on his participation in the Battle of Barnet (1471), where he had been severely wounded.[36] Similarly, in his 1446 abolition letter pardoning multiple pillages, Raymon Chauveteau indicates that he participated in the siege of Aubeterre, "where he had been injured by an arrow in the thigh, because of which he had been ill for five years,"[37] although, unlike Jehan Chauvet, he did not try to frame his crimes as a consequence of this injury.

Although most petitioners did not elaborate on the long-term consequences of their battle injuries, such physical trauma often marked their bodies permanently, as in the case of Pierre Baut, who "was severely injured in the face at the siege of Blaye in 1451" and probably left with several scars.[38] The erratic nature of the medical treatment of battle injuries certainly increased the risk of disability for wounded combatants, as shown in the case of Jehan Colart who, after being seriously injured during a fight

---

**34** AN JJ 204, fol. 58r, no. 94.

**35** John P. Sexton, "Atypical Bodies: Seeking after Meaning in Physical Difference," in *A Cultural History of Disability in the Middle Ages*, eds. Jonathan Hsy et al. (London: Bloomsbury Academic, 2020), 19–34, at 29.

**36** Kew, The National Archives (hereafter TNA), SC 8/251/12527: "Your besecher hath ben at all your victorious feldes sithen the begynnyng of your moste noble reygne and at your last feld of Barnet was grevously hurt and maymed as it is wele understoud among the servicte of your honourable houshold."

**37** AN, JJ 176, fol. 289r–v, no. 436 published in Guérin and Celier, eds., *Recueil des documents*, 8:379–81: "où il fut blecié d'un traict en la cuisse, dont il a esté malade par l'espace de V ans."

**38** AN, JJ 185, fols. 186r–187r, no. 265, published in Guérin and Celier, eds., *Recueil des documents*, 9:262–67: "lequel estant au siège de Blaye fut tres griefvement blecié ou visage."

against English soldiers, "could not find any barber or expert surgeon for his cure" in the nearby town.[39] As Giulia Morosini suggests, there may have been a certain prestige among combatants in acquiring battle scars "that told the story of the soldier's past gestures and his ability to endure pain."[40] Similarly, according to Kenneth Hodges, medieval chivalric literature did not see battle wounds "as failures to achieve a dream of inviolate masculinity," but instead considered them inevitable even for the best soldier, therefore praising "knightly suffering as admirable penance."[41] Yet as Irina Metzler has shown, medieval society maintained a profoundly ambivalent attitude toward disability, viewing it both as a sign of spiritual purity and as a marker of sin, depending on the circumstances.[42] The same ambiguity applied to war wounds. In the fifteenth century, amid widespread mistrust of combatants following the devastations of the Hundred Years' War,[43] serious mutilation could also become a negative social marker beyond the military sphere, making soldiers and veterans easily recognizable and sometimes turning them into outcasts. This is precisely the experience described in the remission letter granted in the early sixteenth century to a combatant named Loys Tyore, who recalled going to a church on June 24, 1528, to offer his prayers

---

**39** AN, JJ 185, fols. 204r–205r, no. 295, published in Guérin and Celier,eds., *Recueil des documents*, 9:316–20: "non povant trouver barbier ne cirurgien expert a sa garison expedier." On military surgery, see Metzler, *Disability in Medieval Europe*, 118–20, and Robert C. Woosnam-Savage and Kelly DeVries, "Battle Trauma in Medieval Warfare: Wounds, Weapons and Armor," in *Wounds and Wound Repair in Medieval Culture*, eds. Larissa Tracy and Kelly DeVries (Leiden: Brill, 2016), 27–56, at 47–52.

**40** Giulia Morosini, "Manly Virtues, Emotions, and Scars: Competition among Italian Renaissance Soldiers through Bodily Practices," in *Gender and Status Competition in Pre-Modern Societies*, eds. Martha Bayless et al. (Turnhout: Brepols, 2021), 79–107, at 90. See also Patricia Skinner, "Visible Prowess?: Reading Men's Head and Face Wounds in Early Medieval Europe to 1000 CE," in *Wounds and Wound Repair*, eds. Tracy and DeVries, 81–101, at 83.

**41** Kenneth Hodges, "Wounded Masculinity: Injury and Gender in Sir Thomas Malory's 'Le Morte Darthur,'" *Studies in Philology* 106, no. 1 (2009): 14–31, at 14 and 15.

**42** Metzler, *Disability in the Middle Ages*, 39–55.

**43** Christopher Allmand, "Changing Views of the Soldier in Late Medieval France," in *Guerre et société en France, en Angleterre et en Bourgogne, XIVe–XVe siècle*, eds. Philippe Contamine et al. (Lille: Université Charles de Gaulle, 1991), 171–88; David Grummitt, "Changing Perceptions of the Soldier in Late Medieval England," in *The Fifteenth Century X: Parliament, Personalities and Power. Papers Presented to Linda S. Clark*, ed. Hannes Kleineke (Woodbridge: Brewer, 2011), 189–202; Claude Gauvard, "Rumeur et gens de guerre dans le royaume de France au milieu du XVe siècle," *Hypothèses* 1 (2000): 281–92.

to St. John, only to be mocked by several men who called him a "one-eyed gendarme and cowardly gendarme."[44]

Furthermore, while the loss of an eye or finger may not prevent a soldier from continuing his military career or pursuing another profession outside the army, the situation was quite different for injuries that resulted in a permanent restriction of senses or mobility. As the contributions by Wendy J. Turner and Michael Depreter in this collective volume show, in the Late Middle Ages, neither England, France, nor the Low Countries had yet developed a global military pension system for retired combatants, and so severely disabled soldiers with little financial resources risked to fall into poverty and thereafter criminality, committing theft and robberies to survive, as already shown with the case of Jehan Chauvet.[45] Another French remission letter granted to a retired combatant of the Hundred Years' War is more revealing of how battle traumas could have a dramatic impact on a soldier's entire family, even among nobility. In 1396, Jehan de la Bothe, a squire aged nineteen or twenty, was pardoned by Charles VI for a series of petty thefts committed in the two or three previous years. Jehan was the son of Regnault de la Bothe, himself a squire and a former soldier who had not only lost most of his money during the wars against the English, but "had also been so severely wounded at [the Battle of] Pontvallain [in 1370] that he became deaf."[46] As his family had no longer any source of revenue, Jehan resorted to stealing several pots, sheets, and money, while also beating a man under the king's safeguard. After being imprisoned for his crimes, he was eventually pardoned by Charles VI, considering the significant harm that war had inflicted on both the body and property of Jehan's father.[47] Far from a triumph of masculine endurance celebrated in chivalric literature, the reality of war injuries often exposed maimed soldiers to great economic and social vulnerability.

**44** Robert Muchembled, *La violence au village: Sociabilité et comportements populaires en Artois du XV^e^ au XVII^e^ siècle* (Turnhout: Brepols, 1989), 114: "gendarme à ung oeul et gendarme failly."

**45** Priscille Aladjidi, *Le roi, père des pauvres: France, XIII^e^–XV^e^ siècle* (Rennes: Presses universitaires de Rennes, 2008), 162–63; Marjorie Keniston McIntosh, *Poor Relief in England, 1350–1600* (Cambridge: Cambridge University Press, 2013), 156–58.

**46** AN, JJ 146, fol. 53r, no. 111: "il fu tant navré a Pont Valain qu'il en est assourdi." My sincere thanks to Sasha Pfau for bringing this case to my attention.

**47** AN, JJ 146, fol. 53r, no. 111: "les grandes pertes que a faictes sondit père, tant de corps comme de biens pour cause de noz dictes guerres."

## Mercy, Charity, and the Recognition of the Military Service

To understand why soldiers chose to disclose their impairment caused by military service, even when their war injuries had little to nothing to do with their crimes, we must take a closer look at the rules that regulated the process of petitioning for pardon. Since the fourteenth century, the pardoning procedure had been the subject of increasing royal and princely legislation, including on how petitions should be drafted and submitted to the monarchs.[48] In England, a royal statute promulgated in 1390 provides that any petition for the pardon of a homicide should clearly indicate if the crime was committed by surprise or premeditation.[49] Similarly, in France, the ordinance promulgated following the Cabochiens revolt in 1413 indicates that supplicants must clearly expose the "manner, quality, and circumstances of the offences," so that the seriousness of their crime could not be concealed.[50] Moreover, whether in France, England, or the Burgundian Low Countries, the text of a petition for pardon followed a predefined structure established in chancery and based on the rules of the *ars dictaminis*, the rhetorical art of writing letters: *salutatio* (address), *exordium* (introduction), *narratio* (narrative of the context for the demand), *petitio* (formal demand), and *conclusio* (final formulae).[51]

To better navigate these rules, petitioners were usually assisted by trained scribes, clerks, or legal advisors who composed the petition for them.[52] A chancery formulary produced in 1426 or 1427 by French clerk

---

**48** Hugo De Schepper, "Het gratierecht in het Bourgondisch-Habsburgse Nederland, 1384–1633, vorstelijk prerogatief en machtsmiddel," in *Symposium over de centrale overheidsinstellingen van de Habsburgse Nederlanden: Tien bijdragen over de staat, de regering en de ambtenaren van de 16de tot de 18de eeuw*, eds. H. Coppens and K. Van Honacker (Brussels: Archives générales du Royaume, 1995), 43–87; Quentin Verreycken, "'*As moost Cristen prynce whos clemens is to be noted*': Tempérer la grâce du roi en Angleterre et en France (XIIIe–XVe siècles)," in *Les discours adressés au(x) pouvoir(s)*, eds. Noëlline Castagnez et al. (Paris: Classiques Garnier, 2024), 249–65.

**49** *The Statutes of the Realm* (London: Dawsons, 1816), 2:69.

**50** Alfred Coville, ed., *L'ordonnance cabochienne (26–27 mai 1413)* (Paris: Picard, 1891), 142: "la manière, qualité, circonstance des délitz."

**51** Gwilym Dodd, "Writing Wrongs: The Drafting of Supplications to the Crown in Later Fourteenth-Century England," *Medium Aevum* 80, no. 2 (2011): 217–46, at 222–29.

**52** Claude Gauvard, "Les clercs de la Chancellerie royale française et l'écriture des lettres de rémission aux XIVe et XVe siècles," in *Écrit et pouvoir dans les chancelleries médiévales: Espace français, espace anglais*, eds. Kouky Fianu and DeLloyd J. Guth (Louvain-la-Neuve: FIDEM, 1997), 281–91; Helen Killick, "The Scribes of Petitions in

Odart Morchesne provides further indications on the principles guiding the drafting of a petition for pardon. According to Morchesne, not only must the narrative of the petition be true to avoid rejection, but it should also feature *causes* or *motives* for which the king was more inclined to grant a pardon, such as pleading self-defence, anger, or the absence of premeditation in case of homicide.[53] Other reasons included "when there is [ground for] pity, like for women and children, or when [the supplicant] is a good person of good reputation."[54] Alongside legal arguments addressing the circumstances of the crime, these appeals to pity therefore encouraged petitioners to emphasize their personal qualities in order to attract the monarch's sympathy. In other words, they were required to make a deliberate effort to declare and define their identity as good, submissive, and repentant supplicants. As with any judicial document, this act of self-enunciation was shaped by established conventions and stereotypes partially addressed by Morchesne's formulary, such as referring to the petitioner's good reputation and family. For example, Jehan Chauvet, presents himself as a man with familial responsibilities, "in charge of a wife and four little children."[55] Similarly, Pierre Baut underscores his moral character by concluding his petition with the assertion that he is a "man of good fame, reputation, and honest conversation."[56]

Considering the importance of these grounds for pity, soldiers held a distinct advantage when seeking pardon compared to other subjects, as they could invoke their military service as a reason to be pardoned.[57] A fourteenth-century English petition illustrates this practice: "To our lord the King, humbly prays Nicholas de Bolton, who had served in your war all

---

Late Medieval England," in *Petitions and Strategies of Persuasion in the Middle Ages: The English Crown and the Church*, eds. Thomas W. Smith and Helen Killick (York: York Medieval Press, 2018), 64–87.

**53** Comparable reasons for being pardoned are to be found in medieval England: Helen Lacey, *The Royal Pardon: Access to Mercy in Fourteenth-Century England* (York: York Medieval Press, 2009), esp. 19–25; Elizabeth Papp Kamali, *Felony and the Guilty Mind in Medieval England* (Oxford: Oxford University Press, 2019).

**54** Olivier Guyotjeannin, Serge Lusignan, and Eduard Frunzeanu, eds., *Le formulaire d'Odart Morchesne dans la version du ms BnF Fr. 5024* (Paris: École des Chartes, 2005), 424: "quant il y a pitié, comme de femme et d'enfans, ou que celui est bonne personne et bien renommé."

**55** AN, JJ 177, fols. 125v–126r, no. 184: "chargié de femme et de quatre petiz enfans."

**56** AN, JJ 185, fols. 186r–187r, no. 265: "homme de bon fame, renommée et honeste conversacion."

**57** Verreycken, *Crimes et gens de guerre*, 265–69 and 160–61.

his time, that it may please you, by your good grace, to grant him a charter of pardon."[58] In this context, invoking war injuries caused by military service further reinforces the idea of the petitioner's loyalty to the monarch. In another remission letter, the knight François de Haneskenke claims having repeatedly served the duke of Burgundy and the king of France in their wars, including at siege of the city of Bourbourg (1383), "where he was harshly and severely wounded."[59] Far from the chivalric ideal of personal achievement in war, military service was consistently depicted by petitioners as a life of hardship and sacrifice. Within this framework, war wounds emerged as a positive marker of such sacrifice, devoid of any moral or religious ambiguity concerning the petitioner. These formulaic portrayals formed the basis of their appeals to their sovereign's mercy, seeking pardon in acknowledgment of their past tribulations.

For the kings of France and England, as well as the duke of Burgundy, issuing a pardon letter was an act of mercy (*misericordia*), intended to soften the rigor of law and justice—"preferring mercy to rigor of justice," as the formula in most French and Burgundian remission letters states.[60] Medieval political thought considered mercy to be a fundamental virtue of the good Christian prince, who should exercise justice with moderation, compassion, and equity, in imitation of God's divine justice. Although royal pardon was frequently criticized for its excesses in allowing too many criminals to escape judicial punishment, the notion that monarchs should balance mercy with justice was never questioned as long as it did not result in inequity.[61] Moreover, in mirrors for princes, this ideal of mercy was expected to manifest in the monarch's treatment of the poorest and most vulnerable among their subjects, echoing another duty inherent to royal power: charity (*caritas*). Thus, in the early sixteenth century, the English Franciscan Stephen Baron described the clemency of a good ruler as "showing compassion to his afflicted subjects."[62] Granting pardons to the most vulnerable fitted into

---

**58** TNA, SC 8/179/8926: "A notre sir le Roi prie humblement Nicholas de Bolton qui ad travaille en votre guerre tout son temps que vous plese de votre bonne grace lui granter chartre de pardon."

**59** ADN, B 1681, fol. 53v: "ou il fu moult durement et griefement navré de son corps."

**60** For instance, AN, JJ 177, fols. 125v–126r, no. 184: "misericorde preferer à rigueur de justice."

**61** Claude Gauvard, *Violence et ordre public au Moyen Âge* (Paris: Picard, 2005), 92–115; Lacey, *The Royal Pardon*, 100–106; Verreycken, "'*As moost Cristen prynce*.'"

**62** Stephen Baron, *De regimine principum (1509)*, ed. P. J. Mroczkowski (New York: Lang, 2005), 85 quoted by Aladjidi, *Le roi, père des pauvres*, 100.

this concept, as illustrated by this standard closing phrase used by English petitioners: "for God and by way of charity."[63] By disclosing their impairment caused by military service, soldiers therefore highlighted their own physical vulnerability to appeal to both the mercy and charity of their monarchs. This also served as a reminder of the king's or duke's duties as a military leader, who was bound to protect and reward those who served him accordingly.[64] This explains the recurrence of similar mentions military service in other sources emphasizing the monarchs' generosity toward their soldiers, such as the Burgundian account books analyzed by Michael Depreter in his contribution to the present volume. Of course, such arguments alone were rarely sufficient to guarantee a pardon, as most military petitioners had to substantiate their requests with further evidence that their crime merited forgiveness. Nevertheless, formulations such as "he had always well and loyally served at war and exposed his body"[65] or "he had continuously used his body and possessions in our service at war"[66] emphasized how military petitioners expected specific considerations given the way they exposed their bodies to the violence of combats.

While references to war wounds lent a personal touch to the petitions for pardon, these descriptions often followed strikingly similar templates from one letter to another, which suggests that chancery clerks likely guided petitioners in using these standardized formulas.[67] By aligning with the common image of the loyal soldier who endured sacrifices at war, these combatants sought to differentiate themselves from petitioners who had not borne arms. In her study of the petitions submitted to the papal chancery, Ninon Dubourg notes that "the standardization of descriptions of impairment allowed for the emergence of a common identity, as

---

**63** Gwilym Dodd, *Justice and Grace: Private Petitioning and the English Parliament in the Late Middle Ages* (Oxford: Oxford University Press, 2007), 283–84: "pur Dieu et en oevre de charité or for the loue of God and in wey of charitee."

**64** Benjamin Deruelle and Quentin Verreycken, "Père du peuple ou roi de guerre? Arbitraire et arbitrage de la grâce des gens de guerre dans le royaume de France (1460–1559)," in *Arbitraire et arbitrages: Les zones grises du pouvoir (XII$^{e}$–XVIII$^{e}$ siècles)*, eds. Benjamin Deruelle and Michel Hébert (Villeneuve-d'Ascq: Presses universitaires du Septentrion, 2024), 261–84.

**65** AN, JJ 203 fols. 18v–19r, no. 33: "tousiours bien et loyaulment servy ou fait de noz guerres et exposé son corps."

**66** AN, JJ 176, fol. 270r, no. 385, published in Guérin and Celier, eds., *Recueil des documents*, 8:130–31: "il se soit continuelment emploié corps et biens en nostre service ou fait de la guerre."

**67** Gauvard, *"De grace especial,"* 857.

petitioners enunciated their unique experiences in a shared formulaic discourse. Indeed, standardized descriptors could offer individuals powerful moments of recognition, as they saw traces of their own lives captured in the administrative phraseology."[68] These observations also apply to the petitions for pardon submitted by soldiers, who described their injuries and impairments as "an essential part of the identity [they] claimed"[69] and leveraged to secure a pardon. The administrative language of the petition enabled recognition of suffering endured in war, making it a source of pride rather than shame, even when a soldier emphasized participation in a major military defeat—such as the French loss at the Battle of Verneuil (1424): "he was at the Battle of Verneuil, were he had been severely injured and captured by the English, our former enemies, and severely ransomed."[70] By detailing their war wounds and disabilities in their petitions, soldiers therefore did not undermine their own masculinity; rather, they emphasized their belonging to a military community with a shared identity and a special bond with their monarch.

In that sense, as Lloyd Bowen reminds us, we should not underestimate the public dimension of petitioning.[71] As we have seen, whether in France, England, or the Low Countries, a pardon letter issued by the royal or princely chancery had to be endorsed by a local court for the pardon to be permanently valid. These hearings were public, often attended by local community members, and required the petitioners to appear in person. Their scars and physical impairment were visible to all, allowing the community to witness firsthand their claims of disability. Similarly, their letters were read aloud by judges, so everyone could hear the account of their military service. The final endorsement of the pardon letter therefore helped for the public recognition of the status of the petitioners as a maimed veteran by the community.

**68** Dubourg, *Disabled Clerics*, 124.

**69** Dubourg, *Disabled Clerics*, 126.

**70** AN, JJ 178, fol. 9r, no. 14: "fut à la bataille de Vernueil, où il fut fort blecié et prins par les Anglois, nos anciens ennemis, et mis à grosse finance et raençon." For further examples, see AN, JJ 169, fol. 69r–v, no. 90 (Battle of Agincourt), and JJ 195, fol. 361v, no. 1515 (Battle of Montlhéry), and Gauvard, *"De grace especial,"* 857.

**71** Bowen, "Genre, Authorship and Authenticity," 48–49.

## Combat-Caused Disabilities as an Argument for Self-Defence

While petitioners occasionally detailed the location of their wounds, the weapon used, or even the battle in which they were injured, the exact circumstances of these injuries often remain vague, seemingly obscured by the chaos of combat. For instance, the squire Anthoine de Langlade mentions being "gravely wounded"[72] at the Battle of Montlhéry in 1465, but omits details about his role or what he was doing on the battlefield at the time of his injury. The study of late medieval military memoirs similarly reveals that the experience of battle was often confusing for its participants, who had no clear view of the overall action.[73] Yet, for petitioners, there was little need to provide a detailed account of their battlefield actions; merely stating that they fought in a specific battle and were injured was usually sufficient to support their claim for pardon. In this respect, pardon letters provide only limited information on soldiers' experience on the battlefield. There is, however, one context in which military petitioners provided a more detailed account of their participation in combat: when their injuries had been inflicted outside the battlefield, in personal brawls that escalated into assaults or homicides, for which they subsequently sought pardon.

In November 1438, Ostelet de Zwynenade, an archer in the duke of Burgundy's personal guard, was in Lille on personal business. One night, he joined Robert de Baufremet and Pierre d'Aucome for drinks at a tavern. Tension suddenly arose when Pierre d'Aucome began harassing a woman, forcing her to sit at their table. Disturbed by his companion's behaviour, Ostelet de Zwynenade intervened, sparking an argument that continued later that night at another tavern. The confrontation quickly escalated into a fistfight, taking an even more violent turn when Pierre d'Aucome drew a dagger and slashed Ostelet de Zwynenade's arm. Both men subsequently exchanged knife blows, parting ways only after they both sustained severe wounds, causing Pierre d'Aucome's death a few days or weeks later. At least, this is the story recounted in the remission letter granted by Philipp the Good to Ostelet de Zwynenade in February 1439. His primary defence rested on the assertion that he had not initiated the fight but had acted in response to the injuries inflicted by his opponent—literally, "feeling himself thus injured."[74]

---

**72** AN, JJ 195, fol. 361v, no. 1515: *griefvement blecié.*

**73** Yuval Noah Harari, *Renaissance Military Memoirs: War, History, and Identity, 1450–1600* (Woodbridge: Boydell, 2004). See also John Keegan, *The Face of Battle: A Study of Agincourt, Waterloo, and the Somme* (New York: Viking, 1976).

**74** ADN, B 1682, fols. 40r–40 bis r: "se sentant ainsi navré."

He further recounted that while recovering from his wounds at the Recollects convent in Lille, a parish priest informed him that Pierre d'Aucome, on his deathbed, had forgiven him and sought his own forgiveness in return. Concluding his appeal to the duke's mercy, Ostelet once again insisted on the "insults and injuries inflicted upon him by the deceased"[75] to support his claim for self-defence.

This case, taking place outside the context of a military campaign, is a good illustration of the typical conflicts and tavern brawls documented in late medieval pardon letters—conflicts in which soldiers were frequently involved. Multiple quantitative surveys show that in fifteenth-century France and the Low Countries, between 60 and 80 percent of remission letters involved homicide cases, including many granted to soldiers.[76] As Odart Morchesne's formulary emphasizes, a critical argument for obtaining a remission letter was to demonstrate that the petitioner was neither the "offender nor the first aggressor"[77] who instigated the fight. This principle applied similarly in England, where claiming self-defence significantly increased the chances of securing a royal pardon.[78] As such, an effective strategy to claim self-defence was to establish that the petitioner had not struck the first blow and had been injured by the victim, as in Ostelet de Zwynenade's case. Although this argument was not exclusive to soldiers and appeared frequently in petitions submitted by non-combatants as well, the emphasis on injuries once again highlights the battered bodies of combatants, weakened by confrontations for which they were not responsible.

In that sense, some petitioners further underscored the permanence of their injuries to amplify the perception of the initial aggression they suffered from their victims. For instance, in the remission letter he obtained in December 1445, the squire Loys du Ton—a regular participant in the king's campaigns against the English—narrates how, a few weeks earlier, he was

**75** ADN, B 1682, fols. 40r–40 bis r: "les iniures et bleceures faictes par ledit defunct."

**76** Beaulant, *Les pratiques de la grâce*, 248; Gauvard, *"De grace especial,"* 242; Verreycken, *Crimes et gens de guerre*, 84–89.

**77** Guyotjeannin, Lusignan, and Frunzeanu, *Le formulaire d'Odart Morchesne*, 424: "n'a pas esté transgresseur ne premier invaseur."

**78** Lacey, *The Royal Pardon*, 22–26; Kamali, *Felony and the Guilty Mind*, 67–77. On the other hand, it is difficult to establish reliable statistics for crimes pardoned in fifteenth-century England, as most of the letters granted at that time were general pardons, likely covering a broad range of crimes, including homicides: K. J. Kesselring, *Mercy and Authority in the Tudor State* (Cambridge: Cambridge University Press, 2003), 76; Verreycken, *Crimes et gens de guerre*, 84.

collecting annuities from his landholdings in Poitou when a dispute arose with another nobleman, Pontenier de Poictiers, who refused to pay him. Their argument quickly escalated into a violent clash during which Pontenier, aided by his servant, severely wounded Loys, striking him in the chest and injuring his hand. Driven mad by these injuries, Loys quickly retaliated and killed Pontenier in revenge. To prove the legitimacy of his reaction, he later insisted in his petition in the seriousness of his injuries, claiming that his left thumb "was almost cut off and was still attached to his hand by a small amount of skin only,"[79] so that according to the surgeons and barbers, "he is at risk of losing his hand."[80] We find a similar statement in the remission letter of Regnault Chabot, a former soldier and lord of Jarnac in Poitou, whose fight against a group of stable workers left him "severely ill and in danger of losing his leg."[81]

Not all petitioners provided injury descriptions as detailed as those by Loys du Ton or Regnault Chabot. In fact, most of them placed more emphasis on the location of the fatal wound they inflicted on their opponent, often aiming to show that they had not intended to kill them outright but rather to bring the fight to a swift end.[82] However, petitioners who insisted on the fact that they were also injured in the confrontation tended to use generic formulations to describe their own wounds, such as *navrure* ("injury") or "mutilation," implying that the wound would leave a scar, a permanent mark, or result in the loss of a toe or finger. In the medieval period, such injuries were considered both insulting and humiliating, particularly when they involved head wounds that caused disfigurement. As Patricia Skinner notes, "visible mutilation was associated with breaches of trust, and thus intimately connected with the codes of honour expressed in the injury tariff lists. To mutilate someone judicially (or politically) carried the same meaning: it was a shaming act, regardless of the actual severity of the bodily injury."[83] In the

**79** AN, JJ 177, fols. 74r–76r, no. 122: "le posse de la main destre coppé avecques autres coups si avant que le dit pousse ne tient que à ung peu de peau."

**80** AN, JJ 177, fols. 74r–76r, no. 122: "dient les cyzurgiens et barbiers qu'il est en adventure d'en perdre la main."

**81** AN JJ 199, fols. 29r–31r, no. 42: "très grandement malade et en danger d'estre perdus de ladicte jambe."

**82** Pierre-Henry Bas, "Entre mouvements intuitifs et gestes techniques : 'poignarder' un homme (xv^e^–xvi^e^ siècles)," *E-Phaïstos* 4, no. 1 (2015): 43–55, at 52; Verreycken, *Crimes et gens de guerre*, 103.

**83** Patricia Skinner, *Living with Disfigurement in Early Medieval Europe* (New York: Palgrave, 2017), 77.

mid-sixteenth century, the Flemish lawyer Joos de Damhouder develops this idea in his *Praxis rerum criminalium*, a legal treaty that dedicates an entire chapter to injuries and mutilations inflicted by others. Damhouder explains that there are two ways of inflicting wounds: through spoken insult or physical blows, connecting physical harm with personal insult. Moreover, he notes that head injuries, particularly those causing mutilation, must be punished more severely.[84] By emphasizing the injuries inflicted by their opponents, petitioners asserted that they killed in self-defence not only to protect their lives but also to preserve their honour by avenging an insult. As Damhouder writes: "If someone tries to slap me, I am justified in stopping him with my sword if I cannot stop him any other way. And if I kill him, it becomes a case of necessary defence, as I cannot accept shame or embarrassment."[85] As such, a detailed account of the confrontation and the petitioner's injuries was crucial evidence for supporting a pardon request, making it both credible and verifiable, as it could be corroborated by witnesses or surgeons, as in Loys du Ton's case, where medical opinions substantiated the risk of losing his hand.

## Conclusion

As this contribution demonstrates, criminal archives, including pardon letters preserved in chancery records, prove to be a valuable source for writing the history of war disability, complementing narrative and medical sources as well as financial accounts. Although the pardon letters granted to impaired soldiers due to injuries acquired on the battlefield remain rare, these documents provide a formidable insight into disability experiences among late medieval combatants, allowing us to better understand the impact of war and combat injuries on soldiers' lives, which weakened them physically and made them more vulnerable to poverty and social exclusion. Far from concealing their impairments, these soldiers chose to acknowledge them in their petitions, adopting the submissive posture of the good and loyal subject, whose injuries served as evidence of good conduct and shaped their masculinity through their commitment to military service. Therefore, wounded soldiers developed a discourse about themselves and their shared

**84** Joos de Damhouder, *La practique et enchiridion des causes criminelles* (Louvain: Wauters et Bathen, 1555), 326–27.

**85** Damhouder, *La practique*, 147: "Quand ung aultre me vault donner ung soufflet, je le puis empescher par mon espée, si je ne le puis aultrement empescher. Et si je le tue, il devient defense necessaire, car je ne doibz pas la vergongne et honte admettre."

military identity that "may have been strategic," but "was also anchored in verifiable and authenticated experience."[86] In that sense, obtaining a pardon letter was also an opportunity for them to obtain public recognition of their status as maimed soldiers, not only in the eyes of the monarch, but also of their local authorities and community. Ultimately, in the absence of an institutionalized military pension and despite their limited numbers, these pardons allowed the kings of France and England, as well as the duke of Burgundy, to remedy, on a case-by-case basis, the challenges faced by those who served them in arms.

**86** Bowen, "Genre, Authorship and Authenticity," 55.

Chapter 5

# TRAUMATIC REPERCUSSIONS

## WARFARE AND DISABILITY IN THE FRENCH COUNTRYSIDE

ALEKSANDRA PFAU

IN 1416, ROBIN LE CRAT from Mons near Gisors sought a letter of remission from the king of France. His crime, as it gradually emerged from the narrative in his letter, was to have wished out loud that the English would conquer them. The letter explains that Robin, who was a labourer and vintner, had a wife who had been bedridden for the last ten years. He had gone to Chaumont-en-Vexin at the end of August, where he stopped to get a drink with his neighbour, Gosse, from Mons, and a group of other men, who all began to complain about the taxes they had to pay. When Robin's friend Gosse said that he had to pay more, and Robin did not have anything to complain about, Robin responded that he should not say that and "he well knows that he would not have anything if he did not gain it with his labour and if the English were in the countryside that they would not be able to be ransomed anymore unless you ransomed me." After these words, the men continued to drink together to the point of drunkenness, when, on their way home, angry about the earlier argument and upset that he had lost all of his inheritance, he said "that he had heard from some people who came from Rouen that the English" demanded much lower taxes and they would get better deals if the English were there. The other men responded that he was wrong, and that the English would kill them if they were there, to which Robin replied that he wished that the English were there (of course, he would get his wish a few years later)! These words came to the attention of the king's procurer and Robin le Crat was held in prison and tried for treason. His letter of remission was granted partly on the grounds that he and

**ALEKSANDRA "Sasha" PFAU** is James and Emily Bost Odyssey Professor of History, Hendrix College. Her research uses medieval legal records to access disability, with a particular focus on mental disability in her book, *Medieval Communities and the Mad: Narratives of Crime and Mental Illness in Late Medieval France* (2021).

his companions were extremely drunk, but also "having pity and compassion for the long illness of his said wife."[1]

There are two key threads that I will draw from this case and weave through the rest of this essay: first, the complexities of loyalties during the Hundred Years' War; and second, the ways that disabilities can exacerbate or, in some cases, arise from those complexities. The works in this collection discuss the challenges of finding evidence of war-related disabilities in medieval archives. Michael Depreter focuses on the difficulty of distinguishing between short-term injury and longer-term disability in records of compensation for combatants.[2] Quentin Verreycken highlights the ways that the evidence from remission letters in particular can be elusive.[3] Even when these oblique or passing references appear, it is impossible to be certain what the evidence tells us. My goal is not to provide any definitive answers, but to ask specific questions about the experience of living in a war-torn countryside, where allegiances were shifting, and change was constant. In pulling apart these complexities and the ways that they impinged on lived experiences, I will examine the impact of war on the level of the king of France himself before considering the more fragmentary evidence for individuals, most of whom like Robin le Crat and his wife were not directly involved in warfare as combatants but were nevertheless harmed by it, illuminating the common experiences of war-related trauma and fear across different levels of society in the face of treason, pillage, and ransom.

---

1 Paris, Archives nationales, JJ 169, fol. 288r–v no. 430, available from the "Himanis–Historical MANuscript Indexing for user-controlled Search Project," http://himanis.huma-num.fr/app/, on pages 591–92. (Henceforth abbreviated as AN, JJ 169, fol. 288r–v, no. 430; Himanis, 591–92): "il savoit bien que il navoit Riens se il ne le gaignoit a ses bras et que se les anglois estoient ou pais quilz ne pourroient plus estre Ranconnez que vous me Ranconnez"; "quil avoit oy dire a gens qui venoient de Rouen que les anglois quictoient les bonn gens du pais pour quatre solz le mois et que cestoit meillieur marche que nous navons"; "aians pitie et compassion de la longue maladie de sadite femme."

2 Michael Depreter, "After Combat: War Wounds, Soldiers' Benefits, and Dynastic Policies in the Burgundian-Habsburg Armies (1363–1506)," in this volume.

3 Quentin Verreycken, "A Vulnerable Military Masculinity: Soldiers and Disability in Late Medieval Pardon Letters (France, England, and the Low Countries)," in this volume.

## The King's Trauma

Perhaps the most famous instance of suspicion, betrayal, and trauma from this period is the case of Charles VI.[4] His first public episode of mad behaviour occurred shortly after he declared war on the duke of Brittany and was embedded within the ceremonies of warfare and larger concerns about treason. Because of the public and unexpected nature of the event, this moment was described in far more detail than any of the king's other periods of madness, which allows for a detailed consideration of how Charles's contemporaries sought to explain the king's actions. Warfare, and particularly the king's command over and control of his armies, plays a central role in the chroniclers' depiction of Charles's madness, allowing an exploration of the importance of war in the process of the king's becoming disabled.[5]

Modern scholars have considered this moment from a number of different perspectives. Penelope Doob uses Froissart's account to argue that Charles VI's friends viewed his disease as morally neutral and stemming from natural causes whereas his enemies explained it through supernatural and moral causes.[6] Judith Neaman, who also depended exclusively on Froissart's account to describe the king's madness, gleans from Froissart's account that "kings and beggars might both suffer madness, but that society treated one with care, the second with abuse, and that a monarch's state of intellect was inseparable from the divine plan of history."[7] However, the madness of the king was the focus of much more complex and varied beliefs than Doob and Neaman discuss. Froissart was only one of the chroniclers who wrote about the king's madness, and there are also many other sources available for considering the political and social effects of a mad king. Richard Famiglietti's conscientious study of Charles VI's reign minutely examines the chronicles and evidence from chancery documents to establish the

---

**4** I considered this episode in my dissertation, Aleksandra Pfau, "Madness in the Realm: Narratives of Mental Illness in Late Medieval France," (PhD diss., University of Michigan, 2008), chapter 2. See also Bernard Guenée, *La folie de Charles VI, roi bien-aimé* (Paris: Perrin, 2004), 7–21.

**5** As I have explained in detail in my book about madness in the Middle Ages, I have chosen to use madness as an umbrella term that encompasses the complexity of medieval French and Latin terms for the condition. See Pfau, *Medieval Communities and the Mad*, 11–12.

**6** Penelope Doob, *Nebuchadnezzar's Children: Conventions in Madness in Middle English Literature* (New Haven: Yale University Press, 1974), 45–49.

**7** Judith Neaman, *Suggestion of the Devil: The Origins of Madness* (New York: Anchor, 1975), 122.

effect of the king's madness on the political scene. His brief introductory study of the king's madness itself is focused on providing a twentieth-century diagnosis for the king's fourteenth-century ailment.[8] Bernard Guenée's study of Charles VI mines all of the available evidence to talk about the social and cultural aspects of the king's madness and provides a complement to Famiglietti's focus on politics. Guenée uses the king's first episode of madness to introduce his book, and points out the ways that the descriptions tell us more about the chroniclers than about the king.[9] The book focuses more on what it means for the French to have a mad *king* than it does on what these descriptions of the king can tell us about *madness*, arguing that "the useless king was not deposed because no one, either outside the realm or within it, had the legal or political means to depose him, nor to govern in his place."[10] In this essay, I will examine the event in terms of madness of an individual, not necessarily of a king, and not as we understand it today, but as it was seen by contemporaries in the fourteenth century.

The events leading up to the king's first episode of madness were complex and controversial. Charles VI came to the throne in 1380 at age eleven, and his powerful uncles governed the kingdom during his minority. As was true for so many medieval child kings, Charles VI struggled to assert his majority, and challenges to his ability to rule were bound up in medieval concepts of masculinity and adulthood.[11] This crisis was part of that conflict, occurring when he was twenty-three and working to separate himself from his uncles' influence. On June 13, 1392, while walking home with a small contingent of guards after a dinner with the king, Olivier de Clisson, Constable of France, was attacked by Pierre de Craon, who reportedly believed that the constable was behind his fall from the position of king's chamberlain. The failed attempt to murder the constable of France, and the repercussions stemming from that event, constituted the first major political crisis that Charles VI approached without the advice of his uncles. The young king was angry when he heard of the attack, considering it a treasonous offense

---

**8** R. C. Famiglietti, *Royal Intrigue: Crisis at the Court of Charles VI, 1392–1420* (New York: AMS, 1986), 1–21.

**9** Guenée, *La folie de Charles VI*, 18.

**10** Guenée, *La folie de Charles VI*, 232: "Le roi inutile n'a pas été déposé parce que personne, ni hors du royaume ni dans le royaume, n'avait les moyens juridiques ou politiques de le déposer, ni même de gouverner à sa place."

**11** This was also true of his contemporary, Richard II of England. These struggles were linked to questions of masculinity. See Christopher Fletcher, *Richard II: Manhood, Youth, and Politics 1377–1399* (Oxford: Oxford University Press, 2008).

against the crown. Although Clisson was left for dead, his wounds were superficial, and he recovered within a few weeks.

Pierre de Craon, meanwhile, escaped his pursuers and sought refuge in Brittany with the duke, Jean IV. The relationship between Jean IV of Brittany and the French kings had been tense for many years, as he vacillated between allying himself with France and with England. Jean also had a particularly fraught personal and political relationship with Olivier de Clisson.[12] The duke of Brittany assured the king that Pierre de Craon had passed through Brittany after committing the crime, but that he had already departed. The young king refused to accept this explanation, particularly since, according to one chronicler, Charles "firmly believed that the duke was an accomplice in the crime."[13] Encouraged by his favoured advisors, the *Marmousets* (a derogatory nickname highlighting their youth and inexperience), Charles decided to go to war against the duke, calling up his liege men and their armies. For the first time, the king had made a decision without the consultation of his uncles, the Princes of the Blood. According to the chronicle accounts, the duke of Burgundy and the duke of Berry were both displeased at Charles's decision. Although they brought their armies to join the king at Le Mans, they took their time arriving, delaying the king as a demonstration of their disapproval.[14] Charles VI's decision to take an army into Brittany was thus the result of a crime that he considered treasonous, and the entire campaign took place under a cloud of paranoia. It was also intended to be a dramatic statement of his majority and his independence from his powerful uncles.

---

**12** Olivier de Clisson and Jean IV of Brittany were both exiles in England during their youths. While Jean IV was able to recover his dukedom, Olivier de Clisson had trouble reacquiring his ancestral lands in Brittany. Jean IV continued to have diplomatic relations with England, calling in English troops whenever he felt threatened by French interests. Olivier de Clisson, in contrast, conceived a hatred for the English and considered Jean IV to have violated his vows of fealty to the French king. See John Bell Henneman, *Olivier de Clisson and Political Society in France Under Charles V and Charles VI* (Philadelphia: University of Pennsylvania Press, 1996); John Bell Henneman, "Reassessing the Career of Olivier de Clisson, Constable of France," in *Law, Custom, and the Social Fabric in Medieval Europe: Essays in Honor of Bryce Lyon*, eds. Bernard S. Bachrach and David Nicholas (Kalamazoo: Western Michigan University Press, 1990), 211–34.

**13** [Michel Pintoin, known as] Le Religieux de Saint-Denis, *Chronique*, ed. M. L. Bellaguet (Paris: Éditions du Comité des travaux historiques et scientifiques, 1842; reprint, 1994), 2:10. "qui conscius sceleris perpetrati...firmiter credebatur."

**14** For more details about the political situation, see Françoise Autrand, *Charles VI: La folie du roi* (Paris: Fayard, 1986), 271–328; Henneman, *Olivier de Clisson.*

It was in the context of this great gathering of force that Charles VI's madness erupted. The three contemporary chroniclers who addressed this event constructed a performance of madness layered within a performance of the martial power of the French kingdom. The onset of the king's madness occurred in public, and the assembled army witnessed his distressing actions. The march of the army was a formalized and ritualized event, in which the king led the aggregate forces of his lords towards the enemy. After the long delay in Le Mans, the king could at last demonstrate his power. His frenetic behaviour disrupted this procession, ultimately forcing the troops to return to Le Mans. Whereas the king's later episodes of madness were generally played out in the confines of the palace, this first event was spectacular, not least because of the ritual performance that it impinged upon.[15]

In retrospect, the three chroniclers who described the king's deployment of his armies found signs that this elaboration of the king's strength was doomed to fail. Although the basic story was the same, there are several details on which they differed. Michel Pintoin, the monk who composed the *Chronicle of St. Denis,* wrote his account in the context of his roles as a monk and as the official royal historian.[16] Jean Froissart, with patronage ties to the English court and the count of Foix and a friendship with Bureau de la Rivière, one of the *Marmousets* who fell from power when the king's uncles took over as a result of his madness, had different priorities.[17] The goals of the anonymous author of the *Chronique des quatre premiers Valois* are less clear, but since he ended his account with the recovery of the king, it seems he sought to create a triumphal conclusion that could alleviate the concerns raised by a king's madness.[18] While Michel Pintoin and Jean

**15** The movement of the army can be imagined in terms of a procession, much like a king's entry into a city. For more on the processionals that took place at king's entries, see Margot Fassler, "*Adventus* at Chartres: Ritual Models for Major Processions," in *Ceremonial Culture in Pre-Modern Europe*, ed. Nicholas Howe (Notre Dame: University of Notre Dame Press, 2007), 13–62; Bernard Guenée and Françoise Lehoux, *Les entrées royales françaises de 1328 à 1515* (Paris: Éditions du Centre national de la recherche scientifique, 1968).

**16** For the attribution of this chronicle to Michel Pintoin, see Bernard Guenée, *Un roi et son historien: Vingt études sur le règne de Charles VI et la Chronique du Religieux de Saint-Denis* (Paris: Académie des Inscriptions et Belles-lettres, 1999), 33–78 ("Michel Pintoin: Sa vie, son œuvre").

**17** See Peter Ainsworth, *Jean Froissart and the Fabric of History: Truth, Myth, and Fiction in the Chroniques* (Oxford: Clarendon, 1990), esp. 192–97.

**18** *Chronique des quatre premiers Valois (1327–1393)*, ed. Siméon Luce (Paris: Renouard, 1862).

Froissart both saw evidence of disturbing behaviour early in the rallying of troops, the anonymous author of the *Chronique des quatre premiers Valois* did not note anything strange until the day that the troops began to march into the forest. As Kristina Hildebrand notes in her contribution to this volume, medieval literature made a connection between madness and wilderness that was echoed in this event.[19] Michel Pintoin recalled that the king had shown signs of being "not of sound mind" for several days before he ordered his armies to depart Le Mans. As evidence, the monk referred to the king's "fatuous words and gestures unbecoming to royal majesty."[20] Michel Pintoin did not describe these gestures in detail, but it is clear that to him Charles's madness was specifically the madness of a king. Kate McGrath has examined the question of royal madness and the link between anger and madness in eleventh- and twelfth-century Anglo-Norman chronicles, noting that "[b]y connecting excessive anger to madness, ecclesiastical historians had an important rhetorical tool that they could use to construct boundaries around what they considered to be appropriate displays of anger and, then, condemn displays that they viewed as excessive."[21] The monk of St. Denis similarly chose to characterize Charles VI's behaviour as outside the bounds of appropriate kingly anger.

Jean Froissart also sought foreshadowings of the king's madness, but he focused on the king's internal physical state, rather than his external actions.[22] Froissart noted that,

> [i]n the city of Le Mans the lords stayed for more than three weeks, because the king was not capable of riding, and was very feverish. And his doctors said to his brother and his uncles: "One makes the king travel; but certainly he should not do it, because he is not in a good state for riding. Resting will go much better for him."[23]

---

**19** Kristina Hildebrand, "Hungry for Love: Disabling the Knightly Body and Mind through Starvation in Sir Thomas Malory's *Le Morte Darthur*," chapter 3 of this volume.

**20** Michel Pintoin, *Chronique*, 2:18: "velut vir non sane mentis, verbis fatuis utendo, gestus eciam majestatem regiam dedecentes exercuerat."

**21** Kate McGrath, "Royal Madness and the Law: The Role of Anger in Representations of Royal Authority in Eleventh- and Twelfth-Century Anglo-Norman Texts," in *Madness in Medieval Law and Custom*, ed. Wendy J. Turner (Leiden: Brill, 2010), 125.

**22** Unlike the monk of Saint-Denis, Froissart was not present for the king's aborted campaign. Based on internal evidence, it seems that he relied on the account of his friend, the lord of Coucy, who was riding with the king. See Famiglietti, *Royal Intrigue*, 207n12.

**23** Jean Froissart, *Œuvres*, ed. J. B. M. C. Kervyn de Lettenhove (Brussels: Devaux-

In Froissart's description of events, Charles VI's eruption into madness should not have surprised anyone. He noted that it was a hot day in mid-August and that the king was wearing heavy armour, suggesting that physical discomfort and over-heating due to the exigencies of preparations for battle caused the king's previous illness to erupt into madness.[24] The king's physicians had expressed serious concerns about his ability to travel, warning the king's close family members to guard him from overexertion, but these warnings were not sufficiently heeded.

These chroniclers' retrospective efforts to find some unheeded warning that the king was going to go mad culminated in the tale of the prophetic beggar, who interrupted the king's procession in order to warn him to beware of treachery in the ranks. The identity of the beggar varies in each of the three chronicle accounts. In Michel Pintoin's narrative, he was a leper, whose words exacerbated the king's already disturbed imagination.[25] The threat of treason, reiterated by the leper, weighed on the king's mind. When one of the *gens d'armes* accidentally dropped his sword, the king turned on him, killing him and then attacking others. In this account the king, who continued to attack his men for over an hour, cried, "'I am delivered to my enemies,' attempting to kill allies as well as unknown men."[26] The king's fear of betrayal and treason thus acted as a driving force, leading him to strike out at all those around him. According to the monk's tally, Charles VI killed four men and would have killed more if his sword had not broken, thus allowing his men to restrain him. The disruptive scene of the king's "fury," introduced

---

Closson, 1867–1877), 15:29: "En la cité du Mans séjournèrent les seigneurs plus de trois septmaines, car le roy n'estoit mie en point de chevauchier et estoit tout fièvreus, et disoient ses médechins à son frère et à ses oncles: 'On fait le roy traveillier; mais certainement il n'en euist que faire, car il n'est point en estat pour chevauchier. Le repos luy vauldroit assés mieulx; car, depuis que il se party d'Amiens où les parlemens furent, il ne fut en si bon estat comme il estoit en-devant.'"

**24** Froissart, *Œuvres*, 15:36–37.

**25** Indeed, literary and figurative wild men were quite fashionable during Charles VI's reign, and the king and several of his friends performed a dance while dressed as wild men in January of 1393. See the description of the dance by Michel Pintoin, *Chronique*, 2:64–70. The performance is analyzed in Susan Crane, *The Performance of Self: Ritual, Clothing, and Identity during the Hundred Years War* (Philadelphia: University of Pennsylvania Press, 2002), 140–174. On wild men, see Richard Bernheimer, *Wild Men in the Middle Ages: A Study in Art, Sentiment, and Demonology* (Cambridge, MA: Harvard University Press, 1952); Joyce Salisbury, *The Beast Within: Animals in the Middle Ages* (New York: Routledge, 1994).

**26** Michel Pintoin, *Chronique*, 2:18: "'Sum ego adversariis tradendus,' nunc amicos, nunc ignotos occidere conabatur."

as it was with the threat of treason and betrayal, highlighted the potential disunity of the realm, which was emphasized further as the king attacked all his men, even those who ordinarily were "allies."

Jean Froissart's narrative concentrated even more on the potential for treason, particularly during a campaign against the duke of Brittany, who had sympathizers among the French armies. He imagined the conversations of the men in camp, who considered the political situation.

> "See," said others, "if there is not treason. Do you think that all those who are [here] and ride with the king are truly enemies of the Duke of Brittany? Certainly not. Who dares to say so? And one can easily see many signs, because they do nothing night and day but counsel, and all to break off and shatter this voyage, and the king has such melancholy of it that he can hardly have wellness or health."[27]

Froissart's vision of the disunity in the ranks of the king's armies allows him to suggest that the king's fear of treason may not have been unjustified paranoia, and indeed that his unease about the loyalty of his troops in general, and his uncles in particular, contributed to his disease. If the threat of treason was real, should he be blamed for reacting excessively in fear of it in a pre-emptive strike? The rest of Froissart's narrative argued that the king's actions were evidence of madness, but his suggestion that the treason the king feared may have been real provided an alternative interpretation of the disruption within the realm. Rather than springing from the king's madness, the power struggles may have contributed to it. In this version, the prophetic figure was described as a man who "showed more of the fool than the wise man,"[28] not a leper, and thus as a direct parallel to the king's own madness. In fact, Froissart suggested that the king's followers made a serious error by ignoring the fool, rather than stopping to enquire whether he "was naturally foolish or wise, and know who made him say such words, or from whence they came to him."[29] Froissart continued to refer to the man as

**27** Froissart, *Œuvres*, 15:29: "Voire, disoient les autres, se il n'y a trahison. Pensés-vous que tous ceulx qui sont et chevauchent aveuc le roy, soient vrais ennemis au duc de Bretaigne? Certes, nennil. Qui l'oseroit dire? Et on en puet bien veir aucuns signes, car on ne fait nuit, ne jour que conseillier, et tout pour rompre et briiser ce voyage, et le roy en a telle mérancolie que à paines peult-il avoir ne bien, ne santé."

**28** Froissart, *Œuvres*, 15:37: "monstroit mieulx que il fuist fol que sage."

**29** Froissart, *Œuvres*, 15:37: "estoit naturellement fol ou sage, et scavoir qui luy faisoit telles paroles dire, ne dont elles luy venoient à savoir."

"the mad man or the sage,"[30] marking the possibility that the king really was in danger of being betrayed.

In Froissart's account, the noise that precipitated Charles's madness was made by his pages, at which point the king, believing himself betrayed, drew his sword. In a much more dramatic scene than that described by Michel Pintoin, Froissart explained that

> [t]he Duke of Orléans was not at that time very far from the king. The king went towards him, holding his naked sword; and already the king, from his frenzy and the feebleness of his head, lost recognition, and knew neither who was his brother nor who his uncle. When the Duke of Orléans saw him coming towards him with a naked sword, he was so afraid, and did not wish to wait (and for a good cause), and he spurred his horse quickly with the king following after. The Duke of Burgundy was riding alongside, and by the fear of the horses, and because already he had heard the cries of the king's pages, he glanced over there, and saw the king, who had a naked sword, chasing his brother.[31]

The rich and personalized image Froissart provided emphasized the deterioration of kin bonds, particularly those between the king and his closest relatives. Rather than attacking the anonymous crowd of his men, as Michel Pintoin suggested, Froissart portrayed the king attacking his brother and uncle. Froissart's focus on the threat of treason and his emphasis on two powerful figures in the king's family as targets of the king's furious rage combined to suggest that Charles's disruptive madness was only part of the troubles disrupting French royal power.

The anonymous *Chronique des quatre premiers Valois* included two separate prophetic figures, combining the narratives that were presumably both current in contemporary rumours. One prophet, a disfigured man, warned the king that if he entered the forest of Le Mans, it would go badly for him. The other, a fool, who also had a disfigured face, told the king that if he went further he would die. According to this version, Charles's response was immediate, and he attempted to kill the fool. He tried to take his sword from his

---

**30** Froissart, *Œuvres*, 15:40: "le fol homme ou le sage."

**31** Froissart, *Œuvres*, 15:41: "Le duc d'Orléans, n'éstoit pour l'eure trop loings du roy. Le roy s'adrecha devers luy, tenant l'espée toute nue, et jà en avoit le roy par sa frénaisie et foiblesse de chief perdu la congnoissance, ne il ne sçavoit qui estoit son frère ou son oncle. Quant le duc d'Orléans le perceu venir devers luy, l'espée toute nue en sa main, si se effréa et ne voult pas attendre et à bonne cause, et poindy le cheval quoiteusement, et le roy après luy. Le duc de Bourgoingne estoit et chevauchoit de costé, et pour l'effroy des chevaulx et que jà il avoit ouy les pages du roy crier, jetta son regard de celle part et congneu le roy qui, à l'espée toute nue, chassoit son frère."

page, but the page, frightened, ran away. When the king finally managed to get his sword, "from ire and from anger, he marvelled or despaired, or he was poisoned or ensorcelled or tormented, as it is held. Because when he had the sword, he turned on those around him, and wounded them greatly."[32] Even within one sentence, this chronicler had difficulty deciding how to ascribe a cause to the king's illness, suggesting on the one hand that the king acted from the internal impetus of anger or despair, but on the other hand that he might have been targeted by the external threats of poison or sorcery. The *Valois* chronicler ended his account with the happy news that the king's physician had cured him, news that other chroniclers who continued their account into the king's many relapses were not able to view with so much relief.

Regardless of the differences in detail, all three chroniclers recorded the fear generated by the king's attacks on his own men. This action was particularly egregious given the ideological framework within which the French monarchy was expected to provide protection in exchange for service. At that particular moment, when the king was in the process of demonstrating his power through the gathering of French forces in an effort to castigate the duke of Brittany, the symbolism inherent in his attack on his own forces must have been clear to all observers.

As this analysis of the first episode of the king's madness demonstrates, the chroniclers understood Charles VI's madness in terms of irrational and warlike behaviour. The king actually appears to be suffering from *pre*-traumatic stress, responding violently to an innocuous sound that mimicked the sounds of warfare long before he engaged in battle. Their descriptions of the onset of the king's madness resonated with concern about the stress of warfare and fears about loyalty. This narrative of the king's fear of treachery was particularly compelling in a moment of conflict, as the king prepared to fight a battle.

## *Chevauchée*, Ransom, and Trauma

Charles VI's reign was part of a long period of instability in France that took its toll on the countryside. The on again, off again conflict between the English and the French known as the Hundred Years' War began in 1337 when the English king Edward III claimed to be the rightful heir to the French throne. When Charles VI came to the throne as a child in 1380,

**32** *Chronique des quatre premiers Valois*, ed. Luce, 324: "d'ire et de couroult, se marvoya ou desespera, ou il fut empoisonnéz ou ensorceléz ou entaraudéz, comme l'en tenoit. Car comme il oult l'espée, il couru sus à ceulx d'entour lui, et moult en navra."

the English also had a child king in Richard II and the two sides negotiated a peace. However, conflicts continued on the ground in France, erupting eventually into a civil war between the Burgundians and the Armagnacs over the question of who would govern the realm during Charles VI's periods of madness. Then, in 1415, the new English king Henry V resumed the campaign to claim the French throne. His efforts were the most successful, and culminated in the Treaty of Troyes in 1420, in which Charles VI disinherited his son in favour of Henry V, who married Charles's daughter Catherine of Valois. Henry V became regent of France until Charles VI's death, but Henry died in 1422, mere months before Charles VI, who left his newborn grandson, Henry VI of England, as king of France. Charles VII set himself up as an alternative monarch in the Loire valley, but was unable to retake Paris and the north until Joan of Arc came to his aid in 1429. Indeed, even with her help, it was not until 1438 that Charles VII finally replaced the English rule. Although some warfare in this period consisted of pitched battles or sieges, much of the violence took place as smaller units rode around the countryside seeking provisions and pillaging in a method known as *chevauchée*. In addition to the officially sanctioned soldiers who participated in such raids, many brigands also took the opportunity to profit, and individuals were often held for ransom.[33]

During all these conflicts, the French king was not the only person perceived as suffering from mental disturbance during warfare. Evidence of the impact of war on the wider population can be found in fourteenth- and fifteenth-century remission letters, like the one for Robin le Crat, many of which viewed war as a potential catalyst of mental disturbance. France was often in a state of turmoil and, in the imaginations of the general public, the pillaging and brigandage surrounding the war with England and the civil wars among the French nobility were detrimental to the livelihoods as well as to the mental stability of the people.

Interestingly, unlike Charles VI whose first episode of madness occurred while he was actively participating in preparations for war, most people described in remission letters as mad due to the war were not active participants but rather "non-combatants" as Christopher Allmand has called them.[34]

---

**33** See Pfau, "Madness in the Realm," chapter 2; Christopher Allmand, *The Hundred Years War: England and France at War c. 1300–c. 1450* (Cambridge: Cambridge University Press, 1988); Autrand, *Charles VI*; Famiglietti, *Royal Intrigue*; Guenée, *La folie de Charles VI.*

**34** Christopher Allmand first proposed this terminology, which he took from contemporary discussion of the Vietnam War, in Christopher Allmand, "The War

This may be due to the particularity of remission letters as sources.[35] These narratives requesting the king's pardon originated in the early fourteenth century, when the French king began to demonstrate his grace and mercy by granting remission for offences that were punishable by death.[36] The criminal, or the criminal's family members, with the help of a royal notary, told the story of the crime, focusing on the details of the event and providing background information as the narrator deemed appropriate. The king's power of grace and mercy allowed him to act above the law, which meant that the remission letters did not need to follow a prescribed storyline to ensure validation,[37] and at least some amount of truth was necessary, since the

---

and the Non-combatant," in *The Hundred Years War*, ed. Kenneth Fowler (London: MacMillan, 1971), 163–83, but it can also be found in Allmand, *The Hundred Years War* and Christopher Allmand, "War and the Non-Combatant in the Middle Ages," in *Medieval Warfare: A History*, ed. Maurice Keen (Oxford: Oxford University Press, 1999), 253–72. See also Nicholas Wright, "French Peasants in the Hundred Years War," *History Today* 33, no. 6 (1983): 38–42; Nicholas Wright, *Knights and Peasants: The Hundred Years War in the French Countryside* (Woodbridge: Boydell, 1998); Nicholas Wright, "'Pillagers' and 'Brigands' in the Hundred Years War," *Journal of Medieval History* 9 (1983): 15–24; Nicholas Wright, "Ransoms of Non-combatants during the Hundred Years War," *Journal of Medieval History* 17 (1991): 323–32.

**35** I have discussed this in Aleksandra Pfau, "Warfare, Trauma, and Madness in French Remission Letters of the Hundred Years War," in *The Hundred Years War (Part III): Further Considerations*, eds. L. J. Andrew Villalon and Donald J. Kagay (Leiden: Brill, 2013), 437–54. Wendy J. Turner has provided a fascinating study of madness during the Hundred Years' War in England, where the legal situation focused considerably more on guardianship than in France. In England, the mad were wards of the crown, so soldiers who returned from the wars in mentally fraught or fragile conditions were of interest to the king. In France, in contrast, the king had no vested interest in the mad, so the legal sources discussing insanity differ. See Wendy J. Turner, "Mental Incapacity and the Financing of War in Medieval England," in *The Hundred Years War (Part II): Different Vistas*, eds. L. J. Andrew Villalon and Donald J. Kagay (Leiden: Brill, 2008), 387–402.

**36** The first remission letter appeared in May of 1304. See Claude Gauvard, *"De grace especial": Crime, état et société en France à la fin du Moyen Âge* (Paris: Publications de la Sorbonne, 1991), 64.

**37** As distinct from the English law courts, where there were strict conditions for proving madness, which caused a certain amount of conformity among cases. See Thomas A. Green, "Societal Concepts of Criminal Liability for Homicide in Mediaeval England," *Speculum* 47, no. 4 (1972): 680; Wendy J. Turner, "'Afflicted with Insanity': The Care and Custody of the Feeble Minded in Late Medieval England" (PhD diss., University of California, Los Angeles, 2000).

letter had to be read aloud by the local judge in the presence of the adverse party, and if they raised an objection the remission could be annulled.[38]

My research has shown that the composers of remission letters seldom chose to frame a crime narrative in terms of madness.[39] Those that do are scattered throughout the registers, suggesting that madness was not a common trope in the genre but a relatively unusual manifestation for the royal notaries who recorded and helped to compose these letters. Letters mentioning madness as a result of pillaging appeared most regularly during the period of English rule and civil war, and many reflect concerns about the shifting boundaries, loyalties, and fears of treason underlying that conflict.

One such war-related case appeared in a letter from May of 1424, when Henriette, wife of Jehan Charnel, committed suicide in the town of Montagny-Sainte-Félicité near Senlis. According to her family and relatives, a company of soldiers had come to Montagny looking for provisions while Jehan Charnel was away in Picardy selling apples. The soldiers found Jehan Charnel's mare and appropriated it and two robes from Charnel's house. Henriette attempted to prevent them, but was so badly beaten for her pains that she lay bedridden for fifteen days afterwards. Eight days later, the soldiers returned and found their second horse. This time Jehan Charnel, who had returned home, tried to prevent them, but he was no more successful than his wife had been. When the bedridden Henriette was told that their second horse was gone, as well, she was so angered and displeased that she became "troubled in her good sense and memory," saying several times each day that they had lost everything by losing their horses.[40] This narrative suggested that Henriette's anger at losing everything provided sufficient cause for her to go out of her mind and hang herself.

Although some men committed suicide due to losses caused by war, in these cases madness was not mentioned as an ancillary reason.[41] While suicide does not seem to have been considered a gendered response to war, madness leading to suicide appears to have been.[42] Men's war-related

**38** Quentin Verreycken, "The Power to Pardon in Late Medieval and Early Modern Europe: New Perspectives in the History of Crime and Criminal Justice," *History Compass* 17, no. 6 (2019), 62.

**39** See Pfau, *Medieval Communities and the Mad*.

**40** AN, JJ 172, fol. 266r–v no. 474; Himanis, 535–36: "troublee en son bon sens et memoire."

**41** See AN, JJ 130, fol. 152v no. 269; Himanis, 314 (in 1387); and AN, JJ 166, fol. 213 no. 317; Himanis, 435 (in 1412).

**42** One study on women's roles during the Hundred Years War uses chronicle

madness was generally described as the "youthful folly" of those men seeking remission for fighting for the "enemy" or becoming a brigand, and the "lack of sense" that caused a man who had lost his livelihood during the war to violate trade sanctions by selling food to the enemy, or in enemy-occupied territory.[43]

For example, in a remission letter from 1422, Pierre de Compans, a twenty-year-old from Paris, explained that five or six years earlier he had "by his folly and youth and by the instigation of Molinet de Compans," his uncle, left Paris and joined the king's enemies and adversaries, including the Lord of Boqueaux whom he served for a few years.[44] He was caught when he went to Hainault to buy some horses and put in prison by the garrison at Beaurevoir from which he was ransomed. However, "considering that he had done badly to have followed our said adversaries" he left their company, wishing to return "to Paris and to our obedience."[45] Pierre insisted that, although he had ridden with the king's enemies, he had never participated in any occasion where someone was pillaged, robbed, or killed, and highlighted his youthful folly as the reason for his actions, an excuse that Charles VI and his council accepted.

The links between pillage, ransom, and mental distress seem to have led men to action as opposed to suicide. In a fascinating case from 1390, the narrative does not explicitly mention mental illness as a possible underlying factor for the crime, but it is difficult to imagine that trauma did not play some role. Jean, lord of Montaurel, knight, was involved in France's failed campaign in August 1388 against Duke William of Guelders. The duke had

---

accounts and some letters to valorize the women in question, without addressing the ways in which these narratives of strong women or of entire communities, including women, joining in to help with the defence of a town may reflect the desires and goals of the chronicler or letter-writer. James E. Gilbert, "A Medieval 'Rosie the Riveter'? Women in France and Southern England during the Hundred Years War," in *The Hundred Years War: A Wider Focus*, eds. L. J. Andrew Villalon and Donald J. Kagay (Leiden: Brill, 2005), 333–61.

**43** For the "folie et jeunesse" leading to joining the enemy's army or brigandage, see AN, JJ 174, fol. 101r–v no. 228; Himanis, 209–10 (in 1428). For the "non sens" or "folie et ignorance" that caused people to sell flour or other foods to the enemy or in enemy-occupied lands, see AN, JJ 172, fol. 261r–v no. 465; Himanis, 525–26 (in 1424); fol. 310r–v no. 558; Himanis, 623–24 (in 1423); AN, JJ 175, fol. 133r–v no. 369; Himanis, 273–74 (in 1434).

**44** AN, JJ 172, fol. 66r no. 131; Himanis, 135: "par sa folie et jeunesse et par lenvortement de feu molinet de campans oncle dudit suppliant."

**45** AN, JJ 172, fol. 66r no. 131; Himanis, 135: "considerant quil avoit mal fait davoir suy nosdiz adversaires"; "de Paris et en notre obeissance."

allied himself with the English against the duke of Burgundy's influence in the Netherlands.[46] During the conflict, Jean, along with many other gentlemen including his squire Pierre de Matringuehen who submitted his own request for pardon, was "taken and put in prison by the Germans in very difficult, diverse, and terrible prisons in which they suffered and withstood many grievances and punishments, both from being tortured and put in irons and from being put in a flying pillory in which the said knight was hung for a long time in the air."[47] As Wendy J. Turner notes in this volume, suffering during imprisonment could be seen as a cause of mental trauma and a justification for later actions.[48] In fact, the pillory in particular was seen as a form of punishment from which the nobility would be exempt, which may have further contributed to Jean's distress.[49] Finally, Jean was ransomed, which in many ways compounded his problems, since he also lost a lot of money.[50] Jean's description of the harshness of German treatment of captives is corroborated by Jean Froissart in his chronicle. When describing the treatment of English captives by the French, he contrasts their leniency with the Germans, "who are harsh and austere to their prisoners and hold and put them in pillories, in irons, in chains, and in fetters, and do them damage and suffering to their bodies so that they can push them to pay more ransom."[51] In his narrative, Jean emphasized the experiences that he had suffered, bodily, mentally, and economically from his imprisonment. Although he did not describe himself as disabled, his description of the tortures that

---

**46** Autrand, *Charles VI*, 161–63.

**47** AN, JJ 140, fol. 159r–v no. 121; Himanis, 169–70: "eussent este par les alemans priz et menez prisonniers en tres dures diverses et mauvaises prisons esqueles ilz souffrirent et soubstindrent plusieurs griefs et peines tant de tirer gehnier et mettre en fers comme ester mis en un cep volant ou quell le dit chevalier fu pendu par long temps en air."

**48** Wendy J. Turner, "Investigating the Lifecycle of the Medieval English Soldier: Disability, Mental Trauma, and Medicine in Connection with War in Late Medieval English Records," in this volume.

**49** Isabelle D'Artagnan, *Le pilori au Moyen Âge dans l'espace français: XII^e^–XV^e^ siècle* (Rennes: Presses universitaires de Rennes, 2024), 89–114.

**50** Michael K. Jones, "Ransom Brokerage in the Fifteenth Century," in *Guerre et société en France, en Angleterre et en Bourgogne XIV^e^–XV^e^ siècle*, eds. Phillipe Contamine et al. (Villeneuve-d'Ascq: Publications de l'Institut de recherches historiques du Septentrion, 1991), 221–35.

**51** Froissart, *Œuvres*, 8:50: "car il sont dur et auster à leur prisonniers et les tiennent et mettent en ceps, en fiers, en buies et en grésillons, et leur font grieftés dou corps souffrir à le fin qu'il en puissant plus presser de finanche."

he had endured was detailed and lengthy. Like the Swiss soldiers examined by Bianca Frohne in this volume, however, Jean did not provide any detail about the long-term effects of these injuries.[52] Nevertheless, his narrative seems to reveal some of the struggles of managing the aftermath of injuries. Because the conflict had ended with a peace treaty, Jean and his companions could not have any redress for their losses. Around the feast of Pentecost 1389, he and some of his companions who had also been ransomed gathered together and attacked a group of German pilgrims, imprisoning them in turn and using torture to attempt to get more ransom money from them. Of the three German prisoners, two died due to mistreatment, but one managed to be ransomed by his family and went to Paris looking for his own justice. In this case, the trauma of imprisonment during warfare was heightened when a peace treaty ended hostilities, since Jean and his squire were no longer able to get retribution for their injuries.

In many ways, these narratives of decisions to attack innocent, or at least indirectly implicated, people in a form of vigilante revenge reflect the general sense of uncertainty of a country riven by civil war and, after the Treaty of Troyes in 1420, ultimately under the control of a foreign king. Lines of allegiance shifted swiftly, and loyalties were not always clear. The need for a letter of remission to allow the bearer to avoid the repercussions of actions that at the local level might have seemed unproblematic reveals both the lengths to which the English king of France was willing to go to solidify these ties and the fragility of the new alliances. Perhaps, therefore, it is unsurprising that there is an increase in the number of letters relating to the war during Henry VI's reign.

A set of four remission letters all dealing with the same crime appear in the chancery records for 1424 and 1425.[53] It is not a story about madness itself, but one that offers insight into how the discourse of madness was deployed and how multiple levels of community were constructed. In these four letters sent to the king, a number of residents of a town in the diocese of Bayeux explained to the English government of France how it came to pass that they had banded together to attack two Englishmen in November of

52 Bianca Frohne, "'What pain I suffered at that time, anyone can well imagine': Experiences of War, Injury, and Pain in Fifteenth and Sixteenth Centuries Germany and Switzerland," in this volume.

53 AN, JJ 173, fols. 22v–23r no. 44, Himanis, 50–51; fol. 88r–v no. 170; Himanis 177–78; fols. 88v–89r no. 171; Himanis, 178–79; fol. 89r–v no. 172; Himanis 179–80. I have also discussed these in Pfau, *Medieval Communities and the Mad*, 169–76.

1417, shortly after Henry V's army had overtaken Caen.[54] No one could understand these strangers, who had decided to lodge at Guillaume le Paumier's *hôtel*. When the two men started to gather together the Paumiers' goods, Alips, Guillaume le Paumier's wife, left the *hôtel* seeking help, and a group of townspeople returned with her and killed the two men.

Their requests for remission were written against the background of national events. In the seven years between 1417, when the act was committed, and 1424, when remission was sought, the political landscape in France had shifted, in part due to repercussions from the king's madness. Charles VI had died in 1422, leaving political confusion and civil war dividing the realm. The dead king's son, Charles, had been officially disinherited, and controlled only southern France. His grandson, Henry, the heir according to the Treaty of Troyes, was just a baby, and with the aid of an English regent and the duke of Burgundy, held Paris and northern France. In such a divisive moment, fundamental questions about the very constitution of the French realm, French identity, and the relationship between the French and the English were at stake.[55] The political situation was so complex in part because of the king's madness, which had left his legacy, shaped through the Treaty of Troyes, open to question.[56] As these four remission letters demonstrate, changes at the level of the realm had real repercussions in local communities. This series of letters moves beyond the general acknowledgement of alternating loyalties, however, considering problems of linguistic differences, communal defence, and the long-term fears that such shifts engender.

Robert le Panomer's letter was recorded in the chancery in December of 1424, and was the first remission letter sought by members of this community in reference to the death of the two strangers.[57] The three other letters relating to this crime were all recorded consecutively in June of 1425, and appear to have been composed in consultation with each other. Indeed, these three

---

**54** Jacqueline Horeau-Dodinau has traced a standard narrative about violence against pillaging soldiers in remission letters. See "La Vengeance du paysan," in *Anthropologies juridiques: Mélanges Pierre Braun*, eds. Jacqueline Horeau-Dodinau and Pascale Texier (Limoges: Presses universitaires de Limoges, 1998), 385–423.

**55** Colette Beaune, *The Birth of an Ideology: Myths and Symbols of Nation in Late-Medieval France* (Berkeley: University of California Press, 1991).

**56** Medieval authors seeking to prove that the Treaty of Troyes was not legally sound often pointed to the mental state of Charles VI. See Nicole Pons, "Intellectual Patterns and Affective Reactions in Defence of the Dauphin Charles, 1419–1422," in *War, Government and Power in Late Medieval France*, ed. Christopher Allmand (Liverpool: Liverpool University Press, 2000), 54–69.

**57** AN, JJ 173, fols. 22v–23r no. 44; Himanis, 50–51.

letters are practically word-for-word exact replicas of each other. The first of these was composed on behalf of Guillaume and Alips le Paumier,[58] who were pardoned together as a married couple. The two others were for Robin Germain[59] and Jehan Germain,[60] perhaps brothers or a father and son, though their relationship to each other was not specified in the letters. These three identical letters with slight alterations in reference to the particular supplicant involved reveal the careful construction that went into these crime narratives. In the essentials, they do not diverge significantly from Robert le Panomer's earlier version, but their narrative is more cautious and considered.

It is tempting to speculate about the exchange of information once Robert le Panomer returned to Normandy with his letter of remission. Guillaume and Alips le Paumier and Robin and Jehan Germain all claimed that they had been hiding "secretly," supported by their neighbours and relatives in the area, for the past seven years. Two possibilities can be imagined. One is that, with Robert le Panomer's letter of remission, the horizon opened for these four fugitives. Here was proof that the English occupiers would not execute them for their crime, but that Henry, like the King of France he claimed to be, would, of his grace and mercy, pardon them. Alternatively, Robert le Panomer's return with a royal pardon might have initiated a legal case against his accomplices, since remission for one participant in a crime did not guarantee remission for the others.[61] Regardless, it is likely that Robert le Panomer's remission letter for this case spurred the others to seek their own. The distance from Paris to the diocese of Bayeux, where their village was located, is around 260 kilometres (160 miles). There was plenty of time between Robert le Panomer's return, probably sometime in late December or early January, and the trip to Paris in May or June by the other four remission seekers. They could get the story straight, ensure that the details matched and that nothing they said had the potential to backfire once they acquired remission.

The first letter, written on behalf of Robert le Panomer, claimed that two strangers arrived in town, "speaking a strange language that they had never heard and they did not know whether they were Bretons, English, Scottish or

58 AN, JJ 173, fol. 88r–v no. 170, Himanis 177–78.

59 AN, JJ 173, fols. 88v–89r no. 171; Himanis, 178–79.

60 AN, JJ 173, fol. 89r–v no. 172; Himanis 179–80.

61 Esther Cohen notes this, although the case she discusses involves people who received remission for crimes for which their accomplices had already been executed. Esther Cohen, *The Crossroads of Justice: Law and Culture in Late Medieval France* (Leiden: Brill, 1993).

other peoples."[62] The letter is a narrative constructing Robert le Panomer's innocence. The men were speaking an incomprehensible language, so no one knew they were English, and, perhaps more significantly, no one knew what they were doing. They were the first aggressors. According to Robert le Panomer's letter, the strangers had threatened the Paumiers by hitting them both several times with the flat of their swords, and gathered all the Paumiers' goods together, planning to steal them in the morning. As if that was not enough to exonerate him, even Alips's decision to call on her neighbours for aid was not done with the intention of attacking the two strangers, but only in a state of temporary madness brought on by fear, loss, and possibly pain, since she had already been beaten by the strangers' swords. According to Robert le Panomer's version of events, Alips "was as if completely out of her good sense and memory because she saw that they wanted to take away their said goods."[63] Thus, her decision to round up the locals to help her prevent these two strangers from stealing from her was not premeditated, but was the result of a temporary insanity brought on by her fear of the loss of their property. In choosing to claim that Alips was mad, Robert le Panomer's letter drew on a wider understanding of the depredations of war as a potential catalyst for mental distress.[64]

However, despite the acceptance of warfare as a cause of mental distress, the version of the narrative agreed upon by Guillaume and Alips le Paumier, Robin Germain, and Jehan Germain departed from Robert le Panomer's in multiple ways, and particularly in their choice not to attribute Alips's behaviour to madness. The supplicants declared that they 'had no memory' of the exact date, just that it was around St. Martin's Day and after the conquest of Caen by the English.[65] By declaring their uncertainty about the date, the composers of these three letters established the uncertain nature of memory. Despite four witnesses who were able to agree on the details to the extent that they presented their cases in almost identical ways, no one could recall the exact date on which these events took place. This reminder of the fragility of human memories, particularly after the passage of time, could

---

**62** AN, JJ 173, fols. 22v–23r no. 44; Himanis, 50–51: "parlans langage estrange que on ne entendoit point et ne savoit ou se cestoient bretons anglois escocoys ou autres gens."

**63** AN, JJ 173, fols. 22v–23r no. 44; Himanis, 50–51: "fut comme toute hors de son bon sens et memoire pour ce quelle veoit quilz vouloient emport leurs diz biens."

**64** For more on these cases, see Pfau, "Warfare, Trauma, and Madness."

**65** AN, JJ 173, fol. 88r–v no. 170; fols. 88v–89r no. 171; fol. 89r–v no. 172: "dont lesdis suppliant ne sont recors."

have been an effort to legitimize their own version of events as opposed to Robert le Panomer's.

The composers of the new narrative of events, unlike Robert, did not choose to provide a list of possible languages that the two men might have been speaking, instead stating it was "English or another language."[66] This version of events also avoided representing the two men with drawn swords during their early interactions with Guillaume and Alips le Paumier. Instead, their threatening actions were directed towards the couple's goods, which they gathered together and seemed to plan to carry away. Indeed, it was because they could not understand these strangers, not because the strangers threatened them with bodily harm, that Guillaume and Alips became frightened and angry. According to their letter, Guillaume went to bed and Alips (without consulting her husband) left the house to complain to the neighbours about these two strangers. Significantly, these three letters did not mention temporary madness as a mitigating factor for Alips's actions.[67] Madness could be a complicated claim to make, since it could lead to a mandate in the letter of remission forcing the family to keep the mad person locked up or under guard.[68] This was particularly true in Normandy where the law codes called for the restraint of the mad to prevent them from causing fires.[69] Clearly, Robert le Panomer did not find it problematic to refer to the temporary madness of his neighbour who called for his aid, whereas Guillaume and Alips le Paumier were hesitant to ascribe her behaviour to madness. Instead, they presented her call for help as an understandable response to the threat of theft that the two strangers represented.

Robert le Panomer, the Paumiers, and the Germains were caught in an awkward moment of transition between political rivals, where alliances shifted and enemies became putative friends. On the ground, in local villages, these shifts engendered confusion, anger, and fear. Caen had fallen to the English forces, but residents of small towns in the countryside could not know in

**66** AN, JJ 173, fol. 88r–v no. 170; fols. 88v–89r no. 171; fol. 89r–v no. 172: "parlans anglois ou autre langage."

**67** AN, JJ 173, fol. 88r–v no. 170; fols. 88v–89r no. 171; fol. 89r–v no. 172.

**68** For example, the letter for Jehan de Moustier in AN, JJ 118, fols. 18v–19r, no. 18; Himanis, 38–39 (in 1380) and one for Jehannecte Troppé in AN, JJ 173, fols. 33v–34r no. 63; Himanis, 70–71 (in 1425). Edited in *Actes de la chancellerie d'Henri VI concernant la Normandie sous la domination anglaise (1422–1435), extraits des registres du Trésor des Chartes aux Archives nationales*, ed. Paul Le Cacheux (Rouen-Paris: Lestraingant-Picard, 1907–1908), 1:181–83.

**69** *L'ancienne coutume de Normandie*, ed. William Lawrence de Gruchy (Jersey: LeFeuvre, 1881), 184.

that moment how changes in policies at the level of kings and princes would colour their own actions, reframing them in unexpected ways. From their perspective, they had banded together as neighbours to defend their community from strangers with whom they were unable to communicate. Within three years, those strangers had, through the Treaty of Troyes, become allies. Within five years, the kingdoms of France and England were joined under a single king. As the first remission seeker, Robert le Panomer sought to emphasize the fear and confusion brought on by the unexplained actions of these two strangers, explaining that the men had drawn their swords and beaten the Paumiers. He described Alips le Paumier as out of her senses in an attempt to recapture the emotional tenor of the moment and explain why her neighbours were so quick to come to her aid. The later letters were more balanced in their portrayal of the two strangers and in their depiction of Alips's actions.

## Conclusion

From kings to knights to villagers, instabilities caused by war had tangible effects on individuals. Just as chroniclers sought to tie King Charles VI's paranoia about treason to his first episode of madness, so too did Robert le Panomer attribute Alips le Paumier's actions against the English soldiers to her mental distress. As all of these remission letters demonstrate, confusion of loyalties on the level of the realm had repercussions in local communities. Treaties made by those in power could rapidly transform actions from legitimate defence to illegitimate private warfare. As Jean, lord of Montaurel discovered, getting revenge on Germans who had tortured him during the war declared by the French king was no longer acceptable when those Germans were now allies going on pilgrimage who could call on the French king for aid. For the Paumiers, with an English king on the throne, actions that might in other contexts have appeared simply as a commendable and heroic defence of the village against enemies of the realm, were suddenly construed as the murder of loyal soldiers and subjects of the king. These conflicts over changing identities and shifting boundaries between enemy and friend were relatively common in this period, and a number of remission letters reflect discomfort and uncertainty on a local level, caused by political events. As Robin le Crat, whose story began this essay, demonstrated, sometimes national loyalty was under significant stress in a time of warfare, particularly when coping with a loved one who was unable to work became more difficult due to the pressures of supporting the war effort through taxation. Themes of treason, paranoia, pillage, and ransom arose for kings, nobles, and peasants alike and contributed to the traumas of a war-torn countryside.

Chapter 6

# INVESTIGATING THE LIFECYCLE OF THE MEDIEVAL ENGLISH SOLDIER

## DISABILITY, MENTAL TRAUMA, AND MEDICINE IN CONNECTION WITH WAR IN LATE MEDIEVAL ENGLISH RECORDS

WENDY J. TURNER

THIS PAPER FOLLOWS the lives of medieval English soldiers from first battle until the end of their careers and into retirement or a lack thereof through the administrative records of the English Crown, such as the close rolls (private correspondence and directives), patent rolls (public letters, announcements, and orders), and inquisitions: both miscellaneous inquiries and postmortem investigations. Several interrelated topics on battlefield trauma and the aftermath, including trauma during or because of ransom, are pieced together from these royal records of England. Battlefield- or captivity-related injuries to bodies or minds could cause fighters to become disabled. And once home as a survivor of war, society managed the care and properties of those who had disabilities from war-affiliated traumas. There are two types of trauma, mental and physical; and while medieval people did not use our contemporary term "trauma" for mental trauma in the Middle Ages, records of persons with mental health issues following war or war-related experiences exist. This paper will look primarily but not exclusively at mental health trauma, which is today defined as a stress reaction to a traumatic event.[1]

1 Many thanks to Kelly DeVries for his insights into battle-related injury. For a definition of our contemporary use of the term "trauma" see "Trauma- and Stressor-Related Disorders," especially sections on "posttraumatic stress disorder" and "acute stress disorder," *Diagnostic and Statistical Manual of Mental Disorders*, 5th ed. (hereafter, *DSM-5*), online at http://dsm.psychiatryonline.org, accessed September 13, 2024.

**WENDY J. TURNER** is Professor of History at Augusta University. She is known for her work on medieval mental health, intellectual disabilities, and medicine. She is the author of a monograph and numerous articles as well as having edited five volumes on topics from trauma to malingering to medicine. Her recent research topics revolve around neurohumanities—emotion, pain, age-related disabilities, and epi/pandemic responses.

The idea of historic post-war trauma is not only difficult to prove but also difficult to research. Obviously, we cannot interview these individuals, but we can look at records that report changes in behaviour, self-reporting of emotional extremes, or complete mental deterioration about which contemporaries associated with reported war-related trauma. Medieval post-battle records sometimes mention changes in an individual's mental health or a head injury and recovery after battle, which gives scholars a glimpse at individual responses, treatments, and recovery strategies following battle injuries or reactions. Fighters were trained to aim their blows at the areas of the body not covered in metal or padding, especially lower limbs and the head.[2] This left many fighters, even those who could afford a good helmet, with head injuries from concussions or penetrating wounds. And, while torture for ransomed gentlemen was frowned upon, evidence exists for the use of torture and imprisonment, which encouraged the rapid payment of ransom but destroyed the mental health of some victims. In 1306 for example, Nigel Coppedene, a landholder, killed his neighbour and was pardoned because of a mental illness following "his sufferings as a prisoner of war."[3] Nigel and other former fighters had a difficult time upon returning home. In all cases, the socio-economic status of each fighter affected his recovery efforts, including the time he might be able to take away from duties or work to try to recover, the funds he had to pay for medications or physicians, and even his choices to stop fighting when injured or ill might be hampered because of financial reasons. This paper will take a closer look at later medieval (1280 to about 1550) English cases of trauma and injury of fighters before, during, and after battle.

**2** In Larissa Tracy and Kelly DeVries, eds., *Wounds and Wound Repair in Medieval Culture* (Leiden: Brill, 2016), see especially Larissa Tracy and Kelly DeVries, "Introduction: Penetrating Medieval Wounds," 1–23, and Robert C. Woosnam-Savage and Kelly DeVries, "Battle Trauma in Medieval Warfare: Wounds, Weapons and Armor," 27–56; Rebecca Redfern, "A Bioarcheological Study of Violence in the Roman World," in *The Routledge Handbook of the Bioarchaeology of Human Conflict*, eds. Christopher J. Knüsel and Martin Smith (London: Routledge, 2013), 203–12.

**3** More on Nigel below. Kew, The National Archive (hereafter TNA), PRO C 260/16/m 5b; JUST 1/934/m 3.

## Childhood Training

Often children of aristocrats and the gentry received formal training for battle with wooden swords and lessons in sitting a horse with armour.[4] There could be injuries as young want-to-be soldiers fought in the practice yard. It was rare that these injuries resulted in any permanent damage, but it could happen. Some young people attended jousting matches (fighting with swords) or tilting competitions (which was in essence strength training and horsemanship). For those individuals wanting to improve their technique, there were combat or fight manuals.[5] Fighters from the upper echelons of society sometimes attended battles for the first time as boys and helped in the background alongside a relative's squire, with the hobelars and the horses, weapons' masters in organizing and cleaning spare weapons, or with the cooks, handing out food and water. Peasant boys did not have the same training, unless they were part of a family that specialized as archers,

---

**4** Pierre Gaite, "Exercises in Arms: The Physical and Mental Combat Training of Men-at-Arms in the Fourteenth and Fifteenth Centuries," *Journal of Medieval Military History* 16 (2018): 99–122; Kelly DeVries, ed., *Medieval Warfare 1300–1450* (London: Routledge, 2017); Kelly DeVries, *Medieval Military Technology* (Peterborough, Canada: Broadview, 1992); and Christina Lee, "Healing Words: St. Guthlac and the Trauma of War," in *Trauma in Medieval Society*, eds. Wendy J. Turner and Christina Lee (Leiden: Brill, 2018), 263.

**5** There were many fight manuals in the Middle Ages and most had few words with mostly images of how to stand and move, appearing much like a graphic-novel-type instruction book. Copies floated around Europe regardless of where they originated. The oldest known manual on swordsmanship is known by its archival shelf number, I. 33. There are debates among historians as to who used all these manuals, but they seem to have been widely consumed by civilian fighters, politicians, tacticians, and even ecclesiastical fighters. Everyone needed to know how to defend themselves, and, with few words and mostly pictures, these were easy-to-follow guides on defence and protection. While there are many versions in archives, a few published examples include Daniel Jaquet, Karin Verelst, and Timothy Dawson, eds., *Late Medieval and Early Modern Fight Books: Transmission and Tradition of Martial Arts in Europe (14th–17th Centuries)* (Leiden: Brill, 2016); Sydney Anglo, *The Martial Arts of Renaissance Europe* (New Haven: Yale University Press, 2000); Publius Vegetius Renatus, *Epitoma rei militaris*, ed. Michael D. Reeve (Oxford: Oxford University Press, 2004); *The Medieval Art of Swordsmanship: Royal Armouries MS I.33*, ed. Jeffrey L. Forgeng (Leeds: Royal Armouries, 2018); Rachel E. Kellett, "Royal Armouries MS I.33: The Judicial Combat and The Art of Fencing in Thirteenth- and Fourteenth-Century German Literature," *Oxford German Studies* 41, no. 1 (2012): 32–56; Hans Talhoffer, *Medieval Combat: A Fifteenth-Century Manual of Swordfighting and Close-Quarter Combat*, ed. and trans. Mark Rector (London: Greenhill, 2000); and Joachim Meyer, *The Art of Combat: A German Martial Arts Treatise of 1570*, ed. Jeffrey L. Forgeng (Chicago: Frontline, 2020).

for example, or in other specialty units.[6] Most peasants, though, learned what they knew of battles from friends, neighbours, first-hand accounts and story-telling.

Young men sometimes took the place of their parent or other relative. Individuals who could not continue a campaign or attend a battle because of illness, injury or disability might "depute" an alternate or "designate a champion," essentially deputize their son or another person as their substitute—especially if the boy were nearing the age at which he would have taken part in his own right.[7] For example, Henry Cobeham of Rondale in 1316 was granted permission to stay at home when summoned by the king of England "to join him with horses and arms at Newcastle-on-Tyne," when royal representatives learned "that he is so infirm and ill that he cannot come in person."[8] The king, though, ordered Henry to send "another of his men-at-arms with [his] horses and arms" to serve in his place. As explained above, this could be his son, but a brother, another relative, or even a retainer could be named. In another example, this one in 1322, Robert Stoke, Guy Breton, and William Sutton were ordered to suspend the assessment and fine of 200 *l.* of Richard de Herthull. While the assessment and same fine to other "knights, squires, and other men-at-arms in the county for permission to attend to their own affairs, and to be exempt from the expedition against the king's enemies" stood, it was learned that Richard de Herthull had sent a deputy. His son, also Richard, attended the battle in his place. It was not until after the expedition that the king learned that young Richard had been in attendance. Richard the elder "was too ill to go in the expedition and sent his son Richard in his place, who," the record is careful to point out, "stayed continuously in the expedition with Ralph Basset, as the king learns from Ralph's testimony."[9] Likely

---

**6** Other specialized occupations included early gunpowder experts, crossbow makers (at times), and those who knew how to repair and/or build machines such as ballistas, drills, or siege engines. Helen J. Nicholson, *Medieval Warfare: Theory and Practice of War in Europe, 300–1500* (Basingstoke: Palgrave, 2004); Jan Frans Verbruggen, *The Art of War in Western Europe during the Middle Ages from the Eighth Century* (Woodbridge: Boydell, 1954).

**7** Honorat Bovet, *The Tree of Battles*, ed. George William Coopland (Cambridge, MA: Harvard University Press, 1949), 199.

**8** *Calendar of the Close Rolls Preserved in the Public Record Office* [hereafter *CCR*], *1313–1318* (London: Eyre, 1893), 431. While I cannot concretely say that Henry the elder became disabled in September 1316, his son "Henry de Cobham, the younger" is called to serve in June 1317 without his father.

**9** *CCR, 1318–1323* (London: Eyre, 1895), 441.

Ralph and the senior Richard had an agreement to keep young Richard, his age unstated, safe and/or to teach him how to fight.

This is not to say that illness was in any way the same as a disability or trauma, but if out on campaign and injured—possibly with a wound that might leave a fighter with a disability—that individual could end his involvement with the campaign and, with permission, leave and return home. Some, though, left their sons behind and, like Richard de Herthull, put them into the care of others on the field. The training a real battle might afford, especially if the commander was in control and succeeding, was a valuable experience and as a deputy, that child would have been able to prove he could be responsible.

## Preparations for Battles in Case of Injury

Individuals—aristocrats, gentry, burghers, and peasants—fought in medieval battles because that was part of their expected duties and training. They were conscripted, or more or less voluntarily joined their company. They were not just there for the day and might be expected to forgo food and bathing as well as to bring their own equipment, possibly constructed at home. People could be dismissed from participation by a lord or commander based on poor health, an impairment such as poor eyesight or hearing, or because their overall stamina was not strong enough (e.g., they were chronically ill, or suffered breathing problems, a bad limp, etc.).

Medieval fighters might suffer physical wounds in battle and live to see another day.[10] A number of individuals experienced other issues connected to their service, including illness or a sense of loss. As Robert Woosnam-Savage and Kelly DeVries write, "There were two principal reasons for the survival of wounded soldiers in the Middle Ages…the effectiveness of military surgery and armor." Most soldiers could not afford the luxury of substantial armour; landholders, generally, had quintessential plate armour while infantrymen wore a varied array of armour, amongst which the padded cloth armour.[11]

**10** As pointed out by Robert Woosnam-Savage and Kelly DeVries, "While the *Chirurgia* was not specifically written for military surgeons, they certainly used it." Woosnam-Savage and DeVries, "Battle Trauma," 49. Guy de Chauliac, *Inventarium sive Chirurgia magna*, eds. Michael R. McVaugh and Margaret S. Ogden, 2 vols. (Leiden: Brill, 1997). For more information on battle surgery and medicine, see the article by Depreter, below.

**11** While most fighters were male in the Middle Ages, there were a few women who fought. For more information on female fighters, see J. F. Verbruggen, "Women in Medieval Armies," *Journal of Medieval Military History* 4 (2006): 119–36.

Yet, some soldiers survived war because of military medicine.[12] Surgeons appear to have had success on the battlefield, however limited. As part of the cost of any campaign, a military surgeon was included in the company as was a priest.[13] Some fighters also experienced battle traumas, something like what we would call PTSD (Post Traumatic Stress Disorder).

Along with a surgeon, the king provided necessary medical supplies like honey and wine to military outposts, especially those fortifications near warzones such as the Marches of both Wales and Scotland and the English castles in those areas. Honey and wine, while often listed among pantry items both now and in the Middle Ages, were stocked in abundance, far more than a garrison would ever consume. These items were costly, and yet, all military ports, castles, and outposts were ordered to keep honey and wine on hand.[14] It was difficult to transport them to some of the remote castles or other fortifications, and yet it was vital if war broke out. The Crown had inventories made at each of his Welsh and Scottish strongholds and ordered them all to stock quantities of wine and honey for medical reasons. Before becoming too old to be of use, the London stockpile of wine and honey were sold at one point, and a new one purchased.[15] As tensions rose between England and France, a new law forbid sale of either product to the French; those goods and all gold was to remain in England. In the event of a battle,

**12** Woosnam-Savage and DeVries, "Battle Trauma," 47 (quote)–48. For more on payment: see M. R. Geldof, "'And to describe the shapes of the dead': Making Sense of the Archaeology of Armed Violence," *Wounds and Wound Repair*, 57–80; Kelly DeVries and Robert Douglas Smith, *Medieval Military Technology*, 2nd ed. (Toronto: University of Toronto Press, 2012).

**13** Medieval surgeons did far more than surgeons today. Certainly, they did surgery, but as Piers D. Mitchell points out, they also treated "weapon injuries, fractures, abscesses, bladder stones, haemorrhoids and anal fistulae." Piers D. Mitchell, *Medicine in the Crusades: Warfare, Wounds and the Medieval Surgeon* (Cambridge: Cambridge University Press, 2004), 5. Before the Lateran Council of 1215, other clergy (monks) served as surgeons, but after the church decided that clergy should not be "drawing blood," civilian barber-surgeons took up the task. Philippe Hernigou, Jacques Hernigou, and Marius Scarlat, "Medieval Surgery (Eleventh–Thirteenth Century): Barber Surgeons and Warfare Surgeons in France," *International Orthopaedics* 45 (2021): 1891–98.

**14** Ilana Krug, "The Wounded Soldier: Honey and Late Medieval Military Medicine," in *Wounds and Wound Repair*, 194–214; Edward Wheatley, *Stumbling Blocks Before the Blind: Medieval Constructions of a Disability* (Ann Arbor: University of Michigan Press, 2010), 11.

**15** *CCR, 1313–1318*, 267.

physicians needed wine and honey—both having antiseptic qualities—on hand to heal injured fighters.[16]

In the first half of the fourteenth century, when this study begins, there was constant monitoring of the stores of honey and wine. For example, in February 1316, the king ordered William Trente, the keeper of the exchange at London, "to buy for the king's use all the honey to be found in the city and wheat up to 1000 quarters, and to cause the same to be guarded safely until further orders…for the munition of his castles in Wales."[17] In the years following, again the Crown provisioned its Welsh castles, including Carnarvon; the king sent his clerk, Robert Wodehous [Woodhouse] to the country of Chester "to buy and purvey 40 tuns of wine and four barrels of honey and to take the same to Kaernarvan, in making such provisions [of aid]."[18] A month later, Robert Wodehouse was ordered to provide every castle "wherein there is no honey to be provided with two barrels of honey."[19] More honey for this same provisioning was requisitioned from Hugh Despenser and the castle and town of Bristol for the northern Welsh castles; Despenser needed to find sixty tuns of wine and six tuns of honey.[20] Nearly all purchase orders for honey were followed in the record for food stuffs, wheat, corn, rye and other provisions to feed the army; yet, while honey was used in cooking, the primary purpose for the military was medical.[21] This took care of the soldiers' bodies—food and medicine—and only their minds in so much as a good diet helps to maintain overall health. Also, during the initial outbreak of the plague in 1348 to 1351,[22] as evident in all levels of records, the Crown was determined that no gold, wine, or honey was to be sold abroad. Furthermore, as in times of war, the Crown at one point asked that the old stockpile be sold, and fresh wine be secured "seeing the mortality increase."[23] It was as if the Crown was treating the plague as an enemy.

**16** *CCR, 1313–1318*, 425.

**17** *CCR, 1313–1318*, 267.

**18** *CCR, 1313–1318*, 291, see also 50, 119.

**19** *CCR, 1318–1323*, 292–93.

**20** *CCR, 1318–1323*, 293.

**21** Krug, "The Wounded Soldier."

**22** Wendy J. Turner, "'They Are All Dead, Except a Few': Social Complications and Royal Reactions to Death in England, 1348–1350," in *Reconsidering Extinction in Terms of the History of Global Bioethics*, eds. Stan Booth and Chris Mounsey (London: Routledge, 2022), 112–135.

**23** *CCR. 1349–1354* (London: Mackie, 1905), 98–99.

## Medical Attention

Archers inflicted a lot of damage, if they were within range of their opponents. An arrow might pierce any part of the body and, so long as the tip and shaft had missed any vital organs, arrows could be removed. As a specialized weapon, it implies that in some cases these occupations and the equipment to accompany the position were inherited. These trained combatants were connected to a particular lord as part of his retinue or were recruited from particular areas of the kingdom that specialized in archery.[24] Archers might be injured at times from enemy shot or from accidental friendly fire, or other such mishaps.[25] Additionally, they could be mutilated if captured; the enemies of the English came to hate the English longbowman who shot the longer arrows. They would cut off the archer's first two fingers on his right hand, preventing him from drawing a bow. There is at least one image that includes a possible former archer with prosthetic fingers on his right hand (figure 6.1).[26]

Other than archers, military positions included everything from knights and foot soldiers (who fought hand-to-hand with edged weapons such as swords, spears, knives, and so on, or blunt force weapons, like a mace or staff) to knights' attendants such as squires, bannerets, hobelars (assisting with the horses) who also might have sustained injuries or died in battle. The archaeological record and any "wound man" points to the various trauma to soldiers in hand-to-hand combat, and most frequently to the head

---

**24** Adam Chapman, "Wales, Welshmen, and the Hundred Years War," in *The Hundred Years War (Part III): Further Considerations*, eds. L. J. Andrew Villalon and Donald J. Kagay (Leiden: Brill, 2013), 217–229; Adrian R. Bell, Anne Curry, Andy King, and David Simpkin, *The Soldier in Later Medieval England* (Oxford: Oxford University Press, 2013), 139–78. For more information on the use of English crossbows, see David S. Bachrach's works in which he establishes that Henry II, Richard, and John preferred crossbows to longbows, including "Crossbows for the King: The Crossbow during the Reigns of John and Henry III of England," *Technology and Culture* 45 (2004): 102–19; "Crossbows for the King, Part II: The Crossbow during the Reign of Edward I of England," *Technology and Culture* 47 (2006): 81–90; "Origins of the Crossbow Industry in England," *Journal of Medieval Military History* 2 (2004): 73–88; and "The Royal Crossbow Makers of England, 1204–1272," *Nottingham Medieval Studies* 47 (2003): 168–97.

**25** Iain A. MacInnes, "Head, Shoulders, Knees and Toes: Injury and Death in Anglo-Scottish combat, c. 1296–c. 1403," *Wounds and Wound Repair*, 102–27, at 111.

**26** London, British Library, Additional MS 42130, Luttrell Psalter (1325–1335), fol. 208v. The quoted caption of figure 6.1 comes from the British Library website, https://imagesonline.bl.uk/asset/14006, accessed February 7, 2025.

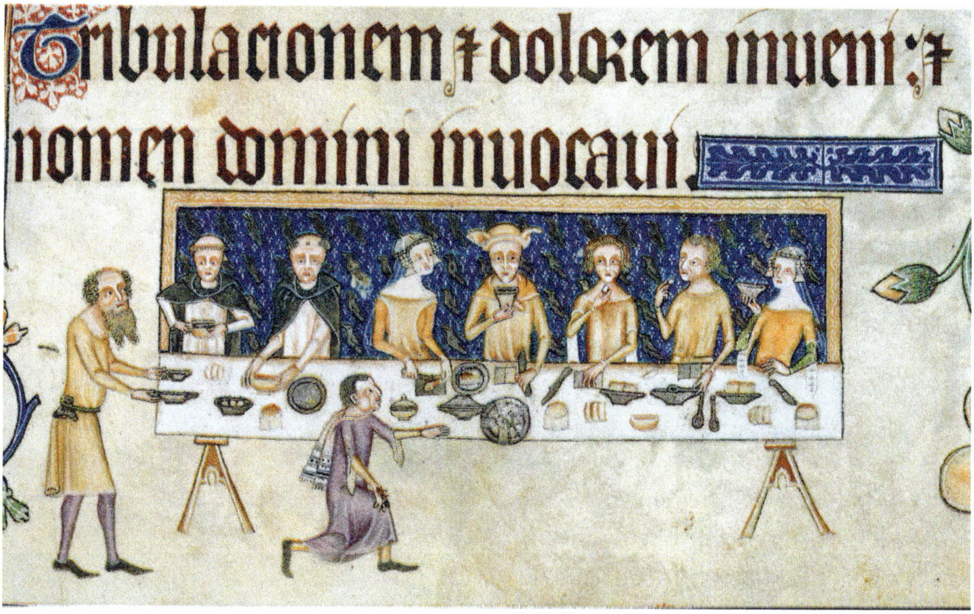


Figure 6.1. Details from the lower marginalia in the Luttrell Psalter. London, British Library, Additional MS 42130, fol. 208v. Courtesy of the British Library.

and limbs.[27] Wound-men always (so far as I know from the fifty images I have seen) include an arrow as do most archaeological battlefields. The archaeological record also has provided the conclusion that many soldiers lived with healed wounds, often for days if not years before finally dying later in battle or from other causes. Those earlier wounds—both from edged weapons and blunt force—healed with the help of battlefield surgeons.[28] All of

---

**27** There are many "wound man" illustrations. For examples see: London, Wellcome Library, MS 49, for a watercolour of a "wound man" from ca. 1420–1430 in a German MS of S. Johannis *Apocalypsis*; or Hans von Gersdorff, *Feldbuch der wundtartzney* (Strasbourg: Schott, 1517), fol. 18v, see Figure 8.1 of this book. For more information on archaeological studies of battle wounds, see (among many articles) *The Towton Battlefield Archaeology Project*, http://towtonbattle.free.fr/, accessed February 6, 2025; Tim Sutherland, "The Towton Battle. A Reinterpretation," *Arms and Armour* 12, no. 2 (2015): 124–35; Alexandra Boucherie, Marie Louise S. Jørkov, and Martin Smith, "Wounded to the Bone: Digital Microscopic Analysis of Traumas in a Medieval Mass Grave Assemblage (Sandbjerget, Denmark, AD 1300–1350)," *International Journal of Paleopathology* 19 (2017): 66–79. On the history of wounds, see Mitchell, *Medicine in the Crusades*; and *Wounds and Wound Repair*. For more information on wound-men, see the chapter by B. Frohne, below.

**28** For a sample of some recent research on wounds, see *Wounds and Wound Repair* and in particular Michael Livingston, "'The Depth of Six Inches': Prince

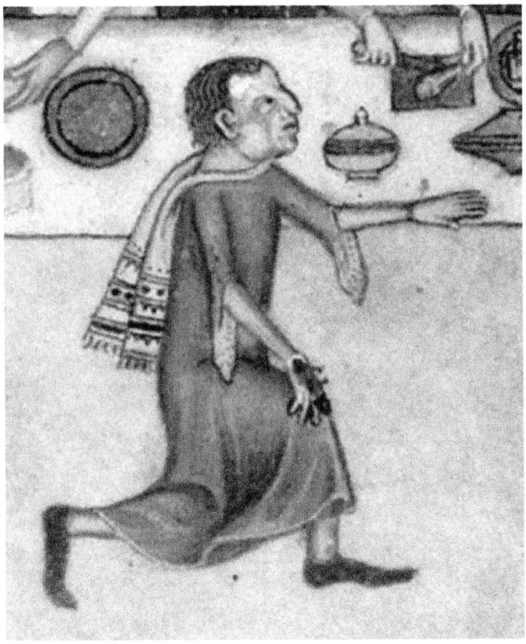

Figure 6.2. The man with the prosthetic hand, dressed in a lavender-coloured tunic and decorated scarf in front of the dining table, genuflecting before the host. Detail from London, British Library, Additional MS 42130, fol. 208v. Courtesy of the British Library.

these military persons could count on the Crown employing a surgeon for any campaign.

If a person in battle sustained a head injury, physicians and surgeons might perform some corrective measures that achieved mixed results.[29] They might save their patient's life but not always his mental capacity. A fifteenth-century commonplace book suggested for "bones broken in a man's head" to draw them out by making a plaster of "betony, vervain and rue" mixed with "honey and flour of rye and of wheat, and the white of an egg."[30] The idea was to get the splinters of bone to work their way out so that the surgeon or physician could then remove them. Today we know that vervain (*verbena officinalis*) is a mild sedative.[31] Rue (*ruta graveolens*) can cause a contact rash but is

---

Hal's Head-Wound at the Battle of Shrewsbury," 215–230; Mark R. Geldof, "'And to describe the shapes of the dead': Making Sense of the Archaeology of Armed Violence," 57–80; Patricia Skinner, "Visible Prowess?: Reading Men's Head and Face Wounds in Early Medieval Europe to 1000 CE," 81–101; and MacInnes, "Heads, Shoulders, Knees and Toes," 102–27.

**29** Erin Connelly et al., "A Case Study of the Ancientbiotics Collaboration," *Patterns* 3 (2022): https://doi.org/10.1016/j.patter.2022.100632.

**30** *A Leechbook or Collection of Medical Recipes of the Fifteenth Century*, ed. Warren R. Dawson (London: Macmillan, 1934), 41, # 89. The editor guesses the date from a mention of John, Duke of Somerset (John Beaufort), who became duke in 1443 and after his recall from Normandy in 1444, died. So, if the text is believed, it was written, if not assembled, sometime in 1443–1444.

**31** Deni Brown, *Herbal: The Essential Guide to Herbs for Living* (London: Pavilion, 2001), 159. See also Minta Collins, *Medieval Herbals: The Illustrative Traditions* (London: British Library, 2000).

rich in iron and minerals and was used as a stimulant and antispasmodic for epilepsy patients.[32] Betony (*stachys officinalis*) originated in Ancient Egypt and was prized in the Middle Ages for all sorts of conditions. It is still used in some herbal tea blends and seems to be good for migraine, asthma, heartburn, diarrhoea, bladder or kidney stones, and stress disorders that (today) might baffle experts. Today, we know that betony decreases blood pressure.[33] Honey, highlighted earlier, has natural antiseptic and antimicrobial qualities. And many people still use egg-whites as a face mask to pull impurities from their skin and tighten pores.[34] This recipe and others like it make some sense to our contemporary audience; medieval physicians were trying to work on the problem with what they had—pain killers, a mild sedative, pull out what is not wanted and keep the area clear of infection until it healed. This 1443–1444 work also suggested a remedy for patients with skulls that had been broken or crushed (bowed) to the point that the patient could no longer speak: "Stamp violet and give him to drink first in wine. And if the right side of the head be hurt, stamp violet and bind it to the sole of the left foot. And if the left side of the head [be injured], lay it to the right foot. And the bone shall rise up, and the patient shall speak again."[35] Medieval physicians knew that the right side of the brain affected the motor control of the left side of the body and vice-versa.[36] The idea behind the pressure to one foot or the other to help the head is something like Chinese acupressure.[37]

*Chirurgia*, a surgical text by Roger Frugard (ca. 1180) that remained popular at least through the fourteenth century, explained "how and when to

---

**32** Brown, *Herbal*, 237–38; Holly H. Shimizu, *Herbs* (London: Dorling, 2002), 124.

**33** Steven Foster and Varro E. Tyler, *The Honest Herbal: A Sensible Guide to the Use of Herbs and Related Remedies* (London: Routledge, 1999); "Betony: Uses, Side Effects, and More," *WebMD*, https://www.webmd.com/vitamins/ai/ingredientmono-587/betony, accessed October 14, 2024.

**34** "Egg White Face Mask for Home Use," *Perfect Image*, https://perfectimage.com/blogs/diy/egg-white-face-mask?srsltid=AfmBOoqYVFHZyLKXl-eYtjy-d4TgLs68neUADTGoDm9BKJfvG5Qqp-ci, accessed October 14, 2024.

**35** *A Leechbook*, 41, # 89. See also Johannes Platearius [Giovanni Plateario il Giovane], "Practica brevis," ed. Tony Hunt, *Anglo-Norman Medicine* (Cambridge: Brewer, 1994), 1:171–84.

**36** As pointed out by the editor of *A Leechbook*, 261, #843.

**37** For more on acupressure, see the article "Acupressure," *Rogel Cancer Center website. University of Michigan Health*, https://www.rogelcancercenter.org/support/symptoms-and-side-effects/alternative medicine/acupressure#:~:text=Acupressure%20is%20similar%20to%20acupuncture,proper%20acupuncture%20point%20is%20pressed, accessed October 16, 2024.

operate on a head injury."[38] This injury he writes could cause "mania or melancholia," both common medieval terms for conditions of mental illness. If the patient has a "cut [broken] head" [*la teste tailleiz*] with a "shard" [skull fragment, *le quir*] afflicting him, Frugard instructed surgeons to:

> first bind the patient. Then, by opening the head with a tool that is called trepan,[39] through removal of the material of the malady, is that which is at issue [causing the problem]. It is the healthy wound, as is truly said, [which] is a cure for the previous wound.[40]

In other words, remove all foreign material—including skull fragments—then bind the wound (the original wound and the new one the physician made to get everything clean). Frugard captures the essence of much medieval English medicine: keep the patient calm, fix as much of the problem as possible, and give the patient time to heal. Certainly, surgeons were necessary and good ones were highly regarded. On the whole, the craft of surgeons and surgery was not considered among the higher arts of medicine in the Middle Ages.[41]

The most famous example of surgery on the field is that for Henry V—written about most recently by Michael Livingston.[42] Sixteen-year-old Henry was not yet king and fought in the Battle of Shrewsbury (1403), taking an arrow to his face. The shaft of the arrow was removed on the field, but the carefully planned surgery took place several weeks later at Kenilworth Castle. What Livingston brings to light is that the tip of the arrow was lodged in the back of Henry's skull, and the skilled surgeon created a contraption to open the wound further in order to be able to insert his pliers into Henry's face and pull out the arrow shaft and point that was stuck. Livingston points out that Henry had a noticeable change to his personality after this event

**38** I have seen this in other places translated "devilry" or "possessed," but I believe it is closer to "thrashing."

**39** Still in use today, a trepan is a saw or chisel used to open the skull.

**40** Roger Frugard, "*Chirurgia*," ed. Tony Hunt, *Anglo-Norman Medicine*, 1:53.

**41** Roy Porter, *The Greatest Benefit to Mankind: A Medical History of Humanity from Antiquity to the Present* (London: HarperCollins, 1997), 11. It was during the time of the Hundred Years' War that "in London a master surgeons' guild had been founded in 1368; [and just after the war] the Mystery or Guild of the Barbers of London received its charter from Edward IV in 1462." These merged into the Barber-Surgeons Company in 1540. Porter, *The Greatest Benefit*, 186.

**42** Livingston, "'The Depth of Six Inches,'" 215–30. For other cases of head injury, see the fascinating study of Towton 16 in Christopher J. Knüsel's chapter in this volume.

and that the described trajectory of the arrow may have damaged his left temporal lobe.

A topic not covered here to any great degree, but one which might prove useful for future work is disease. It was not uncommon for those on campaign to spread illness among their fellows or share illnesses with towns they encountered. For example, in 1322, John Murdac of Fairford had "his lands, goods and chattels, together with the issues received from the lands," taken into the king's custody because he had not shown up to fight against "the rebels"; when the king learned that John had been "so ill and weak that he could not come," his lands and other properties were returned.[43] Thankfully, John had competent and trusted witnesses of his ill health; likely, he should have deputed another to go in his stead, but to be fair, perhaps his illness came on suddenly and he did not have time. At least in his case, he was not permanently disabled and would return to fight another day.

## Post-Battle Trauma

There were other individuals with head wounds who were not so lucky to only have a scar and a change in personality. These individuals suffered unseen mental trauma, just like military personnel today. "Post-Traumatic Stress Disorder" is just that, a stress disorder that appears after the fact following a traumatic event.[44] While there is no diagnosis as such in the Middle Ages, there are glimpses of stress and of individuals who lose their sense of self after battle and, indeed, became disabled. For example, Robert fitz Neel "*by chance* [my emphasis] became of unsound mind."[45] Robert had been in battle and sometime after his marriage and having had several children, he was "struck on the head by a lance at certain jousts [and] has lost his

---

**43** *CCR, 1318–1323*, 436.

**44** Unlike in previous editions of the *DSM*, in the new *DSM-5*, the editors acknowledge that PTSD (Post Traumatic Stress Disorder) has been known by other names, "such as 'shell shock' during the years of World War I and 'combat fatigue' after World War II," and that "PTSD does not just happen to combat veterans." It is nice to see the *DSM* and the American Psychiatric Association evolving to include historic mental health conditions of stress. "Posttraumatic Stress Disorder," *DSM-5*, https://www.psychiatry.org/patients-families/ptsd, accessed October 14, 2024.

**45** Isabel, the "King's eldest daughter," was being granted his guardianship. *Calendar of the Patent Rolls. Edward III* (hereafter *CPR*, London. Anthony, 1909), 10.256. For more information, see: TNA, PRO C 60/151/m 20 and *Calendar of the Fine Rolls* (hereafter *CFR*; London: HMSO, 1921), 6:252.

memory."[46] It seems his contemporaries might have had hope at first that his mental health would right itself and he would not become disabled. Yet, even though he had survived, when he was examined "before the king in the chancery by chancellor and others of the council [he was] found to be in these days insufficient for the rule of himself and his lands."[47] Robert's homage was respited [postponed], and he was made a ward of the Crown with two guardians to care for him and his lands.[48] Even then, there was hope that "he shall recover his memory and be again of sound mind."[49] Two years later (1350), the Crown sent a commission of three men to check on Robert and see if he was still mentally unwell.[50] The guardianship of his lands changed hands several times. By 1350, they were in the care of William Croyser to whom the Crown owed payment.[51] Four years later, the king placed Robert's lands in the joint care of Gerard de Braybrok, *chivaler*, and Geoffrey Lucy.[52] These two men later received permission to lease the lands to Robert

**46** *CPR* (London: Mackie, 1905), 8:413–14.

**47** *CPR*, 8:414.

**48** William was in the hands of two guardians at first, Gerard Baybrok and Geoffrey Lucy, who later put the keeping of the property (leased) into the care of Robert Elbrigge: *CPR*, 10:172, 217. Other parcels of land were placed in the guardianship of other people, such as Robert de Hadham (*CFR*, 6:402) and Thomas de Stiryngham (*CFR*, 6:403). In England by at least 1250, all landholders with severe mental health conditions—meaning they could not attend to their duties—were made wards of the crown. Each individual was given a guardian, who saw to the individual's "maintenance" (food, clothing, shelter) and took over their duties. For a general overview of this system, see Wendy J. Turner, *Care and Custody of the Mentally Ill, Incompetent, and Disabled in Medieval England* (Turnhout: Brepols, 2013), 88, 98, 152–53, 196–98.

**49** *CPR*, 8:414.

**50** This is one of those rare letters of the royal "secret seal." *CPR*, 8:533.

**51** I point in this instance to war trauma since there is no mention of the "pestilence" (Black Death) even though Robert lost his mental health in the years of the initial major outbreak (and most records in the years of 1349 and 1350 point that out if important). Certainly, that is a possibility, but if he faced war and then could not face more death, that too could be attributed to a trauma reaction (*CFR*, 6:252). William Croyser, who got in trouble later for wasting Fitz Neel's property, was part of the investigation commission into Robert's mental status (TNA: PRO C 66/230/m 4d; C 135/111/m 7; and C 66/257/m 3). See also the calendars: *CPR*, 8:533, no. 561; *Calendar of Inquisitions Post Mortem and Other Analogous Documents* (London: HMSO, 1904), 9:409–10, no. 589; in the same volume, 226–27, no. 231, his daughter has died and he is mentioned again as having given her property before his change in mental health.

**52** *CFR*, 6:407; and *CPR*, 10:172, 217.

Elbrigge at 100 s. per year; Elbrigge did all of the work on the land for them, paid them the rent, and made some extra for himself. Ten years later, after Gerard and Geoffrey had been paid, the king transferred the custody of the properties to Robert Elbrigge's eldest daughter, Isabel.[53] Robert fitz Neel's situation provides an example of an individual who fought for the Crown and later, when he could no longer fight, his properties earned revenue for the Crown's continued war, paying the Crown's debts. With residual effects from head injuries or other mental trauma, individuals could not direct their own affairs; and, like Robert fitz Neel, they became wards of the Crown.

Not just Robert fitz Neel, but other landholders who had seen battle and later became mentally ill and disabled, also became wards of the Crown. Bartholomew de Sakeville, for example, became mentally unwell after fighting for the Crown.[54] When he lost his mental health, his father had long-since died and his mother, Matilda, took control of his inheritance in both England and Ireland. The Crown often left the care of mentally incompetent heirs in the hands of mothers if they were alive and capable. Over time, the duties of managing Bartholomew's estate became too much for Matilda to handle, and she hired a couple of attorneys to manage the properties in Ireland. When she finally grew too old "and infirm" to care for Bartholomew's English properties, the Crown assigned guardians to care for Bartholomew's lands from among other family members who were not in line to inherit.[55] This was a common practice for all landholders to have a royal guardian assigned to them, family or not, if and when they became mentally ill. Individuals born with mental health issues, such as intellectual disabilities, would have had a royal guardian at the point at which they were orphaned—as children or adults. Individuals who became mentally incapacitated—either mentally ill or with a diminished memory, or other condition—would also have been provided with a guardian, but only after an interview, as with Robert fitz Neel, and that guardian was in place until they were well or died.[56]

The Crown took all the profit—as if it was the landlord—from lands of intellectually disabled individuals born with their condition as well as any who became mentally disabled for any reason as small children.[57]

**53** TNA, PRO C 66/246/m 17; *CPR*, 10:256.

**54** Turner, *Care and Custody*.

**55** Guardians could not be the direct heirs of their wards for fear that they might harm the wards in order to profit by an early inheritance. See Turner, *Care and Custody*.

**56** Turner, *Care and Custody*.

**57** If a person were born intellectually disabled, the Crown would have the option

It appointed guardians for these individuals, who were to care for the person and their property "without waste," in other words, the guardian could not come in and clear cut a forest or take down buildings. For those people who became mentally ill as adults, the Crown also appointed guardians, but they were most often members of that person's family, so long as they were not direct heirs of the person; this idea, that the mentally disabled landholder might be in danger from someone who might profit from a ward's demise, was quite a progressive one for the time. The guardians of these adults who became mentally disabled did not treat the land as if the Crown was the landlord, but rather as if the individual were injured and might at any moment return to good health. They were to save the general profits from the estate for the person, taking only a fee for the Crown (which the Crown named based on taxes and profit margins) and a small allowance for the guardian. The Crown was not supposed to profit directly or pay for services, but it often did. And there were still inheritance fees once the individual died. It was hard work overseeing someone else's property as well as his own, though, and for his troubles, the guardian did get a stipend and likely this was so that people took the job seriously.[58]

While guardians kept their "allowance," when guarding over someone with an intellectual disability, the fees and profits were given to the Exchequer twice a year near Christmas and Easter. And most often, no matter the mental issue, the Crown chose to place family members that could not inherit in the position of guardian. Of course, the wives and children of a mentally disabled person could not be his guardians, but a mother could be, as in the case of Bartholomew de Sakeville. Husbands could and were guardians of their wives, since those lands were in essence theirs in any case, but wives could not be guardians.[59]

---

of providing a guardian from among the family or outside the family. Often the king used these lands to pay off his debts. Because these heirs sometimes came to their inheritances early in life and remained in the status of ward for all their lives, these were convenient sources of income. This type of action angered many families, but there was little they could do but wait until the intellectually disabled person died. Turner, *Care and Custody*.

**58** Turner, *Care and Custody*, 183–209 (chap. 8 "Guardians").

**59** "Et nullus heredipete suo propinquo vel extraneo (periculosa sane custodia) conmittatur" ("No one shall be entrusted to the care of a person who is claiming his inheritance, whether it is a relative of his or a stranger [a dangerous guardianship indeed]"). *Leges Henrici Primi*, ed. L. J. Downer (Oxford: Clarendon, 1972), 224, no. 70, 19, dated sometime between 1108 and 1118.

## Captives and Ransom

Persons with head injuries or mental trauma from battle were not the only ones who returned home with mental incapacity; a number of individuals who survived battle suffered mental breakdowns following an imprisonment awaiting payment of their ransom. Nigel Coppedene of Sussex, mentioned in the opening of this paper, who murdered a neighbour and was pardoned because he was not mentally aware of his actions following his "sufferings as a prisoner of war" serves as one example.[60] His experiences of "sufferings" early in the fourteenth century parallel those of later captives. An example from France, since he recounted his experiences first-hand, Henriet Gentian, whom his captors seemed to think important to the duke of Bourbon, wrote that there were "'eighteen serpents and other reptiles' in the dungeon in which Francois de la Palu had cast him at Romenay."[61] Maurice Keen points out that this alone would give Henriet a "very sound *prima facie* case," meaning that if possible Henriet could have legally escaped. Certainly, that was true when the expected payment did not arrive, and Francois hammered out several of Henriet's teeth.[62] Although Francois's actions against Henriet would have created stress on his system, there are no records that directly state that he had mental health problems.[63] What stress he or Nigel or other captives endured is hard to say.

---

**60** 1306. TNA, PRO C 260/16/m 5b; JUST 1/934/m 3.

**61** Maurice H. Keen, *The Laws of War in the Late Middle Ages* (London: Routledge, 1965), 180 (from Paris, Archives nationales, X1a 4798, fol. 190r, April 28, 1440), 191 ("Jean le Gastelier, one of Robert Chesnel's men, admitted to the judges at the Chatelet that his job in the company had been to beat prisoners 'until they could stand no more,' to encourage them to promise the largest possible sums."). As Keen notes, this episode is from Henri Duplés Agier, *Registre criminel du Châtelet de Paris du 6 septembre 1389 au 18 mai 1392* (Paris: Lahure, 1864), 2:95. See also William Mark Ormrod, "The Domestic Response to the Hundred Years War," in *Arms, Armies and Fortifications in the Hundred Years War*, eds. Anne Curry and Michael Hughes (Woodbridge: Boydell, 1994), 83–101; Anne Curry, *The Hundred Years War* (New York: St. Martin's, 1993); Jonathan Sumption, *The Hundred Years War*, vol. 1, *Trial by Battle*, 5 vols. (Philadelphia: University of Pennsylvania Press, 1991); David Grummitt, ed., *The English Experience in France c. 1450–1558: War, Diplomacy, and Cultural Exchange* (Ashgate: Aldershot, 2002); and Michael K. Jones, "Ransom Brokerage in the Fifteenth Century," in *Guerre et société en France, en Angleterre et en Bourgogne XIV^e–XV^e siècle*, eds. Philippe Contamine et al. (Villeneuve-d'Ascq: Publications de l'Institut de recherches historiques du Septentrion, 1991), 221–35.

**62** Keen, *The Laws of War*, 180; and Nicholas Wright, *Knights and Peasants: The Hundred Years War in the French Countryside* (Woodbridge: Boydell, 1998), 64–65.

**63** Keen, *The Laws of War*, 243.

Legally, there was a question as to whether a captor could continue to hold his captive if that person became mentally ill. Honorat Bovet in *The Tree of Battles* wrote that, "We find, by written law, and good reason agrees with this, that during his madness, a man out of his senses cannot be considered as an enemy by anyone whatsoever." Bovet's reason was that a person in this condition was just as liable to harm himself or even a close member of his family as to harm a foe because he does not know "whether he does well or ill."[64] Which is exactly the case of poor Nigel Coppedene. Bovet wrote that a captor should not harm a mentally incapacitated person and, in his on-going examination of war added, "consider well what nobility there would be in showing one's courage against a madman, or what gentility in making captive a man sick with so terrible a sickness, which should rouse all gentlemen to have pity and give help towards his cure."[65] Exception was made for a person who regained his senses while incarcerated: he should promise not to make war again, or agree to be ransomed.[66]

## Retirement

Many Crown retirements were offered in the form of corrodies as a way of managing life with a disability. A corrody was normally the retirement—given either as money and dinner once a year, or as room and board for life—offered to older monks and the lay employees of a monastery, meaning those who were not monks. Monasteries or abbeys had non-religious people working there as cooks, stable hands, blacksmiths, or other workers, that would not get to stay in the monastery in their old age, unless the worker had arranged such an agreement with the religious house at the outset. Yet, if a worker had given many years of service to a house of God, the institution might feel obligated to offer some form of care, when possible. As the Crown or lord supported these houses, they often wrote into the foundation or gift that they, too, could have control of one or more corrodies in each institution.[67] The Crown used these corrodies to offer retirements to long-standing

**64** Honorat Bovet, *The Tree of Battles*, ed. Coopland, bk. 4, chap. 91, 182.

**65** Honorat Bovet, *The Tree of Battles*, ed. Coopland, bk. 4, chap. 91, 183.

**66** Honorat Bovet, *The Tree of Battles*, ed. Coopland, bk. 4, chap. 92, 183.

**67** Patricia H. Cullum, *Cremetts and Corrodies: Care of the Poor and Sick at St. Leonard's Hospital, York, in the Middle Ages* (York: Borthwick Institute, 1991); Jenna M. Dittmar et al., "Caring for the Injured: Exploring the Immediate and Long-term Consequences of Injury in Medieval Cambridge, England," *International Journal of Paleopathology* 40 (2023): 7–19.

employees, to manage the care of disabled retainers or fighters, and as payments for services. Recipients could hang onto their corrody or sell it and use the funds as they wanted. In some locations, institutions' leaders figured out that if they, too, made room for a few extra corrodians, they could sell those spaces over time to local parishioners, who in turn would pay into the monastery for the privilege of a guaranteed bed in the hospital or a stipend on which they could live in their old age—giving money or property that supported the monks and the poor.[68]

For those injured in the king's service in battle, this seems to be a great honour and potentially a relief to know someone disabled in battle would be cared for and fed for life. For example, in 1315, the king sent a note to St. John's Hospital at Brakle, to receive Nicholas Russel, "who long served the king and was maimed in his service in Scotland…to receive suitable maintenance in their house."[69] In 1317, "Robert de Maners, hobelar (*hobelarius*), who served the late king in his war in Scotland in divers garrisons there, and who is now so infirm that he can no longer serve the king, is sent to the abbot and convent of Langele to receive his maintenance for life." Or in another 1317 entry, William de Spyney, crossbowman (*balistar*), who served the late king is sent to the abbot and convent of Abbotesbury to receive his maintenance in their house for life.[70]

If a corrodian (loosely trans. "retiree") was unhappy, too far from home, or if there was another issue (finances, trouble between the Crown and the institution leader, etc.), he could be moved. William Blaclowe, who was acknowledged as having "behaved well in several garrisons (*garnisturis*) in Scotland" and "especially in the last siege at Carlisle," was maimed in the king's service there. He was first sent in September 1315 to the prior and convent of Stone (Staffordshire, England) to receive maintenance for life.[71] Then, in December 1315, he was sent to the abbot and convent of Rievaulx (*Ryevall*) (North Yorkshire, England) to receive the same allowance as Peter de Ovinges, now deceased, had in their house by the king's order.[72] This last is common language—one retiree dying and making room for another.

**68** John Robb et al., "Osteobiography: The History of the Body as Real Bottom-Line History," *Bioarchaeology International* 3, no. 1 (2019): 16–31.

**69** *CCR, 1313–1318*, 335.

**70** *CCR, 1313–1318*, 450 (for both cases).

**71** *CCR, 1313–1318*, 311.

**72** *CCR, 1313–1318*, 319.

When an individual became impaired and could no longer serve, depending on his circumstances, a number of different things might happen, but certainly this would today be called "early retirement" or "compensated leave." For example, in 1313, "Simon le Messager, who long served the late king and is now blind" was sent to the "prior and convent of Trinity church, London," with the request that they grant him "suitable maintenance for himself and a groom [a personal assistant since he was blind] in food and clothing, to be received by him whether staying within or without their said house, making letters patent under the seal of their chapter concerning the grant of the same."[73] In other words, if there was no room for him in the priory, he could instead be given a stipend to cover housing and care costs in the local town, having rooms nearby to the monastic community; he could stay in town or move into the community as space became available for him and his attendant.

## Conclusion

Warfare and training for warfare was the job of the medieval *bellatores*, "those who fight." If part of the landed gentry or nobility, they trained from the time they were children. Some peasants trained as children, too, if they would inherit weapons or positions as archers or crossbowmen. All fighters received some training before going to battle and with them went a priest and often a surgeon or barber-surgeon or sometimes a physician. Most armies were supplied with wine, honey, and other lifesaving medicines and medical supplies.

The use of those medical resources was certainly by rank as much as injury. Those with wealth and power would have received the best care and the most attention from the physicians and/or surgeons both on the field and later at home. Other individuals, the infantry for example, would have had less available medical care and few resources off the field of battle to get further treatment or more medication. The differences in economic and social strata would have made clear.

If and when injured or ill, some fighters chose to stop and rest or leave and go home if seriously injured. Again, this was both a matter of wealth—the financial ability to afford the cost of travel home alone—and status—one would need permission to leave the force. A few with the financial means and permission to leave behind a son or other relative or vassal as a deputy,

**73** *CCR, 1313–1318*, 69.

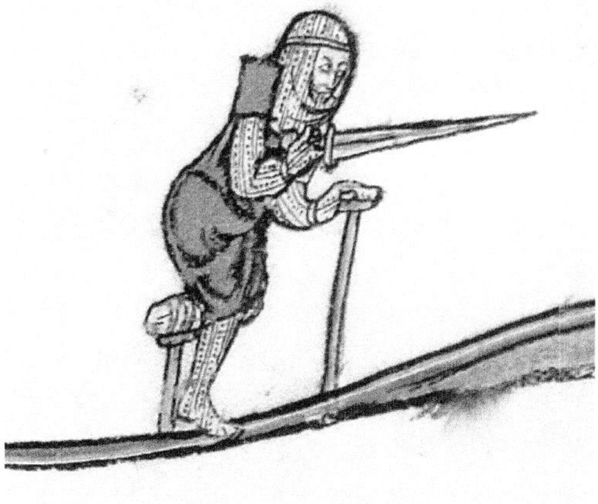

Figure 6.3. This image is of a warrior attempting to continue to fight even while disabled. New Haven, Yale University, Beinecke Rare Book & Manuscript Library, MS 229, fol. 257v. Courtesy of the Yale University, Beinecke Rare Book and Manuscript Library.

a person to give orders, possibly lead troops, and fight in the name of the injured or ill person. Anyone on campaign could also be dismissed by a commander until he had better health, yet many members of the infantry stayed as long as they could, only choosing to leave or rest if absolutely necessary, perhaps because of financial motives or because they did not want to be left behind in enemy territory and did not confidently know the way home. Whatever the reason, most individuals—healthy or not—remained with their company until sent home. And who can say how many injuries happened because the fighters were not at their best?

Mental illness on the battlefield harmed both the fighter and his neighbour. Each individual was to have been concentrating on the task at hand to not only fight but also protect himself and those around him. Injury in this context could lead to mental collapse, capture, or death. A fighter who experienced a head injury might recover, depending on the severity of the injury internally and externally and how quickly medical aid reached him. Some prisoners died under torture or in prison; others, like Nigel Coppedene, found their way back home but had difficulty coping in society. A few hostages, such as Henriet Gentian, made their way home and seem to have been mentally fine, but just because Henriet never broke the law, who can say that he did not experience difficulties in other ways? The impact for families, communities, and, in England, the Crown was two-fold: care had to be found for the mentally incapacitated person and protection be provided to secure his estate. Once more, the level of care and consideration for mental health issues depended entirely on wealth and status. Those fighters with land or family with property were often cared for by relatives in some setting of comfort. Gentry with little land might be granted a royal guardian, but his level of care might be at a subsistence level. Those fighters who were peasants with only moveable goods would end up cared for by family or neighbours; their existence and medical treatment might be very poor.

Those landholders who might have been physically injured in battle could convalesce before they travelled home, yet even while away and certainly once home, they often had the finances and mental wherewithal to arrange matters for themselves. The common soldier, though, might have no time off, no time to recover, and no better food awaiting him. A very different experience from his gentry and noble colleagues on the field. A peasant fighter might fall into depression at the loss of friends or comrades at arms. Once away from the royal surgeon or barber, his medical care may have been poor. A few who came to the attention of their lord or king might have received a corrody—a stipend or even a space with food and shelter at a monastery or other institution where they could convalesce after becoming disabled following war. Overall, war was hard on medieval bodies and minds, but many survived because of their armour and medical care, even if their care and treatment at home was not always the best.

Chapter 7

# "WHAT PAIN I SUFFERED AT THAT TIME, ANYONE CAN WELL IMAGINE"

## EXPERIENCES OF WAR, INJURY, AND PAIN IN FIFTEENTH- AND SIXTEENTH-CENTURY GERMANY AND SWITZERLAND

BIANCA FROHNE

AMONG THE MANY war-related texts and images from the medieval and early modern period, we find detailed descriptions of horrifying injuries: open wounds, loss of limbs, fractures, arrows stuck in bones, chopped-off noses, and smashed-in faces. Many of these are further corroborated by the archaeological evidence.[1] The famous image of the "wound man" in the printed surgery manual *Feldbuch der Wundarznei* by Hans von Gersdorff (d. 1529) gives an idea of the variety of painful injuries that knights and soldiers might encounter on the battlefield in the fifteenth and sixteenth centuries.

In the text above the image, the wounded man is said to be "full of strike and stab wounds / crushed, wounded miserably."[2] The depicted wounds and

1 See Robert C. Woosnam-Savage and Kelly R. DeVries, "Battle Trauma in Medieval Warfare: Wounds, Weapons and Armor," in *Wounds and Wound Repair in Medieval Culture*, eds. Larissa Tracy and Kelly R. DeVries (Leiden: Brill, 2015), 27–56, with many examples.

2 "voll streich vn[d] stich / Zermorscht / verwundet ia[e]merlich". Hans von Gersdorff, *Feldbuch der wundtartzney* (Strasbourg: Schott, 1517), fol. 18v. The image of the "wound man" can also be found in several manuscripts and printed surgery books, for example, Johannes Beris, *Eyn new Wund Artznei M. Johans von Parisijs: Wie mann alle wunden...mit salben/ pflastern vnnd wundttranck/ durch den gantzen leip deß menschens/ vom kopff an biß auff die füß/ heylen sol...jtzunt am newsten auß gangen* (Strasbourg: Jakob Cammerlander, 1539), fol. [IV]v; *Wellcome Apocalypse* (ca. 1420), London, Wellcome Collection, MS 49, fol. 35v (accessible online:

**BIANCA FROHNE** is a lecturer in medieval history at Kiel University. She received her doctorate in 2013 from the University of Bremen and is co-editor of the handbook *Dis/Ability History der Vormoderne: Ein Handbuch = Premodern Dis/Ability History: A Companion*, eds. Cordula Nolte et al. (2017). She is currently working on a project on premodern experiences of chronic pain.

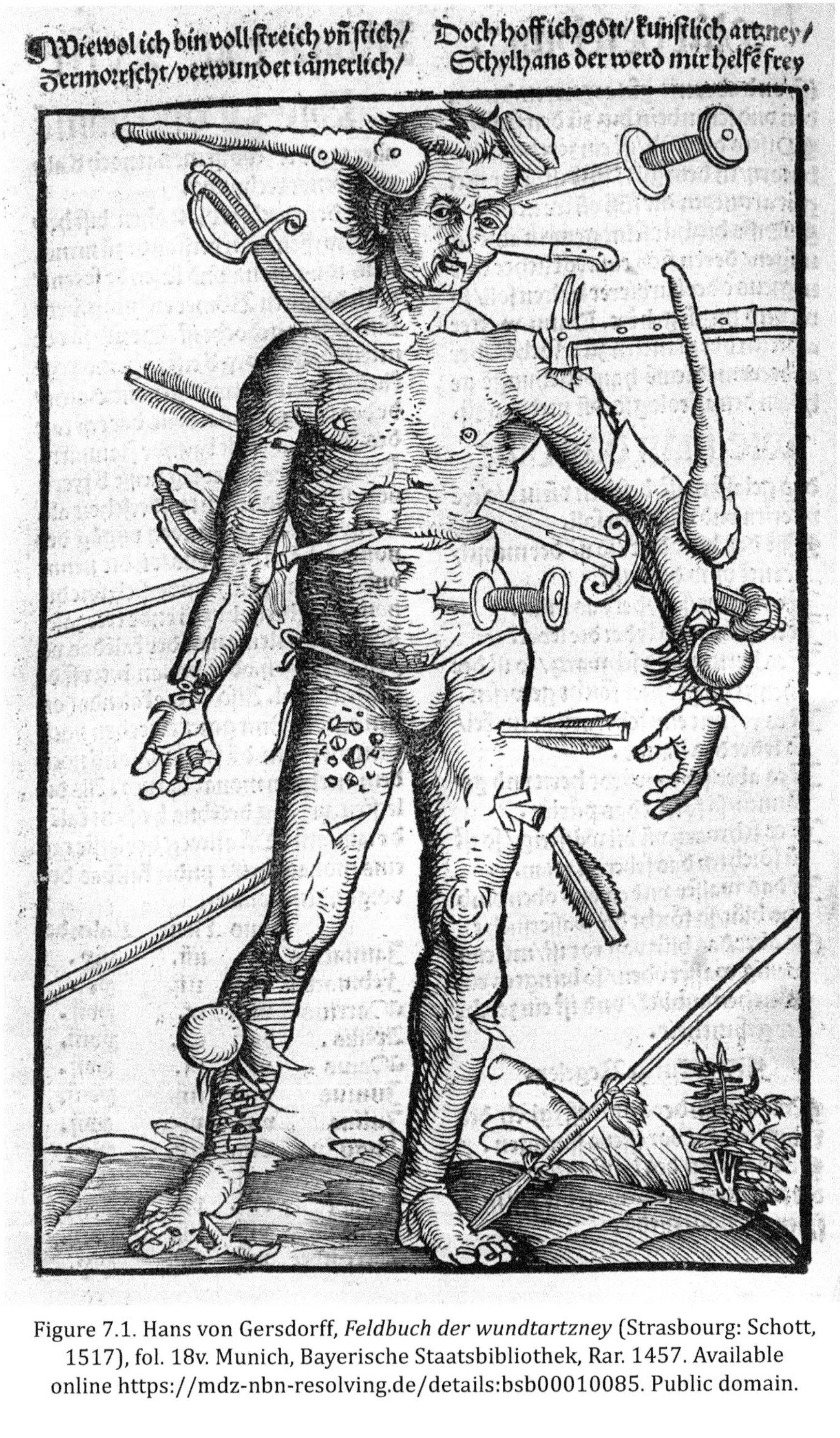


Figure 7.1. Hans von Gersdorff, *Feldbuch der wundtartzney* (Strasbourg: Schott, 1517), fol. 18v. Munich, Bayerische Staatsbibliothek, Rar. 1457. Available online https://mdz-nbn-resolving.de/details:bsb00010085. Public domain.

fractures, combined with the emphatic words focused on the overwhelming destruction of bodily integrity, suggest that the book's intended audience would have an interest in the lasting impact these experiences had on those who survived them. Sources that deal with the long-term consequences of war-related injuries, including lasting illness, impairment, chronic pain, or trauma responses, should therefore be easy to find. Sadly, this is not the case. Several disability historians have remarked on a discrepancy within the surviving source material: on the one hand, premodern epics, poems, chronicles, battle reports, and other sources contain many references to losses, death, captivity, injury, and illness acquired in war. Facing these risks was perceived as central part of the social identities of men-at-arms. On the other hand, war-related injuries and illnesses tend to vanish from narratives and reports as soon as the battle is over, or the conflict resolved. In many instances, the reason for this is that severe injuries are only mentioned because they were also the cause of death. In other cases, however, even life-changing injuries are simply never mentioned again. The long-term consequences of these injuries, such as lasting impairment and chronic pain, as well as lingering psychological wounds, are omitted or mentioned only in passing.[3]

The autobiographical notes of Swiss captain Heinrich Schönbrunner (1498–1537) from Zug are an example. In 1522/23, he sustained a serious head injury during a campaign in the service of the French king, which might have resulted in visual impairment. He gives an overview of the marches and battles, but also mentions scarcity of food and payment by the end of the campaign: "it was a miserable life indeed."[4] According to Schönbrunner, during one of the last battles, which ended in a flight, the Swiss soldiers for hire

https://wellcomecollection.org/works/du9ua6nd/items?canvas=73, accessed February 3, 2025). See Woosnam-Savage and DeVries, "Battle Trauma," 50–52, figure 1.1.

**3** Yuval Noah Harari, *Renaissance Military Memoirs: War, History, and Identity, 1450–1600* (Woodbridge: Boydell, 2004), 48–51, 73–76; Sonja Kerth, "Versehrte Körper: Vernarbte Seelen: Konstruktionen kriegerischer Männlichkeit in der späten Heldendichtung," *Zeitschrift für Germanistik* 2 (2002): 262–74; Oliver Auge, "So solt er im namen gottes mit mir hinfahren, ich were doch verderbt zu einem kriegsmann: Durch Kampf und Turnier körperlich versehrte Adelige im Spannungsfeld von Ehrpostulat und eigener Leistungsfähigkeit," *Medizin, Gesellschaft und Geschichte* 28 (2009): 21–46, at 24–26; Stephan Selzer, "Das Leiden der Krieger: Invalidität und Gefangenschaft in Quellen spätmittelalterlicher Hansestädte," in *Kriegsleiden in Norddeutschland vom Mittelalter bis zum Ersten Weltkrieg*, ed. Ortwin Pelc (Stuttgart: Steiner, 2021), 73–94.

**4** "vnnd was gar ein ellend läben." Bonifaz Staub, "Hauptmann Heinrich Schönbrunner von Zug und sein Tagebuch (1500–1537)," *Der Geschichtsfreund: Mitteilungen des Historischen Vereins der Fünf Orte Luzern, Uri, Schwyz, Unterwalden und Zug* 18

(*Reisläufer*) lost up to six hundred men, "because many were wounded."[5] This number probably refers mainly to those among the contingent of Swiss fighters who had to leave the campaign because of their injuries.[6] At the end of the entry, Schönbrunner resumes: "I, Heinrich Schönbrunner, was also in this campaign, was wounded in the head that I could no longer see in one eye, and was chief forager."[7] We do not learn any more about this injury, and how it affected Schönbrunner, either at this moment or later on in his life: did he receive medical treatment? Did he regain his sight in the affected eye, either partially or completely? Was there any visible tissue damage or scarring? How did he experience the pain such a wound was likely to cause? Did he worry about his future or fear for his capacity to fight and travel? Were there any lasting side-effects, such as chronic pain? Schönbrunner, who was from an influential family in Zug, went on to fight in other campaigns. He also became a councilman of his hometown, held important offices, and served as a military captain. If he retained any visual impairment, it did not seem to have had an impact.[8]

(1862): 205–25, at 211–12; see also Rudolf Hess, *Die zugerischen Geschichtsschreiber des 16. Jahrhunderts* (Zug: Kalt-Zehnder, 1951), 53–55.

**5** Staub, "Heinrich Schönbrunner," 211: "vnnd verlurend ob 600 man, Dann es warend vil verwundt."

**6** There is no mention of any organized medical treatment the wounded received, although it is likely that there were trained surgeons available among the military train; see Clifford J. Rogers, *Soldiers' Lives Through History: The Middle Ages* (Westport: Greenwood, 2007), 224–27; Kelly DeVries, "Medieval Warfare and the Value of a Human Life," in *Noble Ideals and Bloody Realities: Warfare in the Middle Ages*, eds. Niall Christie and Maya Yazigi (Leiden: Brill, 2006), 43–50. Those who were no longer able to fight due to injury or illness made their own way home. Some of them might have stayed in inns and taverns or in private lodgings until they were able to travel. According to legal records, inventories, and other sources, some injured Swiss "Reisläufer" received medical care in inns and taverns during the fifteenth and sixteenth centuries. See Karolina Meyer-Schilf, "'Dazu jch jedem raten wil / er buw vff kriegen nit zu vil': Grundüberlegungen und Forschungsperspektiven zum Umgang mit Kriegsinvalidität im Spätmittelalter," in *Phänomene der "Behinderung" im Alltag: Bausteine zu einer Disability History der Vormoderne*, ed. Cordula Nolte (Affalterbach: Didymos, 2013), 113–23, here 115–17.

**7** Staub, "Heinrich Schönbrunner," 212: "Ich Heinrich Schönbrunner war auch in Disem zug, ward im Houpt verwundt, das ich an einem Aug nüt mehr sach, vnd war Oberster Furier."

**8** Schönbrunner's notes only survive in a seventeenth-century copy which appears to have retained the original text quite faithfully: Renato Morosoli, "Schönbrunner, Heinrich," in *Historisches Lexikon der Schweiz, HLS*, https://hls-dhs-dss.ch/de/articles/025295/2022-06-27/, accessed January 1, 2025; Hess, *Geschichtsschreiber*, 74–77.

So, what can we learn from Schönbrunner's rather laconic remark about having received a potentially life-altering injury? Like many of his contemporaries, he was not interested in relaying his pain in detail or in expanding on the emotional experience related to his injury. From his point of view, the fact that he *had* suffered a serious injury on the battlefield was probably the most valuable information he wanted to provide. We can infer that war-related injuries were noted down in autobiographical writing because they meant *something*. Apparently, they were supposed to be remembered, even if the experience of the injury itself did not take centre stage.

In this chapter, I am going to take this observation as a starting point to examine combat-related injuries from a disability history perspective. I am particularly interested in the medical, social, and cultural significance that was attributed to experiences of physical and emotional pain during and after these events, and the way pain experiences are referred to in different types of sources. Approaching impairment and (chronic) pain from a disability history perspective allows us to study these subjects as socially and culturally constructed phenomena without equating them automatically with tragic fates and unbearable suffering. Diverse phenomena such as chronic illnesses, (chronic) pain, trauma, anxiety, fatigue, and exhaustion have recently become an integral part of critical disability research.[9] Over the last decade, disability theorists have developed an interest in the epistemological value that comes from living with pain over a long period of time. Like many pain researchers today, disability theorists reject the assumption that pain is an uncommunicable and isolating experience.[10] Alison Patsavas, for example, suggests studying how the experience of other's (chronic) pain shapes our own pain experiences.[11] Taking into account that cases of lasting impairment and chronic illness acquired in war were often well-known among the communities of soldiers and knights in the fifteenth and sixteenth centuries, this is an interesting approach to premodern history as

9 Alison Kafer, *Feminist, Queer, Crip* (Bloomington: Indiana University Press, 2013), 10–14; Alison Kafer, "Un/Safe Disclosures: Scenes of Disability and Trauma," *Journal of Literary & Cultural Disability Studies* 10 (2016): 1–20.

10 This view was made famous by Elaine Scarry. For an overview on the arguments against this assumption see Joanna Bourke, *The Story of Pain: From Prayer to Painkillers* (Oxford: Oxford University Press, 2014); Javier Moscoso, *Pain: A Cultural History* (Basingstoke: Palgrave, 2012).

11 Alyson Patsavas, "Recovering a Cripistemology of Pain: Leaky Bodies, Connective Tissue, and Feeling Discourse," *Journal of Literary & Cultural Disability Studies* 8 (2014): 203–18, at 215.

well. What is more: according to medieval and early modern thought, physical and emotional pain were closely connected. Human bodies were thought to be equally susceptible to interior as to exterior sensations and influences. Therefore, they could be affected by injuries, illnesses, and impairment, but also emotional experiences.[12] The question of how the physical and emotional pain of men-at-arms was regarded, and how they interacted with each other in view of this knowledge, can provide valuable insight.

In the following sections, this question will be explored from three different perspectives, drawing on mainly German-language source material from the fifteenth and sixteenth centuries. First, I am going to examine the significance of pain and fear in traumatological treatises. Next, I will take a look at the aftermath of severe injury based on autobiographies and other instances of life writing, paying particular attention to the way physical and emotional pain is referenced as an integral part of the experiences of men-at-arms, and what this can tell us about the social identities of those who chose a life of warfare as their defining characteristic. In the conclusion, battle injuries will be examined with regard to the special significance of pain and trauma within the analyzed sources, leading to some general thoughts on the potential of trauma as a category of analysis within premodern disability history.

## Painful Injury and Medieval Traumatology

What did painful injury mean in the situation on the battlefield and during the first stages of treatment? As shown above, traumatological treatises and surgical manuals, such as *Feldbuch der wundtartzney* by Hans von Gersdorff, can provide some insight. Written by medical practitioners who were often experienced in war surgery, they advise on how to treat a variety of old and new injuries and illnesses, using surgical interventions, potions, syrups, pills, plasters, poultices, ointments, bandages, compresses, and tinctures.[13]

**12** Esther Cohen, "The Animated Pain of the Body," *American Historical Review* 105 (2000): 36–68; Esther Cohen, *The Modulated Scream. Pain in Late Medieval Culture* (Chicago: University of Chicago Press, 2010), 37–43.

**13** DeVries, "Medieval Warfare," 48–49; Karl Sudhoff, *Beiträge zur Geschichte der Chirurgie im Mittelalter: Graphische und textliche Untersuchungen in mittelalterlichen Handschriften*, vol. 2 (Leipzig: Barth, 1918); Ralf Vollmuth, *Traumatologie und Feldchirurgie an der Wende vom Mittelalter zur Neuzeit: Exemplarisch dargestellt anhand der "Grossen Chirurgie" des Walther Hermann Ryff* (Stuttgart: Steiner, 2001); Melanie Panse, *Hans von Gersdorffs "Feldbuch der Wundarznei": Produktion, Präsentation und Rezeption von Wissen* (Wiesbaden: Reichert, 2012).

Combat-related injuries play an important role. Most texts cover wounds left by stabbing or slashing weapons, as well as projectiles made from metal or stone, and a variety of lacerations, fractures, and contusions. From the middle of the fifteenth century onwards, wounds caused by firearms are included.[14] Some elements can be found regularly, such as instructions concerning the treatment of head wounds, particularly fractures of the skull, or the extraction of arrows, a highly specialized and divisive field of work.[15] Many texts deal with the question on how to avoid festering wounds and ulcerations, with a special focus on how to treat painful "wound fluids" that developed soon after an injury. This so-called *gliedwasser* was perceived as highly dangerous and a potential impediment to full recovery.[16] In fact, many of the recipes and instructions show concern about lasting damage or secondary illnesses as a result of inadequate treatment of wounds and injuries.[17]

Moreover, pain itself plays an important part in the segments that explain how to achieve a full recovery with no lasting side-effects. Severe pain was understood as dangerous, even life-threatening, and a possible

---

**14** Ralf Vollmuth, "'Den geschosszenen Wunden': Die Behandlung von Schußwunden in deutschsprachigen chirurgischen Werken des 15. Jahrhunderts," *Orvostörténeti Közlemények: Communicationes de historia artis medicinae* 40 (1994): 5–28, at 6–8, 22. On the use of gunpowder weapons in war, see also Helen Nicholson, *Medieval Warfare: Theory and Practice of War in Europe 300–1500* (Basingstoke: Palgrave, 2004), 96–98; Kelly DeVries, *Medieval Military Technology* (Peterborough: Broadview, 1992), 159–63.

**15** Sudhoff, *Beiträge*, provides an overview that is still useful.

**16** Claudia Richter, *Phytopharmaka und Pharmazeutika in Heinrichs von Pfalzpaint "Wündärznei" (1460)": Untersuchungen zur traumatologischen Pharmakobotanik des Mittelalters* (Würzburg: Königshausen, 2004), 64, 78.

**17** Traumatological treatises regularly include instructions on how to improve on incorrectly healed fractures. The manual by Hans von Gersdorff contains a recipe to prevent pain as a long-term side-effect of broken legs, see Hans von Gersdorff, *Feldbuch der wundtartzney*, fol. 44v: "A good ointment for the time after the fracture if a hardening of tissue remains and hurts from the cold" ("ein gu[o]te salb die geho[e]rt noch dem bruch so ein harter maßer do blibt vn[d] vo[n] kelt we thu[o]t.") Among the recipes for the treatment of lacerations, there is a recipe for "the big red scars that occur on healed wounds" ("für die grossen roten narbe[n] an den geheylten wunden"; Hans von Gersdorff, *Feldbuch der wundtartzney*, fol. 28r–v). See also the specialized treatise focused almost exclusively on leg ulcers, which might have resulted in some cases from older wounds or injuries: Hans-Joachim Peters, *Das "Buch von alten Schäden"* (PhD. diss., Rheinische Friedrich-Wilhelms-Universität Bonn, 1973), which includes the text edition; Ingrid Rohland, *Das "Buch von alten Schäden,"* vol. 2, *Kommentar und Wörterverzeichnis* (Pattensen: Wellm, 1982).

cause of chronic conditions and disabilities.[18] Pain relief was an important step in the treatment of wounds and contusions. The surgery book (*Wundarznei*) by the surgeon and Teutonic knight Heinrich von Pfalzpaint († ca. 1464),[19] written in 1460, warns that excessive pain and heat from wounds and haematomas could cause lasting damage to the muscle tissue and consequently lead to atrophied limbs. The reasoning behind this was that "too much pain and heat from the wounds" (*zu vil wetagen / vnd hitz von den wunden*) can cause blood clotting in the veins, which in turn prevents "fresh blood" (*des newen bluts*) from getting to the wounds. The surrounding tissue is affected because it is not supplied with the fluids it needs.[20] Therefore the flesh will "wither and shrink" (*dörren vnd schwinden*).[21] According to Heinrich von Pfalzpaint, this outcome can be prevented by applying the correct plasters. To prevent further muscle degradation in case of leg injuries, the most effective drugs and treatment methods must be used, for example rubbing the affected areas in a downward direction, away from the body, using a specific leg plaster, and having the patient drink a "wound potion" to soothe the pain. Wound potions can be found in nearly all traumatological texts. They were meant to keep the wounds clean, provide pain relief, and strengthen the affected body parts. Heinrich von Pfalzpaint's wound potion

**18** On the widespread belief that pain could attract humours and harmful matter in medieval medical writing, see also Cohen, "The Expression of Pain," 200–201; Vollmuth, *Traumatologie*, 180–81.

**19** Gundolf Keil, "Heinrich von Pfalzpaint," in *Die deutsche Literatur des Mittelalters: Verfasserlexikon* (Berlin: de Gruyter, 1978–2007), 3:856–62; Sudhoff, *Beiträge*, 531–60.

**20** As described by Richter, *Phytopharmaka*, 77–78.

**21** Halle, University and State Library of Saxony-Anhalt, Cod. 23 G 38, fol. 46v: "Wo von schwinden kompt. Item nu wil ich dir sagen wo von schwinden kompt. Wen einer hart wundt wurt / oder sunst mit trucken schlegen hart geschlagen wurt / vnd wen man jm nicht pflaster dorhindter vnd darauff leget / die dor zu gut sein / vnd jm die adern vnd glider jn guter gewer gehalden mögen alß du bey den wundt salben wol finden wuedest / so kompt zu vil wetagen / vnd hitz von den wunden jn die glider / vnd jn die adern können des newen bluts teglich nicht greaten / vnd wen jn das entgeet so kan das fleysch nicht gedeyen vnd muß dav von dörren vnd schwinden. Wen dy adern mit dem newen blut beholden das fleysch jn guter gewer." A planned critical edition of Pfalzpaint's surgery book has not been published yet (*Editionsbericht: Editionsvorhaben zu mittelalterlichen deutschen Texten*, https://editionsbericht.de/?n=E_Leipold, accessed February 3, 2025). The above-cited manuscript dates from ca. 1495 to 1505 and provides a reliable basis. The nineteenth-century edition derived from a manuscript that is not entirely reliable. The relevant passage can be found in Heinrich von Pfolsprundt, *Buch der Bündth-Ertznei, 1460*, eds. Heinrich Haeser and Albrecht Theodor Middeldorpf (Berlin: Reimer, 1868), 53.

was made of mugwort, comfrey root and daisies. The patient had to drink it warm in the morning and evening.[22]

The impact of shock, fear, and pain was further recognized in a traumatological treatise written by Johannes Beris in the first half of the fifteenth century, which is extensively referenced by Heinrich von Pfalzpaint. One of the printed versions of the text, published in 1539, advises to look carefully after a patient who was wounded in a state of "fright or fear" (*inn eim schrecken oder forcht*). The reason is that in such a situation the blood runs from all extremities to the heart, which turns the blood into an "unnatural" state ("dz blut das es dann gibt ist onnatürlich") and can have fatal consequences.[23] In his study of Beris's work, Georg Purger states that the symptoms of shock are described and correctly classified in terms of their seriousness.[24] Beris's recommendation is to look after the patient very diligently, wait with the bandaging, and to keep him warm so that blood can regain its natural state ("auff das ihm sein natürlich geblüt widerkumm"). Later, the bandages should not be changed very often.[25]

In case of arrow wounds, these harmful changes to the natural balance of the blood are also referenced as the reason for postponing the removal of arrows for three or four days. If necessary, the arrow shaft must be cut down with a saw. Then the wound should be treated with a plaster made from egg whites:

> One should also know that anyone who is shot / his blood gets a fright / therefore one should not draw out the arrow out soon / so that the blood is not frightened or disturbed even more. And the egg white brings back the [good or natural] blood / and kills the evil of the shot / and protects the wound from swelling / because when the wounds swell / it is worrying / because it will become inflamed from it.[26]

---

**22** Richter, *Phytopharmaka*, 53–54, 89–90; Halle, Universitäts- und Landesbibliothek Sachsen-Anhalt, Cod. 23 G 38, fol. 21r–v.

**23** Beris, *Eyn new Wund Artznei*, fol. 13v.

**24** Georg Purger, "'Ein New Wundartzney' des Johannes Beris: Eine Quelle zur spätmittelalterlich-frühneuzeitlichen Traumatologie" (PhD. diss., Julius-Maximilians-Universität Würzburg, 2020), 85.

**25** Beris, *Eyn new Wund Artznei*, fol. 13v: "So einer inn eim schrecken oder forcht wundt wirt / so laufft das geblüt auß allen gliedern züm hertzen / dz blut das es dann gibt ist onnatürlich / vnnd versehenlich zusterben / es sei dann sach das mann sein wol warte nit verbinden / warm halten / auff das ihm sein natürlich geblüt widerkumm / vnnd mann sol ihn selten auffbinden."

**26** "Mann sol auch wissen das ein ieglicher der geschossen wirt / dem erschrickt das geblüt / darumb soll mann den pfeil nit balt herauß ziehen / damit das geblu[e]t

In the sixteenth century, Hans von Gersdorff was also concerned with long-term damage caused by intense pain and fear, but there are some differences. In his chapter on how to avoid an excess of "wound fluid" (*Glidwasser*), his advice is to check if the patient suffers from intense pain or swelling, since this is a common occurrence. If this is the case, it is important to relieve the pain: "So above all soothe the aching and the pain."[27] His recipe "against the pain caused by the wound fluid" (*für den schmertzen des Glidtwassers*) is a warm poultice made from mallow, linseed, and lard. Dissolved turpentine and rose oil, inserted into the wound with cotton, should also still the pain. However, in case of an excess of wound fluid the surgeon should switch from gentle methods to harsher ones. If necessary, the veins and nerves must be corroded and burned to prevent atrophy of the injured limb (*schwi[n]dsucht*).[28]

Similarly, in a chapter on how to staunch bleeding, von Gersdorff advises cauterization, but only if gentler methods are not sufficient. His suggestion is to apply a thin layer of cotton before burning the veins because this procedure is less painful.[29] Throughout the manual, Gersdorff is particularly mindful of pain as a potential cause of chronic conditions. This is evident in his chapter on patients who had received a crushing blow to the head or suffered a skull fracture.[30] According to the text, it is of utmost importance to ensure that there is not too much pain in the *dura mater*, the uppermost membrane of the brain, and no excess of pus, since both lead to long-lasting damage: "Therefore always see to it that you soothe the pain as quickly as you can, and prevent [the forming of] pus, so that no swelling develops in the wrong place."[31] If necessary, the skull must undergo trepanation to ensure

---

nit noch mer erschreck noch gesturt werd. Vnd dz eißweiß bringt das geblu[e]t wider / vnd to[e]dt die boßheit deß schußs / vnnd behu[e]t die wund am ersten fur schwellen / dann wann die wunden schwellent / ist sorglich / dann es wirt dauon entzint." Beris, *Eyn new Wund Artznei*, fol. 11r–v; see also Richter, *Phytopharmaka*, 47n98; Sudhoff, *Beiträge*, 527–28.

**27** Hans von Gersdorff, *Feldbuch der wundtartzney*, fol. 28v: "so lege jm als dan[n] vor allen dingen den schmertzen vn[d] dz we."

**28** Hans von Gersdorff, *Feldbuch der wundtartzney*, fols. 28v–29r, see also further remedies for withering limbs in chap. XII, fols. 36v–37v.

**29** Hans von Gersdorff, *Feldbuch der wundtartzney*, fol. 29v: "vnd thut nit also wee als soltest du vff die blossz aderen brennen."

**30** Hans von Gersdorff, *Feldbuch der wundtartzney*, fols. 23v–24v.

**31** Hans von Gersdorff, *Feldbuch der wundtartzney*, fol. 23v: "Doru[m]b so lu[o]g allwegen dz du den schmertzen stillest als fast du magst / vnd den eyter fürkom[m]est / dz kein apostema werde an d[er] verkerten statt."

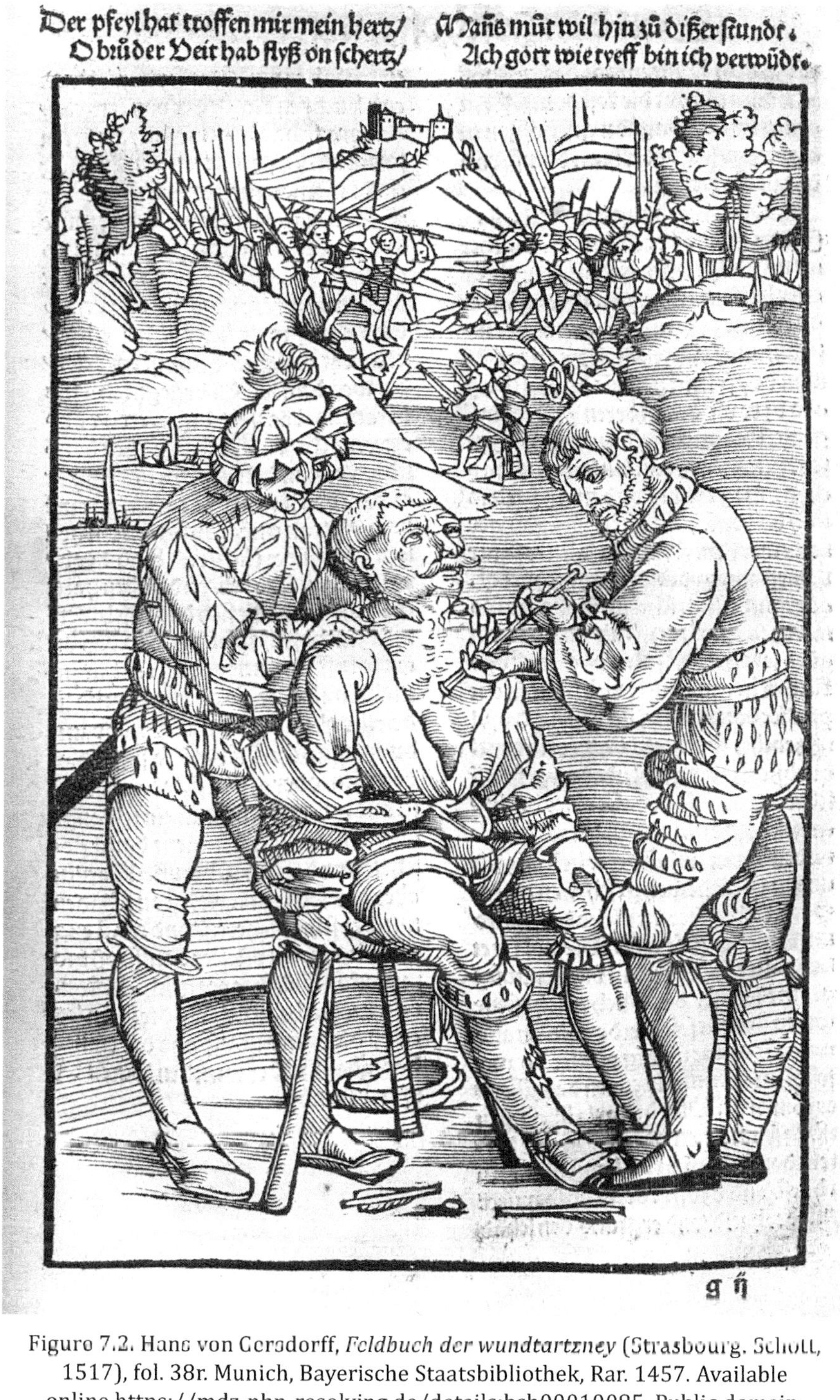


Figure 7.2. Hans von Gersdorff, *Feldbuch der wundtartzney* (Strasbourg: Schott, 1517), fol. 38r. Munich, Bayerische Staatsbibliothek, Rar. 1457. Available online https://mdz-nbn-resolving.de/details:bsb00010085. Public domain.

no bone fragments remain in the wound or hinder the healing process. In general, Hans von Gersdorff insists that head wounds should be treated as "gently" (*senfftigklich*) as possible, particularly shortly after the injury: "this should be a remedy without pain."[32] The wound potion he recommends should be given to the patient as a drink and also be used to wash the wound because it will draw out fragments of bone over the course of two weeks.[33]

Whereas Hans von Gersdorff usually advises to provide as much pain relief as possible and often urges to avoid painful treatment, his advice differs from the traumatological texts from the fifteenth century: unlike the older treatises, he recommends removing arrows and other projectiles immediately, unless the injured person appears to be deadly wounded.[34] Hans von Gersdorff reports that most surgeons allow no waiting time in case the wound was caused by poisonous arrows or gunpowder weapons.[35] Johannes Beris and Heinrich von Pfalzpaint and other writers advised to let arrows stay undisturbed for a few days or even up to two weeks, so that they could be removed without pain. Hans von Gersdorff, in contrast, is willing, although reluctantly, to inflict pain in the process of removing poisoned arrows and projectiles with gunpowder residue.[36] It is interesting that in his surgery manual, the accompanying image to the relevant passage is the only one within the whole printed book that clearly depicts a war scene.

The patient is shown in the process of having an arrow wound treated at the very edge of the battlefield. A surgeon probes the wound in his chest with pliers, possibly to remove any metal or wooden fragments, while a broken arrow lies at his feet. The patient, his face rigid and eyes upturned, sits on a small stool. He is held by the shoulders by an assistant to the surgeon.

---

**32** Hans von Gersdorff, *Feldbuch der wundtartzney*, fol. 24r: "das soll ein artzney sein on schmertzen."

**33** Hans von Gersdorff, *Feldbuch der wundtartzney*, fol. 24r.

**34** Hans von Gersdorff, *Feldbuch der wundtartzney*, fol. 37v. In this case, the surgeon should see to it that the injured receives the sacrament before attempting to remove the projectile. See also Hans von Gersdorff, *Feldbuch der wundtartzney*, fols. 37v–42r; Vollmuth, "Von den geschosszenen Wunden," 24–26.

**35** Hans von Gersdorff, *Feldbuch der wundtartzney*, fol. 38v.

**36** Hans von Gersdorff, *Feldbuch der wundtartzney*, fol. 38v: "Vnd diewyl zu[o]besorgen ist / dz schmertzen do sey / so ist nüt bessers dorfür / dan[n] dz du heissz o[e]le dorin thuest / vnd dz offt." Gunpowder was seen as poisonous; therefore wounds caused by gunpowder weapons were often treated with cauter irons or boiling oil. Ambroise Paré famously argued against this painful practice in his treatise *La methode de traicter les playes faictes par hacqvebvtes et avltres bastons à feu* (1545). Ambroise Paré, *Die Behandlung der Schusswunden [1545]*, trans. Henry E. Sigerist (Leipzig: Barth, 1923).

The accompanying text emphasizes the shock, fear and pain of the patient who faces agonizing treatment and possibly death due to blood loss or infection: "The arrow has struck my heart / O brother Veit, be diligent / [A] man's courage will leave him at this moment. / Oh God, how deeply I am wounded."[37]

These examples from traumatological texts show that pain was understood to have significant impact. Highly painful injuries could lead to permanent damage, chronic states of illness and pain, and to disabilities. We may assume that knights and soldiers were well aware of these general notions, even if they were not familiar with the underlying physiological causes discussed and debated amongst surgeons or learned physicians in any great detail.

## After the Injury: Coping with Impairment and Pain

The *Book of Chivalry* by Geoffroi de Charny († 1356), written in the first half of the fourteenth century, refers repeatedly to the emotional and physical pain men-at-arms had to endure on a regular basis. These hardships are, in fact, what makes their lives exceptionally worthy in the eyes of God, as long as they fight for a noble cause. Charny describes constant physical exertion, bad nutrition, uncomfortable sleep and erratic resting hours. Moreover, he states that men-at-arms have to face "fearful physical perils and the loss of friends whose deaths they have witnessed in many great battles." These experiences have often filled their hearts with great distress and strong emotion."[38] The horrifying situation of witnessing a hall full of dying and injured fighters after a battle was lost is described in emphatic terms in the biography of nobleman and military commander Wilwolt von Schaumberg (ca. 1466–1510). It was written in 1507 by his relative Ludwig von Eyb (1446–1521), apparently to allow young noblemen to learn from his deeds. The passage in question contrasts a terrifying, claustrophobic scene of suffering, screams and prayers inside the hall with the oblivious merrymaking of uninjured soldiers outside:

> and counts, lords, knights and soldiers lay all together in a large hall, one with a pillow, the other with his robe or cloak, whatever anyone might have, placed under his head. Here an arrow was pulled out of one, a lead bullet was taken out from another, one received the holy sacrament, several were

---

**37** Hans von Gersdorff, *Feldbuch der wundtartzney*, fol. 38r: "Der pfeyl hat troffen mir mein hertz / O bru[o]der Veit hab flyß on schertz / Man[n]s mu[o]t will hin zu[o] dißer stundt. Ach gott wie tyeff bin ich verwu[n]dt." See also Panse, *Feldbuch*, 90–91, 134–36.

**38** Geoffroi de Charny, *A Knight's Own Book of Chivalry*, trans. Elspeth Kennedy (Philadelphia: University of Pennsylvania Press, 2005), 47–107, 61 (for the citation).

> shouted at to hold God in their hearts, so the souls went out of some, and everyone was wounded, and it was a terrifying, miserable occurrence. But the soldiers were out in the streets with their drums and pipes, were completely cheerful, and no one, who was not affected, had any compassion for the others.[39]

While the author clearly disapproves of the lack of compassion displayed by the celebrating soldiers, it still appears as if this behaviour was to be expected by some of those who survived without injury. In contrast, the scene was probably meant to evoke "great distress and strong emotion"—as the *Book of Chivalry* puts it—in its anticipated audience. Similar to writings of Charny, witnessing the suffering of others is presented as terrifying and emotionally painful, but also as an integral part of those who chose a life of warfare, something that had to be learned, adopted, and practised compassionately.

Charny describes the constant fear of accidents, injuries and death that accompanied the daily existence during a military campaign as unavoidable. To achieve the highest honours, though, he reminds his readers of the necessity to adapt to those feelings and to learn how to overcome them. To this end, Charny advises men-at-arms to put their trust in God in case of defeat on the battlefield:

> And if you are defeated, does not God show you great mercy if you are taken prisoner honourably, praised by friends and enemies? And if you are in a state of grace and you die honourably, does not God show you great mercy when He grants you such a glorious end to your life in this world and bears your soul away with Him into eternal bliss? And you can see that no one should be too afraid or too overjoyed or too disturbed at such happenings when they occur, but should give thanks and commit everything into the hands of Him who gives graciously more than one can ask for.[40]

---

**39** "vnnd lagenn grauen, herrn, ritter vnnd knecht bey einander in einem grossenn sall, einer hett ein küssen, der annder seinen rock ader cleider, was ein yder haben mocht, vnnter sein haubt gelegt. Da zoch man einem ein pfeill, da gewan man dem andern ein glött, disem gab man das heilig sacrament, da schrey man ettlichem zw, gott im hertzen zwhaben, so gingen ein teillen die selen aus, darnach ein yeder wunth, vnnd was ein erschrockenlich iemerlich handlung. Aber die knecht gingen mit irn trumen vnnd pfeüffenn vff der gassenn, warn gantz frölich, hett keiner, den es nit anging, mit den andern mittleyden." Ludwig von Eyb, *Geschichten und Taten Wilwolts von Schaumberg*, ed. Helgard Ulmschneider (Münster: Waxmann, 2018), 185–86. See also Gero Schreier, *Ritterhelden: Rittertum, Autonomie und Fürstendienst in niederadligen Lebenszeugnissen des 14. bis 16. Jahrhunderts* (Ostfildern: Thorbecke, 2019), 33–34, 173–91.

**40** Geoffroy de Charny, *Book of Chivalry*, 72.

Interestingly, the passage only refers to fighting men dying or being taken into captivity. Although physical and emotional pain that occurs during a campaign are described in great detail in the rest of the text, serious and potentially disabling injuries are not mentioned here. In other passages, the possibility of being wounded is mentioned only vaguely and in passing. The physical, emotional, and social impact experiences of disability could have on a warrior are largely omitted. Only at one point, when Charny praises the members of the "order of knighthood" for their rigorous lifestyle, he states: "and when they would be secure from danger, they will be beset by great terrors, and when they would defeat their enemies, sometimes they may be defeated, or killed, or captured and wounded and struggling to recover."[41] We can infer from these words that the prospect of permanent illness, pain, or disability might have been a common cause of fear. However, these fears are not reflected on in any detail. So how can we know what happened to those who actually survived serious injury?

At this point, I would like to take a closer look at the few descriptions of disabling injury that we have from the point of view of survivors.[42] Archaeological evidence tells us that a surprising number of people recovered from severe injuries, including skull fractures. In his comparative overview on medieval battlefield grave excavations, Piers Mitchell points out that many skeletons show evidence of healed wounds and bone fractures that probably stem from weapons used in war. Apparently, although these men had suffered severe trauma to their bodies, they recovered to such a degree that they were still able to engage in combat later on.[43] Moreover, we know from written sources that knights and soldiers proudly displayed signs of healed battle wounds on their bodies. In a verbal altercation with a non-fighting member of the nobility, German Landsknecht leader Georg von Frundsberg (1473–1528) called his opponent an "armchair knight" (*polster ritter*). He then challenged him to a fight by pointing to his own "crooked foot" (*khrumpen Fueß*), using his long-healed battle injury as proof of his honour and martial

---

**41** Geoffroy de Charny, *Book of Chivalry*, 95.

**42** This section is partly based on Bianca Frohne, *Leben mit "kranckhait": Der gebrechliche Körper in der häuslichen Überlieferung des 15. und 16. Jahrhunderts. Überlegungen zu einer Disability History der Vormoderne* (Affalterbach: Didymos, 2014), 350–57.

**43** Piers D. Mitchell, *Medicine in the Crusades: Warfare, Wounds, and the Medieval Surgeon* (Cambridge: Cambridge University Press, 2004), 108–23; see also Woosnam-Savage and DeVries, "Battle Trauma," and Christopher J. Knüsel's contribution to this volume.

superiority.[44] In contrast, there are few descriptions of the immediate aftermath of an injury from the perspective of the injured themselves. One of them is the—supposedly autobiographical—text that details the life of Gottfried, called Götz, von Berlichingen (1480–1562). To this day, he is famous for losing his right hand in battle, when he was shot with a projectile fired by a culverin during the siege of Landshut, and his use of an iron prosthesis afterwards.[45] The emphatic and lively description of events given in the text, detailing the sympathetic reactions of Götz's peers as well as his emotional struggle to adapt to the new situation, suggest that the loss of a limb and its accompanying circumstances had become the subject of a frequently told narration. While we cannot be sure that this narrative is actually told in Götz's own words—the text was dictated more than fifty years after the incident and probably redacted by several persons after his death—,we can still read it as one of the few texts that engage with the experience of lasting injury and pain due to the loss of limb.[46]

It is particularly noticeable that the text, during the account of Götz's injury, initially does not focus at all on the loss of his hand, but rather on the behaviour of friends, fellow men-at-arms, and high-ranking leaders. At the beginning, the narrator gives a detailed account of Götz's transport from the battlefield. Even then, the focus is not on medical treatment, but on the behaviour of his peers who worry about him and offer support. In describing

**44** Arnold Luschin von Ebengreuth, "Herbersteiniana," *Beiträge zur Kunde steiermärkischer Geschichtsquellen* 25 (1892): 67–122, at 83–84; see also Rogers, *Soldiers' Lives*, 216.

**45** Götz von Berlichingen, *Mein Fehd und Handlungen*, ed. Helgard Ulmschneider (Sigmaringen: Thorbecke, 1981), 75–77. According to the text, the projectile hit the pommel of Götz's sword, pieces of which became embedded in his forearm together with pieces of his armour. On the use of culverins, see DeVries, *Medieval Military Technology*, 152–53.

**46** On the tendency to approach the text as a genuine autobiography, see Tilman G. Moritz, *Autobiographik als ritterschaftliche Selbstverständigung: Ulrich von Hutten, Götz von Berlichingen, Sigmund von Herberstein* (Göttingen: V&R Unipress, 2019), 95–112. While we cannot, with any certainty, estimate the number or the type of interventions that might have occurred during the writing process or as part of later revisions, it is important to note that the text was read and copied predominantly among family members and descendants of Götz, many of whom would have listened to the tales told during his lifetime. Furthermore, even if the text was a complete and accurate reproduction of Götz's own words, this still would not guarantee some form of autobiographical "authenticity." Events would have been shaped and altered in hindsight by the processes inherent to memory retention as well as by contemporary narrative conventions. As with all autobiographical texts, we have to treat the text as a literary construct.

the crowd surrounding his sickbed, the scene is compared to a "pilgrimage."[47] Götz appears to have quizzed his visitors on details about his armour, his horse and his fighting activities to make sure his deeds on the battlefield were appropriately recognized. The text makes his satisfaction known by resuming that they "knew as much as I did about how and what I had been doing for the past two days."[48] Among his visitors are said to have been many of those who fought on the opposing side. While the text provides an excess of details on the sociability and joviality around the sickbed visits, the medical treatment Götz must have received is almost completely omitted. In his surgery manual, Hans von Gersdorff gives instructions on how to deal with arms, hands, legs, or feet which were fractured or shattered by gunpowder weapons.[49] The procedure would have been highly painful, including the sawing off of any projecting bone fragments, and the removal of splinters, using pliers, to make the "stump" (*strumpff*) even. Next, the blood flow has to be stopped, by cauterization if necessary. Hans von Gersdorff also advises to use flax soaked in hemp oil and place it over the stump because it etches and cleans the powder and extinguishes it. When the wounded person is no longer in pain, but there is still blackness to be seen, his suggestion is to make an ointment, spread it on a cloth and place it over the stump to draw out any gunpowder residue.[50] According to the description of Götz's injury, parts of his forearm had been meshed with bits of his armour due to the force of the impact, and his hand was only loosely attached by the skin. It is likely that he required a partial amputation of his forearm. We do not know whether Götz was conscious during initial treatment. In his manual, Hans von Gersdorff dedicates a segment to substances with pain-relieving qualities, among them pills made from opium, mandrake, or nightshade.[51] Since

**47** Götz von Berlichingen, *Mein Fehd und Handlungen*, 75: "es wahr gleich ein walfart zu mir."

**48** Götz von Berlichingen, *Mein Fehd und Handlungen*, 77.

**49** Hans von Gersdorff, *Feldbuch der wundtartzney*, fol. 42r: "Ob eim ein arm / handt / bein / oder fu[o]ß abgeschosszen were[n] in kryegs la[e]uffen / wie du jm wider zu[o] hilff sollest kom[m]en."

**50** Hans von Gersdorff, *Feldbuch der wundtartzney*, fol. 42r.

**51** Hans von Gersdorff, *Feldbuch der wundtartzney*, fol. 51r: "Oppium / ist ein safft magsomen. Mandragora / ist ein wurtzel. Radix solatri mortalis / ist die grossz nachtschatt wurtzel. od[er] dollwurtz. Jusquiamus / ist bylßen sot. Magsomen." On medieval and early modern methods and approaches to pain relief, see also Franz Josef Kuhlen, *Zur Geschichte der Schmerz-, Schlaf- und Betäubungsmittel in Mittelalter und früher Neuzeit* (Stuttgart: Deutscher Apotheker, 1983), 189–212.

these substances could have serious side-effects, they should be used only if the pain is very severe or if the patient is in danger of dying from pain:

> You should know that if the pain cannot be soothed by gentle things, and you are forced by necessity, it is better to use something that might cause a little damage to treat the injury, than that the person dies of pain. And so you have to turn to the strong and anaesthetizing [remedies], as you will find listed hereafter.[52]

Heinrich von Pfalzpaint explains in his surgery manual how to prepare and use a "sleep sponge" in order to "make someone sleep / whom you want to operate on / or otherwise would like to make someone sleep who is ill and cannot sleep."[53] The sponge, which contains opium amongst other anaesthetizing substances, is to be soaked in warm water for about an hour before use, and then held under the patient's nose. It is unknown whether any of these remedies were used on Götz, either during an operation or to allow him to sleep. He probably received at least some treatment aimed at pain relief, in accordance with the understanding of pain as a dangerous factor in its own right. However, whereas the complete account of the events at Landshut takes up ten pages of manuscript, detailing the battle, the injury, the escape from the battlefield, the search for accommodation, and the sickbed visits, there is only one short passage that approaches the physical and emotional pain Götz likely experienced over the course of the next eight months:

---

**52** "Item du solt wissen / wan[n] d[er] smertz nit gestilt mag werde[n] durch die senften ding / vn[d] dich die notturfft zwinget / so ist doch besser das man ettwas bruch das do ein wenig schade[n] bring / den schaden zestraffen / dan[n] das der mensch sterbe von dem schmertze[n]. vnd so mu[o]ssz man als dan[n] gon zu[o] den starken vnd stillmachenden / als du hye noch findest ston." Hans von Gersdorff, *Feldbuch der wundtartzney*, fol. 51r. A very similar passage can be found in *Ein nutzlichs Wundertzney Bu[e]chlein des hochberu[e]mbten Lanfranci aus fu[r]rbit des wolerfarnen Meister Gregorij Fleugaus Chyrurgen vnd Wundartzt zu Strasburg: Dabey viel bewerter Recepten heylsamer salben vnd ertzneyen ein auszug bisher von obgenantem M. Gregorio fur sich selbs yn grossem werd behalten itzt gemeynem nutz zu gut auch ynn druck gegeben Durch Othonem Brunfelss verdeudscht* (Zwickau: G. Kantz, 1529), fol. E1r: "Mag aber der schmertz nicht gestillet werden durch die senfftigungen / vnd dich die not treibt / ist besser das man etwas brauche das ein wenig schadet / den schaden zu straffen / den das der mensch sterb von schmertzen / So mus man starcke vnd stillmachende nemen / wie hernach folget." The manual, published in 1529, is based on the *chirurgia parva* by Lanfranc of Milan (13th c.).

**53** Halle, Universitäts- und Landesbibliothek Sachsen-Anhalt, Cod. 23 G 38, fol. 24v: "wie man einen schlaffen macht / den man schneiden wil / oder sunst gerne schlaffen machen wolte der kranck were vnd nicht schlaffen konde."

> What pain I suffered at that time, anyone can well imagine, and it was my plea to God, which I uttered, that if I was in his divine favour, in the name of God he should take me with him, for I was surely ruined as a man of war.[54]

Despite its brevity, the passage is poignant. It is the narratological highlight and the turning point within this story, as it is immediately followed by a solution that replaces the desperate outlook on life: Götz remembers what his father told him about a warrior who fought with only one hand. At this point, according to the text, he decides to put his trust in God and his own fighting skills, realizing that even if he had twelve hands, but God were not in his favour, he would not prevail as a knight in any case. So, if he had a substitute (*ein behelff*), such as an iron hand, he would be able to prove his value on the battlefield as well as an uninjured person.[55] Götz is presented here in accordance with the ideal image of a God-fearing, steadfast knight.[56] The (auto)biographical episode concludes with an outlook on the future in which Götz prevailed "with one fist" in many battles, feuds, and perils, and remained in God's favour throughout.[57] His words echo those of Geoffroi de

**54** Götz von Berlichingen, *Mein Fehd und Handlungen*, 77: "Was ich die zeitt fur schmertzenn erlittenn habe, das khann ain jeglicher woll erachtenn, vnnd wahr das mein bitt zu gott, die ich thet, wann ich inn seiner gottlichenn gnadt wer, so solt er im namen gottes mit mir hinfarenn, ich wehr doch verderbtt zu einem Kriegsman."

**55** Götz von Berlichingen, *Mein Fehd und Handlungen*, 77: "Der lag mir im sin, das ich gott aber annrufft vnnd gedachtt, wann ich schon zwolff henndt hett, vnnd sein gottliche gnadt vnnd hilff mir nit woll wolltt, so wehr es doch alls vmb sonnst. Vnnd vermeint dernnhalbenn, wann ich doch nit mehr dann ein wenig ein behelff hett, es wehr gleich ein eisenne hanndt oder wie es wehr, so wollt ich demnach mit gottes gnadt vnnd hilff im feld noch irgenndt alls gutt sein, alls sonnst ein heiloss mensch."

**56** At first glance, the religious element within this narrative fits neatly into the "religious model" of disability as developed by Edward Wheatley, *Stumbling Blocks before the Blind: Medieval Constructions of a Disability* (Ann Arbor: University of Michigan Press, 2010), esp. 10–19. Wheatley argues that the social perception and treatment of disabled people in the medieval period were influenced to a high degree by a religious understanding of disability, with a focus on any spiritual impact an impairment could produce. However, the religious model has not been taken up by many disability historians. Götz's narrative, but also many examples in this volume, show that disability experiences were highly variable and complex. While religious understanding certainly played a role, it was not necessarily the most important factor. Furthermore, religious readings of a disability were often highly flexible and situationally adaptive, much like they were regarding other aspects of medieval life.

**57** Götz von Berlichingen, *Mein Fehd und Handlungen*, 77: "Vnnd nachdem ich nun schir sochzig jar mit einer faust krieg, vhedt vnd henndel gehabt, so khann ich wahrlich nit annderst befindenn noch sagen, dann das der allmechtig ewig barmherzig gott wunderbarlich mit großenn gnadenn, bey vnnd mit mir inn allenn

Charny. Similar to the "Book of Chivalry," which acknowledges pain and distress only as part of a warrior's experience on a campaign, the injury practically vanishes from the narration. The missing hand does not play an important role again within the narrative, even though we know that it became somewhat of a public trademark.[58] We also know that he was the owner of at least one iron hand that was used as a prosthesis.[59] Today, two prosthetic hands, which are ascribed to having been in Götz's possession, are kept near his former estate at Jagsthausen. It is unknown who made these hands, at what cost, or in which situations they were used.[60]

In the (auto)biographical text, the material, embodied experience of healing and adapting to living with one hand is not paid any attention. We do not know if the stump of the forearm hurt or required further medical attention, if Götz had any phantom sensations or experienced phantom pain.[61] What is more: even though the (auto)biographical text alludes to an

---

meinen kriegen, vhedenn vnnd geuerlicheitenn gewesenn." In reality Götz did not come close to the knightly ideals proposed by Charny. Several passages of the (auto)biographical text serve as self-justifications within the context of the many violent conflicts he provoked and the crimes he was accused of. Sonja Kerth, "Die letzten taflrunder? Krieg in adligen Autobiographien des 15. und 16. Jahrhunderts," in *Dulce bellum inexpertis: Bilder des Krieges in der deutschen Literatur des 15. und 16. Jahrhunderts* (Wiesbaden: Reichert, 2002), 213–29; Helgard Ulmschneider, *Götz von Berlichingen: Ein adeliges Leben der deutschen Renaissance* (Sigmaringen: Thorbecke, 1974), 92–94.

**58** Ulmschneider, *Götz von Berlichingen*, 151; see also Auge, "So solt er im namen gottes."

**59** Götz von Berlichingen, *Mein Fehd und Handlungen*, 118.

**60** Images are provided by Rachael Gillibrand, "'To Fight as Well as Anyone Else': Medieval Knights and Mechanised Prostheses," *Epoch Magazine* 3 (March 2021). https://www.epoch-magazine.com/post/to-fight-as-well-as-anyone-else-medieval-knights-and-mechanised-prosthesesby, accessed February 3, 2025. See also Heidi Hausse, *The Malleable Body: Surgeons, Artisans, and Amputees in Early Modern Germany* (Manchester: Manchester University Press, 2023), 164–65, figures 5.5. and 5.6, and John Gagné, "Mechanism/Organism: The Premodern Iron Hand as Conceptual Interface," figure 9.6, in this volume. There is no proof that these prostheses had actually ever been in Götz's possession, see Moritz, *Autobiographik*, 96n239: he argues that they might have been acquired by the Berlichingen family after Goethe had made Götz famous in his play, although there is no evidence to support this assumption either. On the interest in the prostheses and the memorabilia focused on the historical Götz in the later eighteenth century, see also Gagné, "Mechanism/Organism."

**61** Phantom limb pain was first described by Ambroise Paré in the sixteenth century. Gundolf Keil, "Sogenannte Erstbeschreibung des Phantomschmerzes von

iron hand being used in battle, modern examinations of the first of the two prostheses ascribed to Götz show that its owner was probably unable to grasp or guide most objects with it.[62] Due to the rigid fixation of the wrist, combat would only have been possible to a very limited extent. It has been suggested that the main use of this iron hand was to enable its owner to ride a horse. Besides that, it probably had cosmetic functions, as traces of flesh-coloured paint were found on it. Götz's handwriting was notoriously difficult to read, suggesting that he had learned how to write with his left hand, which he presumably also used in fights.[63] The (auto)biographical text does not offer any information on the practicalities of Götz's prosthesis. It is likely that it was in frequent use, since the text mentions that he "had [repair] work done on [some part of] the iron hand, which was broken."[64] A more sophisticated prosthesis ascribed to Götz is also kept at Jagsthausen. This iron hand, the more famous of the two today, had a complicated inner mechanism that would have allowed its owner to move digits individually.[65] However, the item does not show signs of extensive use and no traces of paint. It might have been covered with fabric or leather.[66] If it had actually been in Götz's possession, it is possible that he understood it mainly as a prestige object, or even as curiosity to show off its maker's ingenuity. Maybe it was mainly perceived as a symbolic object, focusing attention on resilience and adaptability.[67]

At this point in Götz's life, after he might have acquired the second prosthesis, the experience of his long-healed injury is likely to have already been transformed into the art- and suspenseful narrative that survives today in written form. The (auto)biographical text places the pain and grief

Ambroise Paré," *Fortschritte der Medizin* 108 (1990): 62–66, assumes that even before, phantom pain must have been a well-known phenomenon.

**62** Günter Quasigroch, "Die Handprothesen des fränkischen Reichsritters Götz von Berlichingen. 1. Fortsetzung: Die Ersthand," *Waffen und Kostümkunde* 24 (1982): 17–33.

**63** Quasigroch, "Die Handprothesen."

**64** Götz von Berlichingen, *Mein Fehd und Handlungen*, 118: "etwas ann der eisen handt, so mir zubrochenn wartt, machen lassen."

**65** See Gagné's contribution in this volume.

**66** Quasigroch, "Die Handprothesen," 103–20.

**67** The distinction between "activity objects" and "worth objects" might be useful in this regard: Katherine Ott, "Material Culture, Technology, and the Body," in *Disability History: The Oxford Handbook of Disability History*, eds. Michael Rembis et al. (Oxford: Oxford University Press, 2018), 125–40.

caused by the injury and subsequent loss of a hand firmly within a narrative of *restoration*: not only of Götz's body or his ability to fight, but of his social identity. On a textual level, the process of reclaiming his status as a capable fighter starts at Landshut, immediately after the injury, by repeatedly re-telling the incident amongst his peers during lively sickbed visits. In this process, as becomes apparent by the different phases of the narration, the physical and emotional pain is still suspended, while a socially desirable framework of in-group bravado, solidarity, and mental support takes its place. When the narration finally turns to physical pain as well as feelings of desperation, isolation, and even the wish to die, the text provides only glimpses of an underlying experience. What is more: even the description of Götz's emotional pain is solely directed at the perceived incapability of continuing his existence as a fighter. This narrative focus on a single issue actually serves to strengthen, not weaken, Götz's social position. His fears and doubts regarding his social identity are actually in accordance with an understanding of knighthood as a mental and moral state. As soon as he considers the solution—*ein behelff* in form of an iron hand—his identity as a god-fearing knight is already restored, and then immediately reaffirmed by a glimpse into the future several decades later.

At the same time, Götz's in-group audience, particularly knights and soldiers, probably knew very well how to interpret the brief passage that actually conveys physical and emotional anguish. As the text says: *anyone* could imagine what his experience must have felt like.[68] Within the carefully constructed narrative, this very tentative exploration of disability, pain, and grief would have been enough. Similar to the *Book of Chivalry*, the approach to these aspects of warfare is programmatic. Pain is one of the crucial factors that turn men-at-arms from mere fighters into god-fearing knights whose suffering and mental struggles enhance their self-image. Painful injury and even impairment can be seamlessly integrated into this construction, but only as long as the ability to function in an adequate way is not substantially affected. In Götz's (auto)biography, emotional and physical suffering are only mentioned when the pain is already about to vanish from the narrative. In fact, stories that entail experiences of pain and impairment are only ever told in retrospect. If Götz had been unable to fight again, it is unlikely that his story would have been put into writing at all. Sadly, this means that the testimonies from survivors of severe combat-related injuries that are known to us are usually stories of restoration, of overcoming pain and impairment.

**68** See also Harari, *Renaissance Military Memoirs*, 69.

If Götz suffered from chronic pain or lasting emotional trauma throughout his life, these experiences would probably not have found a place within his stories.

A similar narrative pattern can be found in the autobiography of patrician Ludwig von Diesbach (1452–1527) from Bern. In one passage of his autobiography, he recounts his military deeds to show that he had risked his "body and life" (*leyb unn leben*) and was well worthy of honour like other knights and soldiers.[69] During the time he was serving in the army of King Louis XI of France, "great injury" (*ein grosser schad*) happened to him. Due to a mishap when he tried to bring a horse under control, he fell and accidentally stabbed himself with a spear in the thigh, cutting into an artery. He thought he would die because he bled heavily, but the wound was bound up and the bleeding could be stopped. After three days—probably because it was not safe to move him any earlier—he was brought on a horse stretcher to nearby Compiègne:

> The Queen was now three German miles away. In her service was a surgeon, a German, who was sent to me. He cured me with God's help, but under great pain and with great cost, for I had pierced the artery in my leg. And it was very much feared that I would have to limp with this leg in future. But thanks to God's grace, that didn't happen. I was only two and a half shoes shorter in the long jump, which I was never able to make up for thereafter, but otherwise I was not impaired in any way.[70]

There are several elements here that mirror the story in the (auto)biography of Götz von Berlichingen: both explain how their transport was organized after the injury and mention the support they received from high-standing individuals. Both make sure that the enormity of the pain they had experienced was noted. In both texts, the fear of lasting physical impairment, which would have made them less capable of inhabiting the social roles they aspired to, are voiced. This fear is then immediately allayed within the narrative. In both cases, God's will is referenced and presented as the ultimate

---

**69** Urs Martin Zahnd, *Die autobiographischen Aufzeichnungen Ludwig von Diesbachs: Studien zur spätmittelalterlichen Selbstdarstellung im oberdeutschen und schweizerischen Raume* (Bern: Stämpfli, 1986), 50.

**70** "Nůw wass die ckûngen uff iii ttûttsch mÿll von mÿr. Die hatt ein scherer, was sein ttûscher, ward mÿr geschycktt. Der selb mitt der gocz hÿlff ernartt mich, doch mitt grossem schmerczen unn ckosten; den ich hatt die meÿsterader dûrchstochen im schenkell. Unn entzass man fast, ich mûssttÿ hÿncken werden an dem schenckell. Daß aber nitt beschach von den genaden gocz. Aber woll gÿng mÿr am sprÿngen uff iij schůw ab, die moechtt ich darnach neÿ erffûllen, sûst ttett mÿr ckeÿn arbeÿtt nûcz daran." Zahnd, *Aufzeichnungen*, 52–55. See also Selzer, "Das Leiden der Krieger," 80.

cause of their restoration to their former social state. Both narratives end on a similar note: even if they suffered severe injuries, endured highly painful curative phases, and had to adapt to certain setbacks, they want it to be known that their experiences did not hinder or disable them. Most importantly, both texts are dealing with disability and pain from a position of retrospective storytelling, secure in the knowledge that there had already been visible proof of their continued physical prowess. Maybe this is what allowed both of them to mention their pain in the first place.[71]

There is one example among the writings of injured warriors that stands out in this respect. The account of deeds by the Swabian knight Georg von Ehingen (1428–1508) is focused mainly on his upbringing as a knight, his travels, and martial achievements.[72] During the siege of Granada in 1457, he was injured:

> I was struck by a staff sling on the shinbone, badly wounded. And although I healed well after that, the shinbone broke open again when I got to Swabia and kept a hole in the shinbone and a flow until in my old age.[73]

This account is one of the few in which an injury acquired in war is referred to as a cause of chronic illness and presumably lasting pain or discomfort throughout the life of the affected person. Interestingly, while the "flow" (*fluß*) in his leg is never mentioned again within the text, the injury coincides with a change in Georg's lifestyle: shortly afterwards, he began a successful political and diplomatic career at the Württemberg court. This part of his life, however, together with his marriage and the birth of his children, is omitted from the text. The account concentrates on his knightly journeys only.[74] Although we cannot be sure whether the injury had an impact on Georg's career at all, or if it was even known by others at his point, it is evident that he wanted to be remembered as a knight who not only fought bravely, but damaged his body and his health permanently in pursuit of the

**71** Woosnam-Savage and DeVries, "Battle Trauma," 47, refer to surprising archaeological evidence indicating that warriors with healed fractures and even amputations could apparently still engage in battle.

**72** Georg von Ehingen, *Reisen nach der Ritterschaft*, ed. Gabriele Ehrmann (Göppingen: Kümmerle, 1979), 2:82; see also Kerth, "Die letzten taflrunder," 186–200; Schreier, *Ritterhelden*, 12–14, 155–72.

**73** "Ich ward mit ainer stabschlingen geworffen uff ain schinbain, gar hart wund. Und wie wol ich darnach wolgehailt, brach mir daß schinbain allß ich gen Schwaben kam wider uff und behiellt allso biß in min allter ain löchlin im schinbain und ain fluß." Georg von Ehingen, *Reisen nach der Ritterschaft*, 1:67; see also 2:98.

**74** Georg von Ehingen, *Reisen nach der Ritterschaft*, 2:76.

Christian cause. Once again, painful injury and, in this case, painful chronic illness are placed in a rhetoric framework that strengthened, not weakened, knightly identity. What a life with chronic illness and pain might have meant to him in reality though, remains unknown.

## Concluding Remarks: Disability, Pain, and Trauma

Considering the impact of fear and pain within traumatological treatises as well as the pain narratives studied in the section above, it seems worthwhile to take up the themes of disability, pain, and mental trauma together. It is clear that medieval and early modern traumatological texts connected severe, painful injury with intense, overwhelming shock. Wounds that were received in a state of "fright" were acknowledged as particularly dangerous. In these cases, the wounded men were kept warm, given rest, and treated with special care. Intense pain was understood as harmful and potentially deadly. In many cases, it was to be treated immediately, before any other medical interventions. Surgeons apparently deviated from this principle only to avoid the risk of infection or to treat injuries that required special urgency. Heinrich von Pfalzpaint, Johannes Beris, and Hans von Gersdorff offer physiological reasoning for their decisions. The affective experience of injuries was considered integral to bodily reactions to wounds and injuries. These practices are based on the principles of humoral pathology, which acknowledge the impact of intense emotions on the bodily constitution. Expressions of pain, fear, panic, and shock must have been a common occurrence to which surgeons and other participants in military campaigns must have been exposed. Geoffroi de Charny even understood the permanent fear, the feeling of never being secure or out of harm's way, as a central part of the suffering endured by the "order of knights." In his eyes, living with constant fear, distress, and painful memories deserves higher praise than any achievement within "clerical orders."[75]

With this in mind, can we approach severely painful or life-threatening injury as traumatic events, as experiences that left long-lasting psychological wounds? There are at least a few indicators that mirror typical phenomena connected with Post Traumatic Stress Disorder (PTSD) within the writings of Geoffroi de Charny.[76] Disability historian Sonja Kerth has also found narratives that correspond to our modern understanding of trauma in medieval

**75** Geoffroy de Charny, *Book of Chivalry*, 95–103.

**76** Meyer-Schilf, "dazu jch jedem raten wil," 113.

literature.[77] However, we do not need to establish clinically exact diagnostic criteria to make use of *mental trauma* as a category of historical analysis. These will always remain out of reach.[78] The examples cited in this chapter, as well as in the contributions by Yoav Tirosh, Aleksandra Pfau, and Wendy J. Turner in this volume, demonstrate that battle wounds and injuries were not perceived or treated as mere physical damage. Even though the concept of *trauma* was not used in medieval sources in the same way we use it today, there were similar concepts and a shared understanding regarding the needs of those who survived such incidents. The overwhelming shock and terror that must have accompanied the situation of being severely and painfully injured in a high-risk situation, facing death, imprisonment, or lasting impairment, was acknowledged and incorporated into medical practices and health regimes.

Maybe it is telling that even decades after he had lost his hand, Götz von Berlichingen could likely still describe in excruciating detail how the injury happened, where he had been looking during which moment, and what his arm had looked like immediately after being hit by the projectile. Parts of his narrative, as it survives today, appear as if the injury is relived in slow motion.[79] While this is not necessarily evidence of Götz experiencing flashbacks, it might allow us to assume that he repeatedly retold the incident from memory. It is not out of the question that talking about the injury and crafting an elaborate narrative helped him to process what had happened. The almost unimaginable pain, the fear of being ruined as a warrior, and the wish to die, as cited above, are part of this narrative, yet at the same time they also point us to the mental distress and emotional strain in the aftermath of the injury.

There is much we do not know about the emotional experience of these situations and their long-term impact. Both Götz von Berlichingen and Georg von Frundsberg proudly showed the remains of their healed injuries in public, their pain—and possibly fear—seemingly far in the past. Did these

---

**77** Sonja Kerth, "Narratives of Trauma in Medieval German Literature," in *Trauma in Medieval Society*, eds. Wendy J. Turner and Christina Lee (Leiden: Brill, 2018), 274–97.

**78** Donna Trembinski, "Trauma as a Category of Analysis," in *Trauma in Medieval Society*, 13–38.

**79** Bianca Frohne, "Performing Dis/Ability? Constructions of Infirmity in Late Medieval and Early Modern Life Writing," in *Infirmity in Antiquity and the Middle Ages: Social and Cultural Approaches to Health, Weakness and Care*, eds. Christian Krötzl et al. (Farnham: Ashgate, 2015), 51–65.

acts create distance between themselves and their own vulnerability? Or was this an acknowledgement of trauma and pain, pointing to a shared form of knowledge among men-at-arms? Larissa Tracy and Kelly R. DeVries argue that within medieval sources, psychological wounds and mental traumata "manifest in a variety of ways from melancholy and religious reflection to machismo and ostentatious displays of masculinity."[80]

It is unfortunate that we know even less about the lives of those who were not able, or willing, to return to combat after a serious injury. According to Götz von Berlichingen, there would have been no future for him at all if he had been permanently incapacitated as a fighter. Did others share this sentiment? How did lower-ranking soldiers imagine their futures in comparable situations? To what extent did traumatic experiences shape the understanding of their social identities?[81] We should also look further to include the pain and trauma of those who survived violence, in its many forms, without being active or willing participants of a war situation, as demonstrated by Yoav Tirosh, Aleksandra Pfau, and Wendy J. Turner in this volume.[82] Research on these subjects is still ongoing. To this end, it is to be hoped that pain and trauma will become firmly established as categories of premodern disability history.

---

**80** Larissa Tracy and Kelly R. DeVries, "Introduction: Penetrating Medieval Wounds," in *Wounds and Wound Repair in Medieval Culture*, 1–21, at 4. They point to one of the most famous examples of this kind of bravado: Federico III da Montefeltro (1422–1482), who might have severed parts of his own nose after an injury to his face. On his "corporate identity," see also Auge, "So solt er im namen gottes."

**81** Meyer-Schilf, "dazu jch jedem raten wil."

**82** See also Selzer, "Das Leiden der Krieger," 88–93.

Chapter 8

# MECHANISM/ORGANISM

## THE PREMODERN IRON HAND AS CONCEPTUAL INTERFACE

JOHN GAGNÉ

AN ENGRAVING, NOW well known, of a sixteenth-century prosthetic iron hand hails us from the pages of one of Ambroise Paré's surgery manuals (figure 8.1).[1] Paré, surgeon-general to the kings of France in the 1550s, had honed his craft in the field, tending to wounded soldiers during the Italian Wars of the 1530s and '40s. After attaining his royal charge, Paré later settled in Paris and published a series of vernacular books on field medicine and its lessons, and—as was typical for surgeons to do—he called upon his own patients' cases to illustrate techniques and remedies. In one of Paré's richest volumes, the *Ten Books on Surgery* of 1564, he arranged to illustrate an array of prostheses and surgical techniques: some simple and effective, others remarkably complex.[2] The hand belongs to the more intricate branch, and historians treat it—if they bother to treat it at all—according to that intricacy: as an

1 Claude Menges, "Images et figures de l'anatomie et de la chirurgie: Les éditions illustrées d'Ambroise Paré," in *Ambroise Paré (1510–1590): Pratique et écriture de la science à la Renaissance. Actes du colloque de Pau (6–7 mai 1999)*, ed. Évelyne Berriot-Salvadore (Paris: Champion, 2003), 89–106.

2 Ambroise Paré, *Dix livres de la chirurgie, avec le magasin des instrumens necessaires à icelle* (Paris: Jean Le Royer, 1564). The prosthetic hand appears on fol. 121r.

**JOHN GAGNÉ** is Cassamarca Associate Professor of History at the University of Sydney. He is the author of *Milan Undone: Contested Sovereignties in the Italian Wars* (2021), co-editor of *Shadow Agents of Renaissance War: Suffering, Supporting, and Supplying Conflict in Italy and Beyond*, eds. Stephen Bowd et al. (2023), and co-author with Timothy McCall of *The Fabric of War: The Material Culture and Social Lives of Banners in Renaissance Europe* (2025). This chapter is an adaptation of an essay that will appear in French in *Vie et technique: Perspectives anthropologiques, historiques, et philosophiques*, eds. Leopoldo Iribarren, et al. (Paris: CNRS Éditions). The author gratefully acknowledges the permission to republish here.

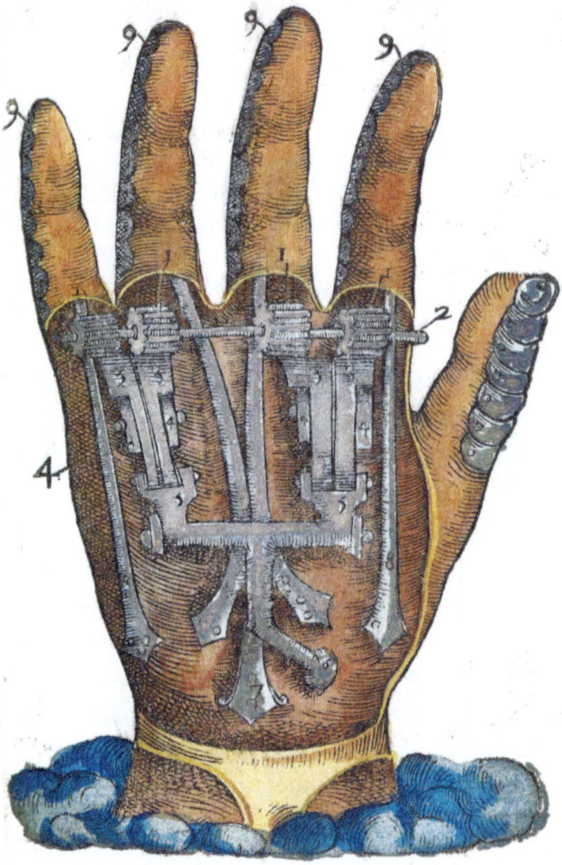

Figure 8.1. "Prosthetic Hand." Ambroise Paré, *Dix livres de la chirurgie, avec le Magasin des Instrumens necessaires à icelle* (Paris: Jean Le Royer 1564). This copy belongs to a set of hand-coloured images titled *Instrumenta chirurgiae et icones anathomicae*, 1564. London, Wellcome Library, EPB/B/4818, fol. 83r. Public Domain.

emblem of the sophistication of mid-sixteenth-century medical technology, or perhaps as an index of the creativity of Renaissance surgeons.[3] It is both of those things.

But let us dwell for a moment on the image of the prosthesis in the *Ten Books on Surgery*. Paré's illustrator slightly misleads us here. He does not show us the true metal edge of the iron hand, but rather conceals it behind a billow of cloud. The image-maker followed a longstanding typology for representing "detached body parts" viewers would otherwise expect to see as part of a larger whole. The conceit aimed to occlude the awkward detachment—to blur the jarringly hard edge—with a literal smokescreen, a representational convention that implied that the rest of a prodigious body

**3** On the historiographical denigration of material culture related to disability, see Katherine Ott, "Material Culture, Technology, and the Body in Disability History," in *The Oxford Handbook of Disability History*, eds. Michael Rembis et al. (Oxford: Oxford University Press, 2018), 129. I thank Bianca Frohne for this reference.

continued outside the image. Medieval illuminators deployed this technique in holy manuscripts when the hand of an unseen God dispensed benedictions from heaven; Paré's illustrator used it in similar ways for his spectacular prosthetics. The reason I say Paré's illustration misleads us is because it softly obscures the most compelling aspect of the prosthetic hand: its interface with humanity. Paré's image makes the object stand on its own; but in every meaningful way, it needs to be seen (and Paré built it to function) in dialogue with a human body. If we blow away the cloud, we finally encounter the strange reality of this object. It straddles the literal and figurative borders between human and machine, between organism and mechanism. It also articulates the link between the technologized body and the disabled person, a multivalent site that was at once physical, political, medical, conceptual, and functional.[4] This chapter invites us to think about these occluded realities.

While I too will reflect in this essay on disembodied iron hands— "in the clouds," as it were—my larger argument is that we should imagine the hand bound to human flesh: in that way, it functions as a conceptual tool for imagining the borders of the premodern body.[5] The prosthetic inhabited a generative frontier for thinking about—and for physically experimenting with the limits of—humanity in preindustrial Europe. For this reason, we must see it as an object with ambitious horizons, even though it was a relative rarity. But the rarity of a piece of history should not inhibit us from drawing cultural meaning from it. Just as historians of ideas seize upon telling passages in political or philosophical texts to point to the development of new intellectual territory, so also can we use the iron hand—itself a telling passage in the history of ideas—as a tool to understand conceptual play and discovery about the living body. It embodies the edge of the possible in the history of premodern human-machine interfaces.

The action that characterizes this zone of play is the grip-release button of the prosthetic hand. Most surviving iron hands between the fifteenth and the seventeenth centuries function according to a shared principle of operation. The fingers of the hand, with varying degrees of complexity, can

---

**4** Alison Kafer, *Feminist, Queer, Crip* (Bloomington: Indiana University Press, 2013), 103–28. I thank Bianca Frohne and Yoav Tirosh for pointing me toward Kafer's work.

**5** More broadly, see Jeffrey Jerome Cohen and Gail Weiss, "Introduction: Bodies at the Limit," in *Thinking the Limits of the Body*, eds. Jeffrey Jerome Cohen and Gail Weiss (Albany: State University of New York Press, 2003), 1–10; Sarah Künzler, *Flesh and Word: Reading Bodies in Old Norse-Icelandic and Early Irish Literature* (Berlin: de Gruyter, 2016), 1–21.

roll into a fist tight enough to hold some kind of object. This rolling action, the mechanics of which I will outline shortly, is never automated: it must be actioned somehow, most likely by the wearer's other hand. To open the iron fist, the wearer presses a button to release the gears and extend the digits, restoring the earlier state. In this single gesture the machine acts out the physics of the body to which it is attached. The button functions as motor impulse; inert matter makes as if to live. The release button, in brief, is the principle of animation at work, a moment of aliveness in which the machine acts in the place of bone and muscle while attached to the human body itself. Where else in preindustrial culture did a simple button unleash such astonishing potentials?

In this chapter, I will first outline the historical background and current state of knowledge about these prosthetic objects. I will introduce a few examples from museum collections in Fribourg, Milan, Paris, and Cambridge to offer a sense of the variety of design but also the commonality of features. Then I will situate the mechanization of the human body in the context of communities of artisans trained in gearwork (gunners, clockmakers, locksmiths) and propose that these objects appeared across diverse class groups, most crucially amongst artisans themselves. Finally, I will conclude with a few remarks on the afterlife of the iron hand. Released from its body, the iron hand attracted new forms of attention and representation. It became a secular relic that demanded fresh modes of display and interpretation. By the eighteenth century, wood had begun to replace iron as the preferred material for prosthetic hands. At that same moment, the metal hand came to be imagined as a symbol of "medieval" ingenuity and had already taken its place in the early modern lexicon as a metaphor to describe unstoppable, impersonal forces. Detached from its body and refigured as a discursive entity, the iron hand lived on.

There are perhaps thirty to forty European metal prosthetic hands that survive from before 1700. In a book published in 1984, Liebhard Löffler catalogued many known exempla ranging from the fifteenth to the twentieth centuries.[6] Here I focus mostly on objects unknown to Löffler as a way to extend our analytical understanding of the objects.[7] The earliest surviving

---

**6** Liebhard Löffler, *Der Ersatz für die obere Extremität: Die Entwicklung von den ersten Zeugnissen bis heute* (Stuttgart: Ferdinand Enke, 1984).

**7** For further recent study of these objects, see Mareike Heide, *Holzbein und Eisenhand: Prothesen in der Frühen Neuzeit* (Frankfurt: Campus, 2019); Heidi Hausse, *The Malleable Body: Surgeons, Artisans, and Amputees in Early Modern Germany* (Manchester: Manchester University Press, 2023).

metal hands appear to date from the fifteenth century: one prosthetic in the Fribourg collection has a particularly strong provenance helping us to date it to 1476, and giving us the identities of both maker and wearer.[8] When I sometimes begin to suspect that all our surviving iron hands are nineteenth-century forgeries masquerading as premodern objects, this one reminds me that we do have objects with solid premodern attributions.[9] It is also an object that unites war and disability, as we will see when I touch on the Fribourg hand in greater detail shortly. The manufacture of these tools long predates the fifteenth century. Pliny's *Natural History* offers the well-known ancient case of the Roman general Marcus Sergius who fought with a right limb made of iron in the second Punic War; from Plutarch we also learn of Archimedes's immense iron claw for sinking enemy ships, sometimes imagined in later centuries as a gargantuan hand.[10] Medieval writers show awareness of these tools as well: in the 1350s, Petrarch listed "wooden feet, iron hands, and wax noses" as examples of the ingenious ways that humankind learns to make up for bodily imperfections.[11] Despite fleeting textual references like Petrarch's, no mechanical prostheses from the fourteenth century appear to survive.

Most of the early extant hands, which include the one in Fribourg and three in the armoury of the Museo Stibbert in Florence, have rudimentary mechanisms in which all four fingers attach to a thin metal rod running along the major knuckle joint at the top of the palm: a central toothed circular wheel rolls with the rod and closes all the fingers together at the same time.[12] The thumb typically remains immobile. Other more sophisticated models permit flexion of two fingers at a time, and still others—including

---

**8** Raoul Blanchard, "Ulrich Wagner: Eiserne Kunsthand des Büchsenmeisters, 1476," *Blätter des MKGF* (2000–2002), four unpaginated pages.

**9** For one example of the nineteenth-century vogue for copying (or inventing) Renaissance metalwork, see Lionello G. Boccia and José A. Godoy, "Una sala d'armi fra scena e istorismo," in *Museo Poldi Pezzoli: Armeria*, eds. Lionello G. Boccia and José A. Godoy, 2 vols. (Milan: Electa, 1985), 1:13–30.

**10** Pliny the Elder, *Natural History*, trans. H. Rackham (Cambridge, MA: Harvard University Press, 1942), bk. 2, chap. 28, at 2:574–75; Plutarch, *Lives*, trans. B. Perin (Cambridge, MA: Harvard University Press, 1917), at 5:474–75 ("Life of Marcellus, XV").

**11** Francesco Petrarca, *Remedies for Fortune Fair and Foul*, trans. Conrad H. Rawski, 5 vols. (Bloomington: Indiana University Press), bk. 2, dialogue 93, at 3:227

**12** For these prostheses, see Vittorio Putti, "Protesi antiche," *La chirurgia degli organi di movimento* 9, nos. 4–5 (1925): 495–526, at 509–15.

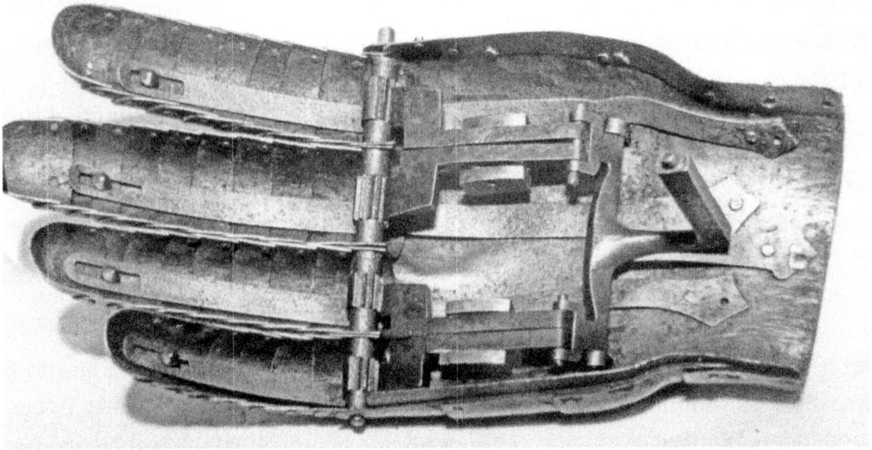

Figure 8.2. The interior of the "Paré hand" during its restoration in 2000. Paris, Musée de la médecine. Photograph by author from restoration file image.

Paré's hand—equip each finger with its own toothed gear, allowing joints and minor knuckles to curl or articulate separately.[13]

The Medical Museum in Paris houses an exact replica of Paré's hand (figure 8.2).[14] It is so close in appearance and mechanical contrivance to the Paré woodcuts as to be almost uncanny. Its provenance is uncertain. The museum itself dates the hand to the sixteenth century, although it was almost certainly constructed in later centuries as a retrospective fabrication based on the published woodcut design or even as a forgery.[15] Photographs prior to its restoration in October 2000 show it rusted and non-functional. During that process the restorer dismantled it, removed the rust that caked it, and reassembled it, no doubt in hopes of testing its functionality. But even after the cleaning, the hand remains difficult to manoeuvre, as I had the opportunity to recognize for myself with the generous permission of the museum in April 2017. The toothed wheels do not catch properly, meaning it is impossible for the hand to form and retain a fist. Moreover, unlike the woodcut in

---

**13** Heidi Hausse, "The Locksmith, the Surgeon, and the Mechanical Hand: Communicating Technical Knowledge in Early Modern Europe," *Technology and Culture* 60, no. 1 (2019): 34–64, especially 44–47.

**14** Paris, Musée d'Histoire de la Médecine, undated, Inv. MHM 90-151-1 ("Main de fer de Paré").

**15** Paris, Musée d'Histoire de la Médecine, Provenance and restoration file of the "Main de fer de Paré." The file makes no mention of forgery but dates the hand to the sixteenth century.

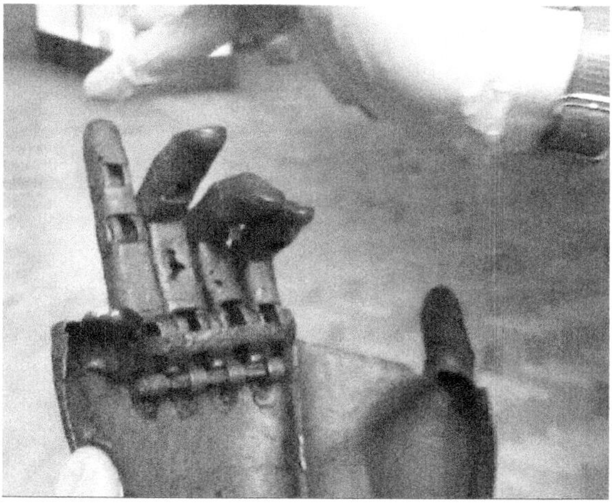

Figure 8.3. Interacting with the Cambridge, Fitzwilliam Museum hand, ca. 1550. The hand has been opened to show the internal mechanism, now broken. The fingers move only by virtue of the hinged knuckles. Photograph by author.

Paré's surgery manual in which the thumb sits alongside the four fingers, the prosthesis itself has an opposable thumb. That placement theoretically offers a more useful design for enclosing objects in a fist, but the thumb's placement in fact impedes the full movement of two fingers, blocking their path of movement and preventing them from curling forward. The design is in so many respects visually perfect, but at the same time it is less than functional in operation.

Experimentation in the zone between functionality, appearance, and movement characterizes many of the surviving hands. The unopposable thumb on one of the two sixteenth-century hands in the Fitzwilliam Museum in Cambridge is all but useless (its knuckle pivots impotently just a few millimetres), but the fingers—even with the hand's mechanism now emptied out—show a remarkable range and fluidity of movement that surprised the curator Victoria Avery and me as we tugged and folded them (figure 8.3).[16] Those Fitzwilliam fingers moved with unsettling smoothness and vivacity; at times they seemed almost to move without much prompting from us. In these and other examples, the nearly universal features of the prosthetic hand in the fifteenth and sixteenth centuries included the toothed wheel (to close the fist) and the release button (to open it). But in their diversity and particularity, they also show us how various makers developed a range of ways to solve the question of how best to manage internal action and scope of movement.[17] Careful observation of the human hand generated ways to

**16** Cambridge, Fitzwilliam Museum, ca. 1550, Inv. M.23-1942 ("German hand").

**17** See also Hausse, "The Locksmith," 53–56.

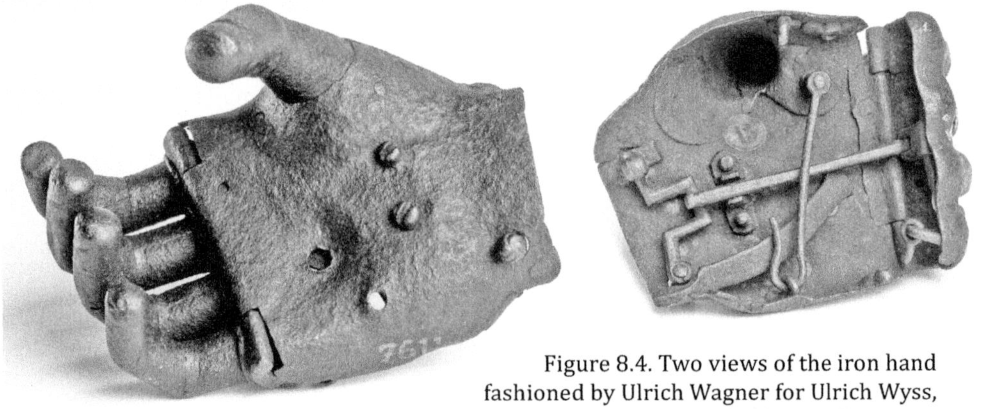

Figure 8.4. Two views of the iron hand fashioned by Ulrich Wagner for Ulrich Wyss, 1476. Fribourg, Musée d'Art et d'Histoire, MAHF 7611. Used with permission.

conceptualize—and to reproduce—ingenious mechanical facsimiles of its physiology using the technical *savoir-faire* of Renaissance metalworkers.

Who were the makers of these instruments? Scholars have often assumed that they must have been armourers, since the prostheses employed the same iron and sometimes—as in the fingers of Paré's hand made just like the lames of an armoured gauntlet—the same techniques. It should not surprise us if armourers took part in conceiving or fabricating these objects, but to my mind the key lies in Ambroise Paré's mention that in order to find someone who could fashion the mechanism of his hand he approached a locksmith in Paris, the man he called "le petit Lorrain."[18] Here we are not far away from the metalcrafts of the armourer, but we are more squarely in the world of artisans who worked with small metal parts—this group includes gunsmiths, clockmakers, and forgers of surgical tools. That cluster of artisans had been in dialogue at least since the fourteenth century as they developed communities of technique that overlapped fruitfully—gunsmiths borrowed trigger technology from lock-makers, and the prosthetician imported ideas from the entire fraternity. These artisans often came into contact during the wars of the fourteenth and fifteenth centuries, as their metalcrafts came to be employed in an array of military applications.[19] The vast majority of wearers of iron hands we see in these

18 Paré, *Dix livres de la chirurgie*, fols. 118v–119r.

19 John Gagné, "Emotional Attachments: Iron Hands, their Makers, and their Wearers, 1450–1600," in *Feeling Things: Objects and Emotions through History*, eds. Stephanie Downes et al. (Oxford: Oxford University Press, 2018), 137–42.

centuries were warriors, especially gunners, whose manual dexterity was their prime asset. While it is true that some prosthetic recipients of the sixteenth century were elite knights—like the renowned Swabian captain Götz von Berlichingen (1480–1562), his near-contemporary the Alsatian Hans von Mittelhausen († 1564), or the French Huguenot commander François de la Noue (1531–1591)—others were much less illustrious, a fact that should help us to see the iron hand not just as a luxury object for wealthy fighters maimed in battle, but also as the product of a fraternity of metalworking professions that could use their skill to aid their comrades.[20] Simply put, it could be a case of smith helping smith.

The case that establishes this possibility is the Fribourg hand (figure 8.4). In 1476, at the Battle of Murten between Burgundy and the Swiss Confederacy, the Fribourg artillery master Ulrich Wyss lost his hand in an explosion. Because he was maimed in the service of the city, the Canton's governing council asked one of its own members for help. That man was Ulrich Wagner, a metalworker originally from Munich. Wagner became a citizen of Fribourg in 1465 and died in 1485. During those twenty years, he offered his services on several occasions to his adopted home. He fashioned clocks for both religious and state buildings, wrought-iron grills for the cathedral choir and for the state chancery, forty-four cannons for civic defence, and the iron hand for Ulrich Wyss.[21] The mechanical skill of one artisan remade the body of another, at the cost to the city of £22.[22]

Many prospects emerge from the Wyss-Wagner exchange, including the notion that a prosthetic could function as a gift; in this case, a grateful municipal council wished to compensate one of its servants for his sacrifice with a form of reincorporation.[23] A similar agreement appears to have been reached in the 1490s between the Venetian senate and some hired gunners who had their hands amputated when they were captured by an enemy captain at Pisa, and they later presented themselves to the Venetian senate hoping to petition for aid. "They gave their word to the Senate," Pietro Bembo tells us in his *History of Venice*, "that once they had artificial iron hands they

**20** For more on Götz, see Bianca Frohne's chapter in this volume.

**21** Marianne Rolle, "Wagner, Ulrich," in *Historisches Lexikon der Schweiz. HLS*, https://hls-dhs-dss.ch/de/articles/010796/2012-07-02/, accessed July 10, 2022.

**22** For the price, see Blanchard, "Ulrich Wagner," [2]. Symbol: £ = 1 livre.

**23** For similar cases of fighters gaining privileges for physical sacrifices made in state service, see the chapter by Quentin Verreycken in this volume.

would return to their trade and make themselves useful to the Republic and, if sent back to Pisa, would avenge their injuries."[24]

The artisan's hand, it hardly needs to be said, was the site of his most precious asset.[25] An artisan's honour inhered in his hands, and a disabled hand threatened his livelihood. Feuding artisans might even attack each other's hands, as happened in 1496 in Milan, when a dispute between court embroiderers culminated with three of them attacking their rival in the street where the armourers plied their trade, cutting three fingers off the victim's left hand.[26] The craftsman's hands operated not just as his tools but as a site of knowledge, and this in part explains the impulse to equip injured artisans with artificial limbs: to endow them with an implement just as marvellous as the one they had lost.

The hand was also one of the chief avenues into knowledge about the human body: Aristotle and Galen had both forwarded the hand as the best example of Nature's ability to form human anatomy suited to its purpose.[27] It was perhaps for this reason that the sixteenth century's most celebrated anatomist, the Flemish surgeon Andreas Vesalius, had his author-portrait engraved for his 1543 textbook so as to draw attention to his hands: the twenty-eight-year-old surgeon looks at us as he pauses from his dissection of a flayed arm (figure 8.5).[28] With pen and paper nearby, he has just scribbled his findings on the "mobile muscles of the fingers." He holds the flayed arm-muscle with one hand, and with the other he draws out the veins and tendons from within the corpse's open palm. The anatomist above all knew how hands could produce knowledge, both his own as a master surgeon and those of the corpse, offering up secrets from within their workings. The tendons of the hand had interested many earlier anatomists as

**24** Pietro Bembo, *History of Venice*, trans. R. W. Ulery Jr. (Cambridge, MA: Harvard University Press, 2007), bk. 4, § 27, at 1:278–79. See also Gagné, "Emotional Attachments," 135–37 for further archival references to these gunners.

**25** Pamela H. Smith, *From Lived Experience to the Written Word: Reconstructing Practical Knowledge in the Early Modern World* (Chicago: University of Chicago Press, 2022), 20–42.

**26** Milan, Archivio di Stato, Carteggio Sforzesco 1135, Milano Città, settembre–ottobre 1496: letter of September 12, 1496.

**27** Aristotle, *Parts of Animals*, trans. A. L. Peck and E. S. Forster (Cambridge, MA: Harvard University Press, 1937), bk. 4, at 370–73; Galen, *On the Usefulness of the Parts of the Body*, trans. M. Talladge May (Ithaca: Cornell University Press, 1968), at 1:68.

**28** Andreas Vesalius, *De humani corporis fabrica libri septem* (Basel: Johannes Oporini, 1543). See the author portrait just before sig. A r.

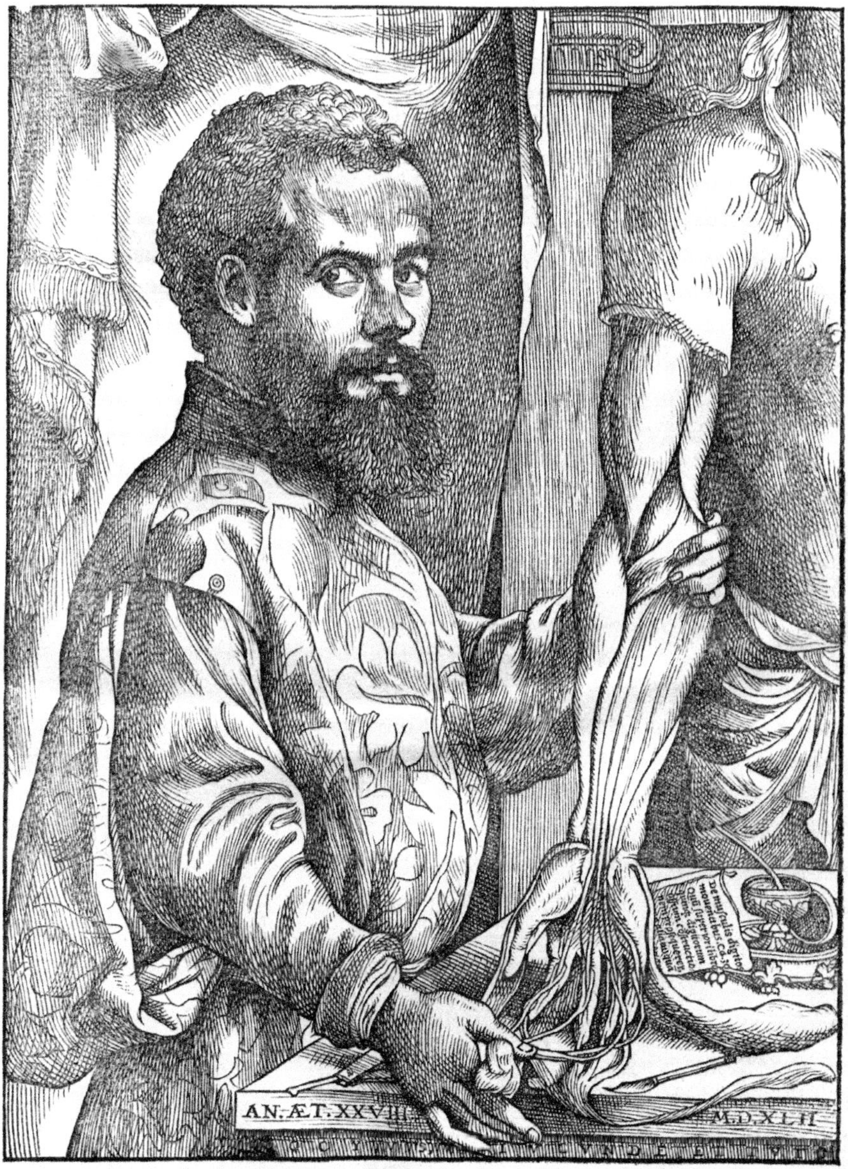


Figure 8.5. "Portrait of Andreas Vesalius," in Vesalius' *De humani corporis fabrica libri septem* (Basel: Johannes Oporinus, 1543). Courtesy of the Wellcome Library, London.

well, not least Leonardo da Vinci who studied them around 1510.[29] In Paré's 1564 woodcut we may even see echoes of the Leonardo-Vesalius tradition: the hand has been opened in a cut-away illustration to display its elegant internal machinery. One of the questions the sixteenth-century iron hand permits us to ask is how it fused the practical identification of organism with mechanism: if we think ahead to the next century and the rise of Cartesian ideas of the mechanical body, these were notions inspired at least in part by Descartes's own experience with machines. Can we see the roots of the philosophical program of seventeenth-century mechanism in tools such as these, machines that artisans had already developed to show the body reimagined as a mechanical simulacrum? An artificial hand in Paris dating to the seventeenth century experiments with the fusion of organic and mechanical by using cotton or hemp strings as tendons and by padding the finger-tips with minuscule pillows of leather.[30] In so doing it makes an argument for the blurred space between the mechanical and the natural that would become increasingly central to the medical discourse of early modernity.

While the prosthetic could be a tool for thinking about life, it also survived its wearer's death: when the church of Balbronn was being restored in 1908, the only body part that workmen discovered in Hans von Mittelhausen's 1564 tomb was his rusted iron hand.[31] Such objects became secular relics in their own right, tokens of wonder or testimonies to ingenuity. Two iron hands ("with springs in them to hold firmly whatever they grasp") appear in the collection of Ferdinando Cospi in Bologna, the inheritor of the vast collection belonging to the sixteenth-century naturalist Ulisse Aldrovandi—one of them hangs in the arches of Museo Cospiano in the engraving published in 1677.[32] Similar hands found their way into the massive armour collections of nineteenth-century collectors like Frederick Stibbert in Florence, Richard Zschille in Großenhain, and Karl Gimbel in Baden-Baden, or into medical collections assembled by doctors like Noël

**29** Windsor, Royal Collection Trust, RCIN 919009. Folio from Leonardo da Vinci, *Anatomical Manuscript A: The Bones, Muscles and Tendons of the Hand*, ca. 1510–1511.

**30** Paris, Musée d'Histoire de la Médecine, Inv. MHM-2022-84 ("Main de fer du XVIIe siècle").

**31** Robert Forrer, "Die eiserne Hand von Balbronn (Elsass)," *Zeitschrift für historische Waffenkunde* 7, no. 1 (1915–1917): 102–7, at 103.

**32** Lorenzo Legati, *Museo Cospiano, annesso a quello del famoso Ulisse Aldrovandi e donato alla sua patria dall'illustrissimo Signor Ferdinando Cospi* (Bologna: Giacomo Monti, 1677), 252, item 2.

Hamonic in Paris (later purchased by Henry Wellcome in London) or Howard Dittrick in Cleveland.[33]

I will only briefly touch here on the interest in metal hands in the years around 1800, an era when, perhaps not coincidentally, they had largely been replaced by prostheses made of materials more amenable to the wearer, especially wood.[34] In this time when iron hands had almost entirely disappeared as bodily tools, they could be reimagined as historical artefacts. The era of the late Enlightenment and early industrial revolution became fascinated with tales of late-medieval warriors and their technology of war, most centrally Johann Wolfgang von Goethe's 1773 drama about Götz von Berlichingen, who died in 1562.[35] That play stimulated curiosity about Götz's surviving two prosthetics still held at his castle in Jagsthausen, an inquisitiveness evidenced in the small book of engravings that revealed the ingenious components of Götz's hand as incised by Goethe's friend, the Swiss engraver Christian von Mechel and published on the occasion of the Congress of Vienna in 1815 (figure 8.6).[36] Goethe's influence may also explain why the Edinburgh novelist Sir Walter Scott told of dismembered hands in his *Fair Maid of Perth* of 1828, a tale set in early fifteenth-century Scotland. Scott had in fact translated Goethe's play into English in 1798–1799, and it set him on a hunt for Scottish antiquities of a similar vintage.[37] In his historical guidebook, the *Border Antiquities of England and Scotland* of 1817, he and his co-authors included the "steel hand of Carslogie," a prosthesis that

---

**33** For Stibbert, see Putti, "Protesi antiche," 509–15; for Zschille, see Robert Forrer, *Die Waffensammlung des Herrn Stadtrath Rich. Zschille in Grossenhain (Sachsen)*, 2 vols. (Berlin: Mertens, 1894), 1:4, item 86, and image on table 19; for Gimbel, see Rudolph Lepke's Kunst-Auctions-Haus, Berlin, *Waffen- und Kunst-Sammlung Karl Gimbel* (Berlin: Lepke, 1904), 12, item 111, and table VII; for the hand at Dittrick's Museum, see Löffler, *Der Ersatz für die obere Extremität*, 38–39.

**34** The reasons for this shift are unclear and require further research. It is also possible that wooden hands existed in earlier centuries, although most of our textual references are to iron ones (as opposed to wooden legs). Wooden hands would naturally have a much lower chance of survival over many centuries.

**35** Johann Wolfgang von Goethe, *Götz von Berlichingen mit der eisernen Hand: Ein Schauspiel* (Frankfurt-Leipzig: s.n., 1775 [3rd edition]).

**36** Christian von Mechel, *Die eiserne Hand des tapfern deutschen Ritters Götz von Berlichingen, wie selbige noch bei seiner Familie in Franken aufbewahrt wird* (Berlin: Georg Decker, 1815). See also Andreas Otte, "Christian von Mechel's Reconstructive Drawings of the Second 'Iron Hand' of Franconian Knight Gottfried (Götz) von Berlichingen (1480–1562)," *Prosthesis* 3 (2021): 105–09.

**37** Michael Wood, "On Form and Feeling: German Drama and the Young Walter Scott," *German Life and Letters* 71, no. 4 (2018): 395–414.

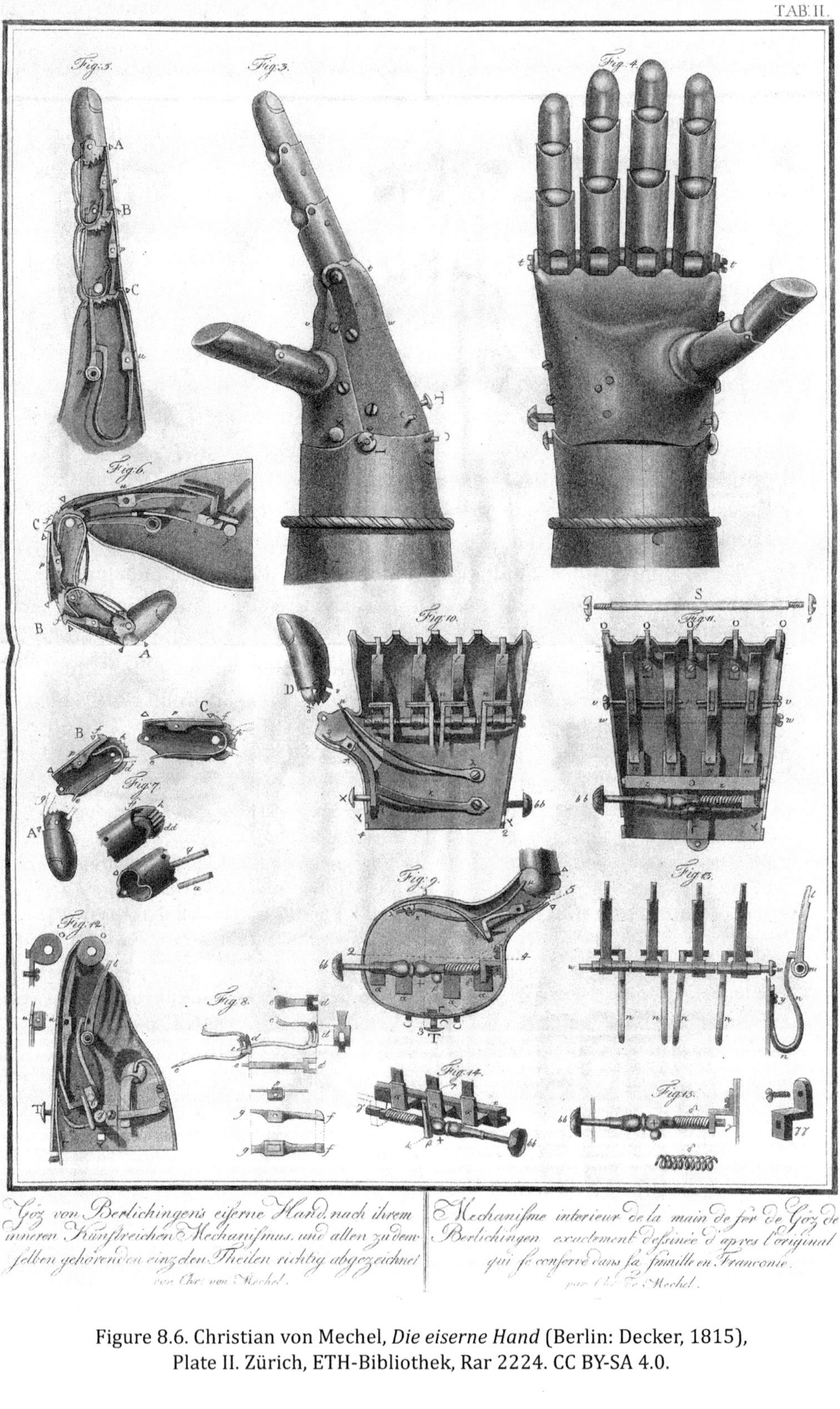

Figure 8.6. Christian von Mechel, *Die eiserne Hand* (Berlin: Decker, 1815), Plate II. Zürich, ETH-Bibliothek, Rar 2224. CC BY-SA 4.0.

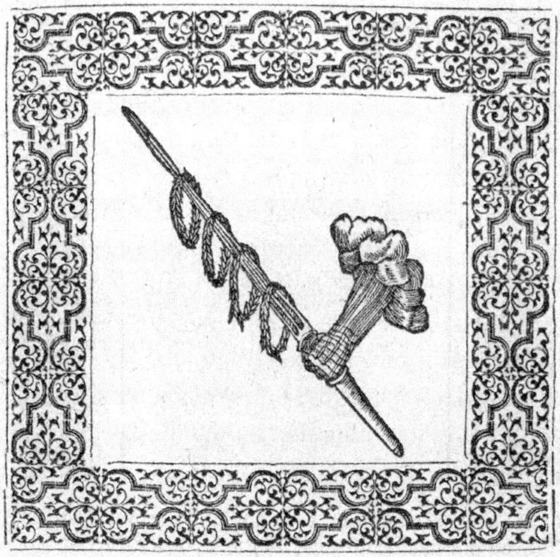

Figure 8.7. "Strongly and bravely." The iron hand of Marcus Sergius in Geffrey Whitney's *Choice of Emblemes* (Leiden: Plantin, 1586). Courtesy of The Huntington Library, San Marino, CA. Public domain.

had belonged since "time immemorial" to the Clephane family, was photographed in the early 1930s, and now seems to belong to the private collections of the Marquess of Northumberland.[38] The early nineteenth-century fascination with the old steel hand pointed to an artisanally ingenious and militarily virtuous European past that seemed to be disappearing in an age of ubiquitous mechanization.

By way of concluding, let us return to those earlier centuries and appreciate the ways that the iron hand survived and transcended its wearer by assuming a discursive function in early modernity as a descriptor of implacable and impersonal forces. Seventeenth-century English writers, for example, used the phrase "iron hand" to refer to God, love, time, war, justice, law, death, age, necessity, heaven, and nature. While the phrase initially struck me as a generic metaphor for firmness of resolve, with further reading I began to see deeper possibilities. The metaphor of the iron hand may possibly have had origins in the evocatively tight grip of the metal prosthetic. The first printed appearances of the phrase "iron hand" in English date to the last three decades of the sixteenth century: they mostly invoke the metal hand of Pliny's Marcus Sergius, as non-Latinate readers could have gathered as early as 1566 with John Alday's English summary of Pliny.[39] After that date, references to Sergius become more frequent, such as Samuel Rowland's

**38** Walter Scott, *The Border Antiquities of England and Scotland*, 2 vols. (London: Longman, 1814), 2:206–7. For the photographs, see London, Wellcome Collection, Wellcome Trust Corporate Archive, "M Series" glass plate negatives M0001978-M0001978.

**39** John Alday, *A Summarie of the Antiquities, and Wonders of the Worlde, Abstracted out of the Sixteen First Books of the Excellent Historiographer Plinie* (London: Henry Denham, 1566), sig. C iii v.

*Choice of Change*, a book of memory which uses the principle of triplicity to associate three facts with every item to be remembered ("Marcus Sergius had the use of 3 hands: A right hand. A left hand. An iron hand in stead of his right hand.")[40] Geffrey Whitney's 1586 *Choice of Emblemes* even illustrated Marcus Sergius's hand as a device with the motto "strongly and bravely" and a free-floating metal gauntlet wielding a lance bedecked with laurels (figure 8.7).[41] In Whitney's image, the disembodied hand once again returns to the clouds, finding a metaphorical significance that we might almost call cosmic: by taking on a life of its own, the iron hand could function as an idea of inanimate and inexorable power, an unliving thing that nonetheless exercised vital dynamism.

Such cultural frameworks for metaphorizing disability, moreover, have been explored by literary scholars. In their book *Narrative Prosthesis*, David T. Mitchell and Sharon L. Snyder trace a much-used traditional discursive pattern that is also a paradox: disabled people have long been socially and politically invisible, but storytelling has regularly relied upon their bodily differences as a potent symbolic tool.[42] In their analysis, Mitchell and Snyder offer examples ranging from ancient Greek myth to contemporary American literature, illustrating disability's extensive use as a cultural idea across time and space. The extraordinary body, and its divergence from norms, has frequently served to generate narrative energy and produce novelty by "posing disability as an 'alien' terrain that promises the revelation of a previously uncomprehended experience."[43] Mitchell and Snyder focus mostly on literary narrative, but their analysis seems capable of encompassing the kind of semantic ideation that the iron hand occupied from the sixteenth century onward. Seeing the iron hand metaphor through their interpretive lens helps to explain how and why the prosthesis became its own concept. Uncoupled from the bodies it existed to service, it could assume new life as a discursive entity and exemplify the paradox *Narrative Prosthesis* proposes to uncover.

---

**40** Samuel Rowland, *Choise of Change: Containing the Triplicitie of Diuinitie, Philosophie and Poetrie...* (London: Roger Warde, 1585), unpaginated, entry 77.

**41** Geffrey Whitney, *A Choice of Emblemes, and Other Deuises, for the Most Parte Gathered out of Sundrie Writers, Englished and Moralized* (Leiden: In the house of Christopher Plantyn, by Francis Raphelengius, 1585), "Fortiter et Feliciter," 115.

**42** David T. Mitchell and Sharon L. Snyder, *Narrative Prosthesis: Disability and the Dependencies of Discourse* (Ann Arbor: University of Michigan Press, 2000), 47–64. I thank the anonymous reviewer for pointing me in this direction.

**43** Mitchell and Snyder, *Narrative Prosthesis*, 55.

Finally, the iron hand also seems useful as a bridge between two strands in thinking the body that seem only sometimes to intersect: first, the future-oriented concept of transhumanism, whose aim is to imagine the evolution of humanity alongside technology; and second, critical histories of disability, devoted to recovering and interpreting a fuller spectrum of past bodily experiences. Both of them are often casually, and erroneously, thought to emerge in the nineteenth century, though we know they are many more centuries in the making.[44] The iron hand belongs to both of those strands, and its history reveals not only transhumanism's late medieval instantiations, but also that era's ambitions to imagine and practice embodiment in all its multifarious realities.

**44** For transhumanism's deep histories, see Peter Harrison and Joseph Wolyniack, "The History of 'Transhumanism,'" *Notes and Queries* 62, no. 3 (2015): 465–67.

Chapter 9

# AFTER COMBAT

## WAR WOUNDS, SOLDIERS' BENEFITS, AND DYNASTIC POLICIES IN THE BURGUNDIAN-HABSBURG ARMIES (1363–1506)

MICHAEL DEPRETER

OVER THE PAST fifty years, the history of war has been considerably renewed. Beyond strategy and tactics, war is now studied in a wider context, in relation to the societies wherein it was embedded and which it contributed to shaping. Reputed historians such as Philippe Contamine, John R. Hale, and Frank Tallett laid the foundations for studies in *War and Society*, paying new attention to how military institutions were shaped by social structures, cultural norms, economic constraints, and political action.[1] Initially, a renewed history of war largely focused on organizational aspects such as financing, recruitment, and logistics, rather than on the experience and fate of soldiers during and after conflicts in which they partook. Hence, when considering soldiers' care, historians of early modern and modern times, especially, have given substantial attention to institutions developed by different polities to

---

* I would like to express heartfelt thanks to Ninon Dubourg and Christophe Masson, editors of this volume and initiators of a very stimulating seminar series on Disability and War in the Middle Ages, for associating me with this collective endeavour, as well as to all participants in the series and subsequent workshop for thoughtful and engaging discussions. Special thanks are due to Bianca Frohne and Christopher J. Knüsel for detailed written feedback on a first full draft. Symbol: £ = 1 livre of 40 Flemish groats.

1 Philippe Contamine, *Guerre, État et société à la fin du Moyen Âge: Études sur les armées des rois de France, 1337–1494* (Paris: Mouton, 1972); John R. Hale, *War and Society in Renaissance Europe, 1450–1620* (Montreal: McGill-Queen's University Press, 1985); Frank Tallett, *War and Society in Early Modern Europe, 1495–1715* (Abingdon: Routledge, 1992).

**MICHAEL DEPRETER** (UCLouvain campus Saint-Louis Bruxelles / University of Oxford) is a historian of war specializing in the social, economic, and political organization of warfare in the late medieval and early modern Low Countries. His PhD thesis (Université libre de Bruxelles, 2014) examines the role of gunpowder artillery in Burgundian-Habsburg state-formation processes.

care for soldiers who incurred often severe injuries in military service. Their studies usually rely on archival material produced by or for institutions such as the renowned Hôtel des Invalides, founded in Paris by Louis XIV in 1670, or the less reputed royal military hospital founded in Mechlin by the Spanish monarchs during the Eighty Years' War (1585, founded again in 1637).[2] The nature of those sources most often led to focus on the institutional and day-to-day workings of these military establishments, leaving the reader in the dark regarding the main beneficiaries.[3]

During the later Middle Ages, such specialized foundations taking care of soldiers having suffered long- or short-term injuries in combat did not, or barely, exist.[4] Late medieval combatants from all social classes were not spared, however, from all sorts of injuries.[5] Benefitting from cross-fertilizing exchanges with specialists in disability history, this article aims to contribute to the history of those soldiers who, waging war in service of late medieval authorities, saw their bodies injured in warfare. Whereas the medical staff hired and the equipment acquired by English kings or Burgundian princes to treat their soldiers' wounds are not unknown,[6]

**2** John Childs and Jean-Pierre Bois, "Invalids," in *A Dictionary of Military History and the Art of War*, eds. André Corvisier and John Childs (Oxford: Blackwell, 1994), 398; André Corvisier, "Medical Services," in *A Dictionary of Military History*, 496; Eugeen van Autenboer, "De eerste stichting van het Spaanse Gasthuis, 1567–1568," *Mechelse Bijdragen* 10 (1943): 99–108; Lucienne van Meerbeeck, "L'hôpital royal de l'armée espagnole à Malines en l'an 1637," *Bulletin du Cercle royal archéologique, littéraire et artistique de Malines* 54 (1950): 81–125; Lucienne van Meerbeeck, "Le service sanitaire de l'armée espagnole des Pays-Bas à la fin du XVIe et au XVIIe siècle," *Revue internationale d'histoire militaire* 20 (1959): 479–93; Fanny Verslype, "L'hôpital royal militaire de Malines (1585–1701): Une 'machine à guérir'?," in *Actes du 11e congrès de l'Association des cercles francophones d'histoire et d'archéologie de Belgique et 58e congrès de la Fédération des Cercles d'archéologie et d'histoire de Belgique*, ed. Jean-Marie Cauchies (Tournai: Hannonia, 2024), 2:381–94.

**3** See also: Antoon Hubert Marie Kerkhoff, *Over de geneeskundige verzorging in het Staatse leger* (Nijmegen: Katholieke Universiteit te Nijmegen, 1976); Matthew Neufeld, "Neither Private Contractors nor Productive Partners: The English Fiscal-Naval State and London Hospitals, 1660–1715," *The International Journal of Maritime History* 28 (2016): 268–90.

**4** Childs and Bois, "Invalids," 397.

**5** Alain Mounier-Khun, "Blessures et chirurgie de guerre au Moyen Âge en Occident," *Revue historique des armées* 239 (2005): 4–17; Robert C. Woosnam-Savage and Kelly DeVries, "Battle Trauma in Medieval Warfare: Wounds, Weapons and Armor," in *Wounds and Wound Repair in Medieval Culture*, eds. Larissa Tracy and Kelly DeVries (Leiden: Brill, 2015), 27–56.

**6** George Ernest Gask, "The Medical Services of Henry the Fifth's Campaign of the

long-term practices and policies of care beyond immediate treatment on or off the battlefield have barely received attention.[7] Beyond a campaign, why, how, and how frequently did late medieval authorities intervene for further care? In other words, can we uncover the perceptions late medieval authorities and their subjects had of injuries incurred in war, and how these possibly fluid perceptions affected policies towards temporarily or enduringly disabled combatants?[8]

To examine these questions, the Burgundian Low Countries offer a rich testing ground. First, from the late fourteenth to the early sixteenth century, the Valois dukes of Burgundy and their first Habsburg successors repeatedly waged war to consolidate what progressively became a composite state ruled by one single dynasty. Indeed, the principates of Philip the Bold (1363–1404) and Philip the Fair (1494–1506) constitute sensible *termini post* and *ad quem*, respectively, both in terms of military and administrative organization: despite progressive territorial aggrandizement and corresponding army growth as new principalities were incorporated to the Burgundian dominion, patterns of army recruitment and mechanisms of pay remained fairly consistent but for the brief period of Charles the Bold's reforms (1467–1477) which, as will be examined, prompted temporary changes in policy towards injured soldiers too. The acquisition of the Spanish and Imperial crowns and

---

Somme in 1415," *Proceedings of the Royal Society of Medicine* 16 (1923): 1–10; Francis Pierrepont Barnard, "Edward IV's Army Surgeons," *British Medical Journal* 1 (1926): 960–61; Joseph Balon, "Un train sanitaire namurois durant le siège de Calais en 1347," *Annales de la Société archéologique de Namur* 39 (1931): 269–99. For Burgundy, see most recently Rabah Ali Bacha, "Les blessures de guerre à la fin du Moyen Âge," 2 vols. (PhD diss. Université Lille III–Charles de Gaulle, 2010), which uncovers particularly rich source material up to 1477. See also, in this volume, Wendy J. Turner, "Investigating the Lifecycle of the Medieval English Soldier: Disability, Mental Trauma, and Medicine in Connection with War in Late Medieval English Records."

**7** A notable exception on Swiss soldiers is Karolina Meyer-Schilf, "'Dazu jch jedem raten will / er buw uf kriegen nit zu vil': Grundüberlegungen und Forschungsperspektiven zum Umgang mit Kriegsinvalidität im Spätmittelalter," in *Phänomene der "Behinderung" im Alltag: Bausteine zu einer Disability History der Vormoderne*, ed. Cordula Nolte (Affalterbach: Didymos, 2013), 113–23. Special thanks are due to Bianca Frohne for pointing me to this article.

**8** Irina Metzler, *A Social History of Disability in the Middle Ages: Cultural Considerations of Physical Impairment* (New York: Routledge, 2013), 1–11; Bianca Frohne and Klaus Peter Horn, "On the Fluidity of 'Disability' in Medieval and Early Modern Societies," in *The Imperfect Historian: Disability Histories in Europe*, eds. Sebastian Barsch et al. (Frankfurt am Main: Lang, 2013), 17–40. In this volume, see also Ninon Dubourg and Christophe Masson, "Disability and War: Becoming, Surviving, Managing."

territories by Charles V (1506–1555), on the other hand, not only led to an unprecedented geographical and military scale-increase but also prompted administrative changes which, already apparent during Philip the Fair's Spanish voyages in terms of expenditure, reflected a progressive geographic shift away from the Low Countries, the latter becoming part of a wider empire stretching well-beyond the scope of this contribution.[9] Secondly, the substantial financial records left by the Burgundian administration allow us to examine the nature of existing policies in the absence of official regulatory texts revealing measures taken for injured soldiers. An almost continuous series of accounts (1363–1506) provided by the receiver responsible to pay out pensions and monetary gifts at a central, courtly level, the *Recette générale des finances*, is complemented by the more fragmentarily preserved accounts of the *Argentier*, in charge of gift-giving and pensions from 1468 to 1477, and again from 1484 to 1492. Although local and regional receivers regularly paid out gifts and pensions for practical, logistical reasons of cash-flow within the Burgundian administrative system, the records issued from central bookkeeping allow us to discern both general patterns of relief oriented towards Burgundian soldiers and its motivations.[10] Occasionally, these accounts can be complemented by narrative sources such as military memoirs to understand perspectives on injury and disability among soldiers, despite the difficulty to put experienced physical and mental trauma into

---

**9** Most recently on the Burgundian polity, see Robert Stein, *Magnanimous Dukes and Rising States: The Unification of the Burgundian Netherlands, 1380–1480* (Oxford: Oxford University Press, 2017), and Élodie Lecuppre-Desjardin, *The Illusion of the Burgundian State* (Manchester: Manchester University Press, 2022). Although both studies tend to consider Mary of Burgundy's principate as an endpoint, Wim Blockmans and Walter Prevenier, *The Promised Lands: The Low Countries under Burgundian rule, 1369–1530* (Philadelphia: University of Pennsylvania Press, 1999) and Jean-Marie Cauchies, *Philippe le Beau: Le dernier duc de Bourgogne* (Turnhout: Brepols, 2003), convincingly argued for the survival of Burgundian forms of government and state structures beyond the passing of Charles the Bold (1477) and Mary of Burgundy (1482).

**10** An almost complete series of accounts of the *Recette générale des finances* is kept at Dijon, Archives départementales de la Côte-d'Or (hereafter ADCO), Série B, covering 1363–1380, 1382–1397, 1398–1413, and at Lille, Archives départementales du Nord (hereafter ADN), Série B, covering 1414–1428, 1431–1455, 1457–1459, 1460–1469, 1471–1477, 1479–1482, 1484, 1486, and 1488–1506. For the *Argenterie*, on the other hand, only a few accounts are preserved, respectively for 1468, 1469, 1470, all published in: *Comptes de l'argentier de Charles le Téméraire, duc de Bourgogne*, eds. Valérie Bessey et al. (Paris: De Boccard, 2001–2008), and 1488 (Brussels, National Archives of Belgium (hereafter AGR), Chambres des comptes, no. 1926).

words.[11] Overall, complementing financial records with memoirs sheds light upon the ways in which Burgundian princely authorities and, indeed, different social groups considered war wounds and responded to their effects beyond the immediate theatre of war.

Both the adopted institutional and socio-political angle and the available source material primarily highlight financial support given to combatants who had suffered physical and mental injuries in war. Other forms of support, including but not limited to medical help beyond first aid and immediate follow-up given by surgeons pensioned by the dynasty,[12] will largely elude us here. Nevertheless, both the terminology used in the accounts and the patterns of gift-giving itself reveal perceptions of war lesions as they were defined at court where injured combatants petitioned the prince, whether the language reflected accepted, remodelled, or imposed self-identification. Indeed, although this article primarily addresses dynastic policies towards combatants, the latter assuredly had some agency in adopting and adapting discourses on disability to further their case, contributing to fashion representations in collaboration with legal advisors providing help to craft their petitions addressed to the princely administration, even when such petitions could be presented orally.[13]

## Injured, Ill, Disabled, or Mad: Finding and Qualifying Physical and Mental Impairment

Strikingly, analysis of granted gifts and pensions in the corresponding sections of Burgundian central account books reveals a relative dearth of combatants receiving compensation for injuries incurred in martial service of the dukes. Overall, between 1363 and 1506, surviving registers include a total of 138 men compensated for physical or mental damage suffered in warfare.[14] On average, then, less than one soldier per year would have benefitted

---

**11** Anna Katharina Heiniger, "The Silenced Trauma in the Islendingasögur," *Gripla* 31 (2020): 233–65. Special thanks to Yoav Tirosh for this reference.

**12** See for instance: Ali Bacha, "Blessures," 200–17.

**13** On petitions beyond pardons, see William Mark Ormrod, "Medieval Petitions in Context," in *Medieval Petitions: Grace and Grievance*, eds. William Mark Ormrod et al. (York: York Medieval Press, 2009), 1–11; Richard Huzzey et al., "Petitions and Petitioning in Historical Perspective," in *Petitions and Petitioning in Europe and North America from the Late Medieval Period to the Present*, eds. Richard Huzzey et al. (London: British Academy, 2024), 1–30.

**14** Calculation based on Ali Bacha, "Blessures," 390–93 (listing gifts between 1365 and 1477) and on my own analysis of the chapters of gifts and pensions in

from financial compensation provided by the central ducal treasuries for incurred impairment. Despite significant gaps in the account series during the civil strife in the 1470s and 1480s, and exceptional years such as 1468 when, after successive campaigns in France and Liège, no less than sixteen cases can be listed,[15] both average and overall counts seem quite low, especially considered against the regularity of warfare and the growing size of princely armies.[16]

What exactly, then, were these combatants compensated for? As pointed out by both Eyler and Turner,[17] particular attention must be paid to the terminology used in medieval sources to comprehend the ways in which injury and disability were understood. Significantly, Burgundian accounts rarely specify the nature of incurred physical lesions which were being compensated. Most frequently, the relatively vague umbrella term "blessure" is used in its different orthographic and grammatical variants ("bleschure," "bleceure," "blecheure," "blechié") to indicate injury.[18] Occasionally, such injuries were further qualified as particularly nasty or severe, as in the case of Pierre Lambart, suffering "several nasty injuries" at the final assault of Melun in 1420,[19] or Jehan le Prévôt, squire and man-at-arms "severely injured" at the Battle of Guinegatte in 1479.[20] Less frequently used, the term "navrure" still regularly appears, most often in combination with "blessure."

---

the preserved *Comptes de l'argentier* (1468, 1469, 1470, and 1488), and in the *Recette générale des finances* between 1477 and 1506. Amending Ali Bacha's sum, combatants benefiting from successive gifts for the same injury are here counted only once. Prior to 1468, a few occurrences of compensation for mental harm may have to be added to Ali Bacha's listed war lesions, but would only marginally affect the overall picture provided here.

**15** *Comptes de l'argentier*, vol. 1.

**16** Contamine, *Guerre*, 136–39, 222–23, 313–19; Bertrand Schnerb, *L'État bourguignon, 1463–1477* (Paris: Perrin, 1999), 264–69. English armies remained comparatively small: Michael Prestwich, *Armies and Warfare in the Middle Ages: The English Experience* (New Haven: Yale University Press, 1996), 336.

**17** Joshua R. Eyler, "Introduction: Breaking Boundaries, Building Bridges," in *Disability in the Middle Ages: Reconsiderations and Reverberations*, ed. Joshua R. Eyler (Farnham: Ashgate, 2010), 1–8, at 7; Wendy J. Turner, *Care and Custody of the Mentally Ill, Incompetent, and Disabled in Medieval England* (Turnhout: Brepols, 2013), 5–7.

**18** For instance: *Comptes de l'argentier*, vol. 1, art. 694, 812, 1788, 1792, 1897, 1898; ADN, B 2121, fol. 284v, fol. 385v; ADN, B 2144, fol. 179v.

**19** ADN, B 1923, fol. 98r (quoted in Ali Bacha, "Blessures," 255: "plusieurs villaines bleceures").

**20** ADN, B 2121, fol. 312v–313r ("griefvement blechié").

According to modern dictionaries of late medieval French, both words almost synonymously referred to wounds and injuries.[21] At the 1421 Battle of Mons-en-Vimeu, for instance, David de Brimeu, lord of Humbercourt, incurred "some severe wounds and injuries."[22] By the early sixteenth century, vocabulary to distinguish between injuries may have become more precise, as two occurrences of open wounds ("playes") appear, one of them in combination with "blessure." This incidence may indicate that the now disappeared "navrure," here seemingly replaced by "playe," referred to open wounds as opposed to other injuries.[23] One single earlier occurrence of the word however attests to the fact that, for now, our evidence is too scarce to be conclusive.[24]

Beyond injuries and wounds, incurred illness, too, was compensated for. Indeed, soldiers suffering from undefined "illnesses" ("maladies") recurrently appear among the beneficiaries of princely munificence.[25] Although the word could serve as an umbrella term for all types of critical change in health condition,[26] "maladie" [illness, disease], often used in conjunction with "blessure" [injury], seems to indicate a condition endured over a longer time-span. Such illness then appears in relation with or stemming from injuries inflicted in combat, perhaps provoking fever or other, longer-lasting, consequences. Hence, in 1389, Guillaume de Mornay was given 200 francs to help him "in the illness in which he remained since the king's campaign in Flanders…when he was hit in his leg by a crossbow bolt."[27] Similarly, in 1441, Jacotin Le Seure, nick-

---

**21** Both words are modernized as "blessure" [injury] in the online *Dictionnaire du Moyen Français (1330–1500)*, https://zeus.atilf.fr/dmf, last accessed April 7, 2025. Our source material does not provide further clarifications regarding possible distinctions between "blessure" and "navrure." Perhaps, they meant to indicate a difference between open and closed wounds, but this must remain hypothetical in the absence of conclusive proof.

**22** ADN, B 1925, fol. 67v (quoted in Ali Bacha, "Blessures," 255: "certaines grandes navrures et blecheures"). Further examples include: ADN, B 1925, fol. 63r (quoted in Ali Bacha, "Blessures," 247); *Comptes de l'argentier*, vol. 1, art. 1890; ADN, B 2121, fol. 387r–v, fol. 425r, fol. 479r; AGR, CC 1926, fol. 106r; ADN, B 2144, fol. 179v.

**23** ADN, B 2191, fol. 291r, fols. 307v–308r.

**24** ADN, B 1923, fol. 111v ("pluseurs playes et navrures," 1421).

**25** Among others, see: *Comptes de l'argentier*, vol. 1, art. 1789, 1890, 1909; *Comptes de l'argentier*, vol. 2, art. 944, 979; ADN, B 2121, fol. 273v, fol. 375r, fols. 442v–443r.

**26** Pierre Cromer, "Maladie," in *Dictionnaire du Moyen Français (1330–1500)*, http://www.atilf.fr/dmf/definition/maladie, last accessed April 8, 2025.

**27** ADCO, B 1475, fol. 65r–v, quoted in Bertrand Schnerb, "Aspects de l'organisation militaire dans les principautés bourguignonnes (v. 1315–v. 1420)," 4 vols. (PhD diss.,

named Gobart, received a gift compensating a leg injury as well as a, possibly related, long-term illness.[28] In 1480, Johannes le Blanc, guard of the duke's oratory, benefited from a gift as he had been "heavily injured and wounded by the French [at Guinegatte], after which he fell in such severe illness as to be bedbound for six weeks."[29] A year later, the case of Georis Karghels further illustrates the longer time-span associated with such illness as this ducal gunner was given financial aid for the "illness in which he had lain for a long time and still was, as the prince was well-aware of."[30]

Occasionally, the accounts briefly specify the affected body part of an injured combatant. We already mentioned how Guillaume de Mornay was hit in his leg by a crossbow bolt.[31] Similarly, in 1411, two illnesses ("maladies") struck Pietrequin Laubegeois, respectively affecting his cheek ("joe") and his arm ("bras"),[32] whereas Antoine de Vaudrey suffered a lance-inflicted injury to the leg at the 1436 siege of Calais.[33] In 1480, both Gherardin de Hulen, squire and provost to the princely artillery, and Estienne Chatart, squire and breadmaster of Maximilian's household, received gifts after having been hit, respectively by a crossbow bolt in the head at the Battle of Guinegatte and by a arquebus shot breaking an arm at the siege of Asperen.[34]

Whereas wounds and illness were considered curable,[35] in a few cases, the wounded combatant is revealed to be injured so severely that a part of

---

Université de Paris–Sorbonne, 1988), annex 3: "en la maladie en quoy il a esté depuis l'armée que le Roy fist en Flandres...en laquelle armée ledit Guillaume fut trait d'un vireton en la jambe."

**28** ADN, B 1972, fol. 191r (quoted in Ali Bacha, "Blessures," 252: "maladie qu'il a eu [de] long temps").

**29** ADN, B 2121, fol. 387r–v ("il fut par les Franchois fort bleschié et navré a laquelle cause il enchey en telle et sy griesve maladie qu'il en a esté six sepmaines au lit").

**30** ADN, B 2124, fol. 209r ("la maladie en laquelle il avoit longuement esté et encoires estoit comme de ce estoit bien adverty icellui seigneur").

**31** ADCO, B 1475, fol. 65r–v (quoted in Schnerb, "Aspects," annex 3: "fut trait d'un vireton en la jambe").

**32** ADCO, B 1570, fol. 18r (quoted in Schnerb, "Aspects," annex 3).

**33** ADN, B 1959, no. 57417 (already quoted in Ali Bacha, "Blessures," 250).

**34** ADN, B 2121, fol. 385v ("en la teste"), fol. 379r–v ("attaint d'une hacquebusque au bras tellement qu'il en est rompu").

**35** John M. Theilmann, "Disease or Disability? The Conceptual Relationship in Medieval and Early Modern England," in *The Treatment of Disabled Persons in Medieval Europe: Examining Disability in the Historical, Legal, Literary, Medical, and Religious Discourses of the Middle Ages*, eds. Wendy J. Turner and Tory V. Pearman (Lewiston: Mellen, 2010), 197–229.

their body would no longer appear or function as it used to. After the 1436 siege of Calais, Geoffroy de Thoisy, squire in the ducal household, obtained financial support in compensation for one of his arms which had been paralysed and mutilated.[36] By 1463, Laurens de Leurins, an archer from the company of the duke's bastard son Anthony, had lost an arm at war.[37] In 1479, after Guinegatte, Jehan de Savoye, a squire from Burgundy, is said to be forever disfigured, a physical alteration which, depending on its (unspecified) nature and interpretative context, could signal martial virtue or bring shame.[38] From the 1460s onwards, the adjective "affolé" seems most frequently used. The word can be translated as maimed, crippled, mutilated, or disabled. Implying a visible form of permanent impairment, a translation as disabled might be preferred.[39] Hence, Pierrequin de Morenghes, a gunner, was disabled in one of his legs.[40] Similarly, the aforementioned Estienne Chatart, shot in the arm by an arquebus at Asperen, was eventually disabled "for life."[41] In both cases, the use of past, present, and future tenses signifies a perception of permanence beyond cure.

Finally, although soldiers, unlike non-combatants, would usually not appear mentally affected by combat trauma in the French remission letters studied by Aleksandra Pfau,[42] a few rare occurrences of combatants diagnosed with "madness" or translated more literally, loss of one's senses,

---

**36** ADN, B 1959, no. 57441 (quoted in Ali Bacha, "Blessures," 250: "un bras que naguere j'ai eu reti et fus mutilé").

**37** ADN, B 1959, no. 57417 (quoted in Ali Bacha, "Blessures," 250: "en la guerre…il perdit un de ses bras") ; ADN, B 2048, fol. 228r.

**38** ADN, B 2121, fol. 412r–v ("fut sy fort blechié ou visaige qu'il en est et demoura a tousjours desfiguré"). On contrasting perceptions of scars and disfigurement for combatants, see Patricia Skinner, "Visible Prowess? Reading Men's Head and Face Wounds in Early Medieval Europe to 1000 CE," in *Wounds and Wound Repair*, 81–101, and Giulia Morosini, "Manly Virtues, Emotions, and Scars: Competition among Italian Renaissance Soldiers through Bodily Practices," in *Gender and Status Competition in Pre-Modern Societies*, eds. Martha Bayless et al. (Turnhout: Brepols, 2021), 79–107. More generally, see Patricia Skinner, *Living with Disfigurement in Early Medieval Europe* (New York: Palgrave, 2017), and Emily Cock and Patricia Skinner, "Situating the Different Face," in *Approaching Facial Difference: Past and Present*, eds. Emily Cock and Patricia Skinner (London: Bloomsbury Academic, 2018), 1–8.

**39** Metzler, *A Social History of Disability*, 4–8.

**40** *Comptes de l'argentier*, vol. 2, art. 116 ("il a esté et est affolé en l'une de ses jambes").

**41** ADN, B 2121, fol. 479r ("il en est demouré et demoura *affolé* toute sa vie").

**42** Aleksandra Pfau, "Warfare, Trauma and Madness in French Remission Letters of the Hundred Years War," in *The Hundred Years War (Part III): Further Considerations*, eds. L. J. Andrew Villalon and Donald J. Kagay (Leiden: Brill, 2013), 437–54. See also,

may signal some limited degree of responsibility assumed by Burgundian-Habsburg authorities. In 1480, a former captain of German foot soldiers is given some cash to keep him away from court, where, "having lost his senses," he had been screaming daily after the prince—possibly making oral bids for the prince's generosity.[43] Two years later, another German, most likely a *landsknecht*, received financial aid as, he too, was "weakened in his common sense."[44] Interestingly, both men remained anonymous, unnamed, in the account books. Overall, this only occurs four times among our 138 cases (the third and fourth occurrence will be addressed in relation to existing socio-economic solidarity networks). Could such anonymity signal a (perceived) loss of identity or did it constitute a protective measure for the men who had "lost their mind"? In any case, whether the two German combatants incurred a form of post-traumatic stress disorder in war seems likely but remains hard to establish with certainty given culturally specific perceptions of mental health conditions and, hence, the risks of anachronism associated with retrospective diagnosis.[45] Nevertheless, although neither is explicitly tied to a combatant's war experience, both cases suggest that the Burgundian-Habsburg dynasty could occasionally take care of soldiers experiencing mental trauma. Unlike in England, however, no wardship policy for the mentally incapacitated, whether former combatant or not, seems to have existed.[46]

## The Charitable Rationale of Dynastic Gift-Giving: Reward Service, Mitigate Hardship

Whether wounded ("blessé," "navré"), ill ("malade"), disabled ("affolé," "retif"), or mad ("debilité de ses sens"), these combatants could benefit from the prince's magnanimity. Assuredly, an ideal of religious charity underpinned this gracious generosity.[47] Such religious sentiment is regu-

in this volume: Aleksandra Pfau, "Traumatic Repercussions: Warfare and Disability in the French Countryside."

**43** ADN, B 2121, fol. 414v ("debilité de ses sens, qui estoit journelement criant après lui [le prince] et afin qu'il fust enmené d'illec sans plus retourner").

**44** ADN, B 2127, fol. 234r ("debilité de son bon sens").

**45** Pfau, "Warfare, Trauma and Madness," 441–42.

**46** Wendy J. Turner, "Mental incapacity and the financing of war in medieval England," in *The Hundred Years War (Part II): Different Vistas*, eds. L. J. Andrew Villalon and Donald J. Kagay (Leiden: Brill, 2008), 387–402.

**47** Beyond general Christian justifications for charity, later medieval writings underscore important criteria to benefit from charity. Among these criteria, some may well have inspired the dukes. Indeed, as we will see, several beneficiaries did face an

larly explicitly referred to, as expressed by the recurring turn of phrase that financial aid was given "for God and in alms" ("pour Dieu et en aulmosne"). Laurens de Leurins, an archer having lost an arm in battle, Hacquinet du Bois, an archer from Charles the Bold's ducal bodyguard suffering illness, Jooris Brauwart, a German soldier having lost a hand in Maximilian's service, and the anonymous German soldier who had lost his senses all benefitted from this charitable motive.[48] Sometimes, a whiff of compassion or pity was explicitly added to the mix. In 1389, Guillaume de Mornay, ducal squire injured at the siege of Damme, benefited from ducal munificence "for the great pity and compassion our lord the duke had towards him."[49] Similarly, in 1463, Laurens de Leurins was granted a monetary sum "considering and pitying that, during the war, he had lost an arm."[50]

Such charitable compassion was, however, rarely the sole or main motive registered in the Burgundian account books.[51] Significantly, notwithstanding a few exceptions, financial benefits were recorded as gifts in the corresponding section, and not in the alms section. Indeed, throughout the examined period, princely generosity was largely based upon the explicit recognition of service rendered to the dynasty. In another recurrent and quite formulaic turn of phrase, often cited as the first grounds for awarding a gift and possibly mirroring the language used by petitioners requesting the prince's appreciation, combatants could benefit from ducal largesse for "good and

---

imminent threat to their lives or well-being, whereas preference was systematically given to relations over strangers, and those of higher caste who were at risk of falling in social status were given preference to those of the lower social orders. On these criteria, see James W. Brodman, *Charity and Religion in Medieval Europe* (Washington, DC: Catholic University of America Press, 2009), 33–35.

**48** ADN, B 2048, fol. 228r (quoted in Ali Bacha, "Blessures," 258); ADN, B 2121, fol. 273v; ADN, B 2124, fol. 241r; ADN, B 2127, fol. 234r.

**49** ADCO, B 1475, fol. 65r–v ("pour le grant pitié et compassion que mondit seigneur a de lui," already quoted in Schnerb, "Aspects," annex 3).

**50** ADN, B 1959, no. 57417 (quoted in Ali Bacha, "Blessures," 258 : "en consideracion et pitié de ce que, en la guerre…il perdit un de ses bras").

**51** On varied motivations for charity beyond religion, see the introductory comments in: Anne M. Scott, "Experiences of Charity: Complex Motivations in the Charitable Endeavour, c. 1100–c. 1650," in *Experiences of Charity, 1250–1650*, ed. Anne M. Scott (Farnham: Ashgate, 2015), 1–14, at 9–11. On the value and limits of understanding premodern disability through charity associated with (extreme) poverty, see: Frohne and Horn, "On the Fluidity of 'Disability,'" 17–40; N. Dubourg, "European Medieval Disability History: An Overview," in *Handbook of Disability: Critical Thought and Social Change in a Globalizing World*, eds. Marcia H. Rioux et al. (Singapore: Springer, 2024), 89–106, at 94–97.

pleasing service," whether in general or on a particular campaign.[52] Rewarding such loyal service was not just a turn of phrase, though, and regularly referred to specific, confirmed service. Hence, in 1470, Jacques de Mussen, a man-at-arms, and eight archers serving under his command, some of whom were injured in combat, were compensated "considering several pleasing services done to the duke in pushing back some French troops, enemies of our duke, who had reached the outskirts of Amiens."[53]

Rather than to compensate for specific injuries or disabilities, princely generosity was most often aimed at mitigating financial loss incurred by combatants while they were treated towards survival and eventual recovery. In 1395, Guillaume des Bours already received 200 francs to help him support the substantial costs and expenses which he had to make in his incurred illness.[54] Similarly, in 1411, Pietrequin Laubegeois was given 100 francs to help him sustain the costs of injuries both to his cheek and to his arm.[55] In 1505, a ducal rider, having been injured during the conflict in Guelders, received £6 to help him pay his doctors.[56] Under the first three Valois dukes, gifts ranged from 4 francs to a ducal messenger to 500 francs to a knight and courtier of the duke whose injury and potential subsequent recovery remain unknown.[57] Similarly, under Charles the Bold, Maximilian, and Philip the Fair, they ranged from a sheer 54 sous to the German captain who had lost his senses, to a vast £1,320 to Martin of Polheim, knight, counsellor, and close friend to Maximilian after he came back "ill" from Guinegatte.[58]

---

**52** ADN, B 1925, fol. 63r (quoted in Ali Bacha, "Blessures," 247: "pour consideracion des bons et agreables services que longuement et loyalement il lui [the duke] a faiz et faisoit encores de jour en jour"); *Comptes de l'argentier*, vol. 2, art. 944 ("en consideracion d'aucuns aggreables services qu'il luy [the duke] a faiz"); *Comptes de l'argentier*, vol. 1, art. 1890 ("en consideracion des services qu'il luy [the duke] a faiz en son armee").

**53** *Comptes de l'argentier*, vol. 3, art. 1796 ("en consideracion de pluseurs aggreables services qu'il luy [the duke] ont faiz au reboutement d'aucuns Franchois, adversaires de mondit seigneur, qui sont nagaires venuz es fauxbou[r]s dudit Amiens").

**54** ADCO, B 1503, fol. 91v ("pour lui aidier a supporter les grans frais et missions qu'il avoit convenue faire en la maladie qu'il a eue").

**55** ADCO, B 1570, fol. 18r, quoted in Schnerb, "Aspects," annex 3 and in Ali Bacha, "Blessures," 249 ("pour l'aidier a soustenir les frais qu'il a du faire a cause de deux maladies, tant en la joe comme au bras").

**56** ADN, B 2191, fol. 287v ("pour lui aidier a paier les medecins").

**57** Ali Bacha, "Blessures," 390–93.

**58** ADN, B 2121, fol. 414v, fols. 442v–443r ("aussi pour le garir de sa maladie en laquelle il estoit escheu depuis son retour de la derreniere bataille de la Viesville").

Even more than social status and (our?) perceived severity of incurred lesions already accurately pointed out by Rabah Ali Bacha,[59] financial costs incurred for medical treatment contribute to explain the wide variety of monetary sums granted to wounded combatants. As costs would vary over time and new forms of compensation appeared (see below), establishing a scale of financial aid corresponding to a typology of injuries proves difficult, pointless even given both the apparent absence of such a scale in Burgundian governmental practice and the lack of detail provided in the accounts. Moreover, to allow for any comparison, beneficiaries of ducal munificence should come from similar social backgrounds and have incurred their wounds at (approximately) the same moment in time. One example will suffice here. At the 1436 siege of Calais, Geoffroy de Thoisy and Antoine de Vaudrey, both squires from important noble families from Burgundy, were injured, respectively at the arm and at the leg. Whereas Antoine was expected to recover, Geoffroy would remain disabled. Geoffroy's compensation, however, only amounted to £32 livres, a sum equivalent to that paid out to Antoine despite Geoffroy's loss of limb (arm).[60] Financial loss, rather than any specific typology of injury or disability, was key.

Indeed, although we have so far tended to separate those combatants who incurred physical and mental damage in war from other beneficiaries of princely gifts, our modern categories of analysis should not obscure the rationale followed by the princely authorities as they appear in the Burgundian account book chapters for gift-giving. In this respect, it is noteworthy that combatants could be compensated for all sorts of financial hazards incurred in warfare. This entailed losses of land, warhorses, military equipment, or even being ransomed. Such material loss would be estimated to a financially higher amount than most physical or mental damage suffered by a combatant, as attested by a comparison between two exceptionally high cases of compensation involving war injuries. After the 1479 Battle of Guinegatte, Jehan le Prevost, squire and man-at-arms from Maximilian's household, benefitted from no less than £1,000, compensating for lands lost in now French-controlled territory as well as for his service at the battle where "he lost everything he had, including military equipment, cash money, horses and armour, and was severely injured and taken prisoner by the

**59** Ali Bacha, "Blessures," 259–61.

**60** ADN, B 1958/9, no. 57279, no. 57441 (both gifts to Geoffroy de Thoisy, amounting to 32 livres de Flandre), no. 57 417 (gift to Antoine de Vaudrey, 40 francs of 32 gros, which is equivalent to 32 livres de Flandre, quoted in Ali Bacha, "Blessures," 250: "pour moy faire guerir d'un coup de lance que j'ay eu naguaire en la jambe").

French to whom he had to pay 200 golden écus in ransom."[61] The already mentioned Estienne Chatart, squire, breadmaster to Maximilian and hence also a member of the duke's household, on the other hand, first received £80 to ensure his healing, then just another £120 when it became apparent that he would never recover the use of his arm after suffering a wound from an arquebus shot.[62] Similarly, the £20 received by Jehan de Savoye, a Burgundian squire who lost all his belongings – not that highly valued ? – and was disfigured at Guinegatte, contrast with the £300 given to Martin Zwarts, a German squire compensated for unspecified (financial) loss and damage including some horses gone missing since he joined Maximilian's service in 1482.[63]

In any case, even when often consisting of much lower sums, financial aid was ideally granted to help wounded combatants cover medical costs towards their prospective physical recovery ("guérison," "guerir," "garir"). In 1441, Jacotin Le Seure was hence given 16 francs to advance the healing of his leg.[64] In 1480, Urbain de La Penne, squire, received £24 to help him recover from a wound incurred at the taking of the castle of Beaumont.[65] In 1505, Jehan de Strasbourg and Jehan le Barbier, both squires and brothers, received £37 10s. (£1 = 20 sous) to help them heal from some injuries and open wounds incurred at [the assault of] a bulwark defending Arnhem, in Guelders.[66] Such recovery would, of course, guarantee the dukes further "good and loyal service" from the beneficiary.[67]

It is often uncertain whether combatants would indeed fully recover from incurred injuries. The financial records rarely inform us about soldiers' long-term condition beyond a granted gift. Some lesions with more permanent consequences did not prevent future participation in military operations. Hence, the (nick)name of a squire to Philip the Bold, receiving monetarily support for a newly incurred arm wound in 1378, suggests that

---

**61** ADN, B 2121, fols. 312v–313r.

**62** ADN, B 2121, fols. 379r–v, fol. 479r.

**63** ADN, B 2121, fol. 412r–v; ADN, B 2127, fol. 190r.

**64** ADN, B 1972, fol. 191r ("pour lui *faire guerir* d'une jambe," italics are mine).

**65** ADN, B 2121, fol. 425r ("pour soy *aidier a garir* de certaine blessure et navrure qu'il lui a esté faicte a la prinse et reddicion du chasteau de Beaumont," italics are mine).

**66** ADN, B 2191, fol. 291r ("aidier a garir de certaines blessures et playes qu'ilz avoient eues en ung bolewerch devant la ville de Aernhem").

**67** Explicitly stated in ADN, B 1920, fol. 92v ("bons et agreables services qu'il... esperoit que encores lui deust faire ou temps advenir") and fol. 100r ("bons et agreables services qu'il...esperoit que encores feist ou temps advenir").

he never fully recovered from a previous injury: assuredly, and although the circumstances in which he lost an eye are unknown, *Le Borgne* de Sovillier was a one-eyed soldier who had kept living from his trade.[68] Although a rare explicit occurrence in our records, Le Borgne must not have been an exception. Indeed, both archaeological data and narrative accounts suggest that combatants having suffered even severe injuries in previous combat sometimes recovered sufficiently to resume their martial activities, becoming "recidivists" as Christopher J. Knüsel qualifies them.[69] Assuredly, muster rolls would provide invaluable additional evidence on both presence and perception of long-term effects of war injuries through combatants' nicknames.[70]

In some cases, however, incurred injuries could lead to an inability to make a living, which could be recognized as such. Laurens de Leurins, the archer who lost an arm in battle and hence became unable to live from his trade—one which had required many years of training—, received £6 in 1463 as a charitable gift "to help him live."[71] Similarly, the German foot soldier captain, said to have lost his senses, and Jooris Brauwart, a German who lost a hand, received 54s. and £6 respectively.[72] Whether this was sufficient to help them out in the long run is highly doubtful: considering an (un)qualified labourer's pay at 2 to 3 sous a day, a total equivalent of 120 sous would only cover between forty and sixty working days in a best-case scenario.[73] Given the higher living standards of noble families, this reasoning

**68** ADCO, B 1452, fol. 66r (quoted in Ali Bacha, "Blessures," 390).

**69** Christopher J. Knüsel and Anthea Boylston, "How Has the Towton Project Contributed to Our Knowledge of Medieval and Later Warfare?," in *Blood Red Roses: The Archaeology of a Mass Grave from the Battle of Towton AD 1461*, eds. Veronica Fiorato et al. (Oxford: Oxbow, 2000), 169–188, at 172–173; Iain MacInnes, "'One man slashes, one slays, one warns, one wounds': Injury and Death in Anglo-Scottish Conflict, *c.* 1296–*c.*1403," in *Killing and Being Killed: Bodies in Battle. Perspectives on Fighters in the Middle Ages*, ed. J. Rogge (Bielefeld: Transcript, 2017), 61–77. See also, in this volume, Christopher J. Knüsel, "The Recidivists: Healed Cranial Trauma from Conflicts in the Late Medieval Period."

**70** On the value of onomastics to disability history: Irina Metzler, "What's in a Name? Considering the Onomastics of Disability in the Middle Ages," in *The Treatment of Disabled Persons*, 15–50. On Burgundian muster rolls: Bertrand Schnerb, "Les montres d'armes, source de l'étude de la société militaire de la fin du Moyen Âge: L'exemple bourguignon," *Revue du Nord* 99, no. 4 (2017): 671–90.

**71** ADN, B 2048, fol. 228r (cited in Ali Bacha, "Blessures," 258: "pour Dieu et en aumosne pour soy aidier a vivre").

**72** ADN, B 2121, fol. 414v; ADN, B 2124, fol. 241r.

**73** Monique Sommé, "Que représente un gage journalier de 3 sous pour l'officier d'un hôtel ducal à la cour de Bourgogne au XV^e siècle?," in *Les niveaux de vie au Moyen*

can, to a certain extent, also be applied to the higher sum of £32 received by Geoffroy de Thoisy in 1436, covering no more than a full year's pay of a qualified labourer, even when discounting the many religious holidays! Whereas Thoisy's regular income, including but not limited to landed property, is harder to evaluate, one can imagine how his revenue from warfare, including pay, loot, and ransoms, could be affected by the loss of an arm.[74] Hence, although recognition of injury, illness, madness, and disability at the Burgundian court, as reflected in the account books, was foremost a matter of compensating financial loss due to the hazards of war, those combatants whose livelihood was at risk to be permanently affected would only receive limited, if any, compensation.

Despite the absence of serial evidence beyond 1470 as the accounts of the *Argenterie* were not preserved, a few cases suggest that, under Charles the Bold (1467-1477), the Burgundian authorities may have adapted this rationale. Indeed, to some extent echoing more lasting retirement schemes occasionally provided by the English Crown to its disabled veterans and other servants in the early fourteenth century in the form of housing and board with a monastic institution (corrodies),[75] a few Burgundian combatants whose means of living had been affected by the hazards of war started to benefit from regular pensions instead of a lump sum granted once by the prince. From September 1, 1469 onwards, Pierrequin de Morenghes, a gunner disabled in one of his legs, would receive a lifelong daily pension of ½ sous "in order for him to live more comfortably and maintain his livelihood in his old days."[76] Another gunner and beneficiary of a pension granted on the same day and amounting to 1 sous per day "to maintain his livelihood and help him live," Coppin Caulier is not explicitly said to have been disabled. Proximity in place, time, and occupation, however, suggests this might well have been the case.[77] A third and last example under Charles the

*Âge: Mesures, perceptions et représentations*, eds. Jean-Pierre Sosson et al. (Louvain-la-Neuve: Bruylant-Academia, 1999), 297–315.

**74** On the rewards of martial activity, see Prestwich, *Armies*, 83–113.

**75** See in this volume, Wendy Turner, "Investigating the Lifecycle of the Medieval English Soldier: Disability, Mental Trauma, and Medicine in Connection with War in Late Medieval English Records."

**76** *Comptes de l'argentier*, vol. 2, art. 116; *Comptes de l'argentier*, vol. 3, art. 118 ("affolé en l'une de ses jambes...afin qu'il ait mieulx de quoy vivre et soy entretenir en ses anciens jours").

**77** *Comptes de l'argentier*, vol. 2, art. 117 ("pour soy entretenir et aidier a vivre"); *Comptes de l'argentier*, vol. 3, art. 119. Although Coppin's grant does not state the

Bold is provided by Adrienet Denis, an archer who benefited from a lifelong daily pension of 2 sous after the 1471 siege of Amiens.[78] With daily pensions ranging between ½ sous and 2 sous, and considering that non-working days were hence paid at the same rate as working days, such benefits were a considerable improvement for disabled soldiers. Indeed, in all three cases, the reasoning behind the grant stresses the former combatants' inability to make a living and autonomously sustain themselves through their labour after incurring impairment in princely service.[79] In two cases, the nature of the injury is explicitly stated as leaving them powerless ("impotent") and disabled ("affolé").

In examining the rationale for granting these pensions, one last element appears noteworthy. Whereas Adrienet Denis is explicitly mentioned as a "young companion," all three men are designated through the diminutive of their given name, respectively Adrienet (for Adrien), Pierrequin (for Pierre), and Coppin (for Jaques/Jacob). One can wonder whether the understanding of impairment and disability was different for men perceived to be of a young age. Although they do not tend to dwell on disabling—or any other—injuries incurred in combat, possibly because of the impossibility to narrate experienced loss and trauma,[80] chroniclers and memorialists, too, seem to emphasize the young age at which a combatant could be impaired and, perhaps, disabled from sustaining himself. In a rare occurrence, Jean de Haynin (1423–1495), a nobleman serving Philip the Good and Charles the Bold in war throughout the 1460s and 1470s, tells the story of Jacques de Jeumont, Lord of Fagnolle, whose left leg was hit by a cannon ball at the Battle of Montlhéry (1465). Suffering the blow just above his foot, Jacques, who did not benefit from any financial compensation in the surviving central accounts (!), was amputated on the battlefield. Haynin stresses the disabling of a man who was perceived to be a "noble, courageous, beautiful and powerful knight."[81]

---

explicit reason behind the gift, both gunners requested and received their ducal pension at the same moment, suggesting that, Coppin too, had been injured.

**78** ADN, B 2085, no. 66115 (quoted by Ali Bacha, "Blessures," 258).

**79** *Comptes de l'argentier*, vol. 2, année 1469, art. 116 (Pierrequin: "afin qu'il ait mieux de quoy vivre et soy entretenir en ses anciens jours"); *Comptes de l'argentier*, vol. 3, année 1470, art. 117 (Coppin: "pour soy entretenir et aidier a vivre"); ADN, B 2085, no. 66115 (Adrienet: "sans ce que jamais il puist son pain gaigner").

**80** See Heiniger, "The Silenced Trauma," 233–65.

**81** Jean de Haynin, *Mémoires*, ed. Françoise Vieillard, collab. Marc H. Smith, Catherine Bébéar (Paris: Société de l'Histoire de France, 2023), 47–48 : "il avient que le boulet de une des serpentines des Franchois ala fraper et ataindre monsieur

In medieval discourse, such an evocation of beauty and strength in the male body, reflecting both physical and moral perfection, was strongly associated with an idealized youth which, manifesting around the age of fifteen, could last into one's early thirties.[82] According to Haynin, Jacques's fate hence provoked great sorrow. Indeed, beyond the prospect of a lengthy life to live in infirmity, disability incurred by these combatants in war at a relatively young age may have affected both their capacity to sustain a family-unit or, to a certain extent, fall back upon the latter in case of (prolonged) celibacy. Indeed, princely gift-giving and pensions only complemented and, in fact, participated in the mechanisms of pre-existing socio-economic solidarity networks.

## Gift-Giving and Pensioning: Ducal Policies and Socio-Economic Solidarities

Although not insignificant, the overall count of 138 combatants compensated for mostly physical or, on a few occasions, mental damage incurred in dynastic warfare is strikingly low considering the thousands of men-at-arms, archers, gunners, and other military personnel partaking in ducal armies. Under Charles the Bold (1467–1477), numbers even went up to a few tens of thousands.[83] Whereas other regional and local treasurers may have paid out gifts to injured combatants who lived nearby, or even delivered the cash for the occasional pension, the central accountancy of the dukes does provide a solid sense of overall patterns. Beyond the charitable rationale motivating gift-giving and pensioning, the relatively rare occurrence of cases compared to both numbers of combatants and expected casualties, strongly indicates that no systematic policy towards compensation to physically or mentally affected combatants was implemented by the Burgundian princely authorities.

---

Jaques de Jeumont, segneur de Fagneulles, secon fis du senescal de Haynau, en la senestre janbe en desous du cras, environ eune pame deseure le pié et li ronpit tout l'os tellement que le pié demora pendant à ung bien peu de piau, et dudit cop il chut a terre et se bailla ung tres grant flat au choir…et là se confessa, et on ala querrir ung mestre hastivement qi le vient viseter, car il en y avoit pluseurs en l'ost et là endroit ledit mestre venu, *il li parcopa le piet tou jus, car il faloit qu'il fut ; dont che fu tres grant damage de che qu'il fu ensi affollé, car il estoit noble, hardi, biau et poisant chevallier. Et eüt tres grant plainte.*" Italics are mine.

**82** Robert Grout, "Concepts of Youth," in *A Cultural History of Youth in the Middle Ages*, ed. Daniel T. Kline (London: Bloomsbury Academic, 2022), 25–44.

**83** Contamine, *Guerre*, 136–39, 313–19; Schnerb, *L'État bourguignon*, 273.

As Rabah Ali Bacha rightly pointed out in his unpublished PhD thesis covering the principates of the Valois dukes, most men benefitting from a form of compensation were members of the ducal household.[84] Indeed, when charitable action was taken, loyal service rewarded, and financial hardship mitigated, this was primarily the case for those men who, as members of the prince's household, were included in a courtly social environment upon which they could fall back. Before wounding, and although income and employment varied according to each man's social status and were not always his main source of livelihood, this environment already provided them with a stable source of revenue and, in some cases, permanent employment, whether as chamberlain,[85] squire at the ducal stables,[86] meatcutter,[87] cupbearer,[88] breadmaster,[89] usher,[90] ducal messenger,[91] or member of the ducal bodyguard company.[92] In this regard, it should be emphasized that combatants were not treated differently from other members of the princely household who were injured or disabled while serving the

---

**84** Ali Bacha, "Blessures," 248–51.

**85** ADCO, B 1461, fol. 113v (Pierre de la Trémoïlle, "chevalier chambellan," 1384); ADN, B 2124, fol. 249r (Antoine de Salenove, knight, counsellor, and chamberlain, 1480).

**86** *Comptes de l'argentier*, vol. 1, art. 1890 (Jacques du Mas, "écuyer d'écurie," 1468).

**87** ADCO, B 1503, fol. 91v (Guillaume des Bours, dit Sauvage, "escuier tranchant de mondit seigneur," 1395).

**88** ADN, B 1959, no. 57417 (Antoine de Vaudrey, "escuier et eschanson de monseigneur le duc," 1436).

**89** ADN, B 1959, no. 57441 (Geoffroy de Thoisy, "escuier et pannetier de monseigneur le duc," 1436); *Comptes de l'argentier*, vol. 1, art. 1906 (Zweer de Ypembrouck, "pannetier du duc"), art. 1909 (Jehan de Vaultravers, écuyer pannetier, 1468); ADN, B 2121, fol. 379r–v, fol. 479 (Estienne Chatart, "escuier pannetier de mondit seigneur," 1480).

**90** ADN, B 1925, fol. 63 (Jehan du Cerc, "huissier d'armes," 1421); ADN, B 2121, fol. 375r (Estienne Waignon, "huissier d'armes," 1480).

**91** AGR, CC 1926, fol. 106r (Bertrand Longhespée, "chevaucheur de l'écurie," 1488); ADN, B 2191, fol. 287v (Jacotin le Maire, "chevaucheur de l'écurie," 1505).

**92** ADN, B 1972, fol. 191r (Jacotin le Seure, "archier de corps de mondit seigneur," 1441); *Comptes de l'argentier*, vol. 1, art. 446 (Bertoulet Willocq, "archer de corps", 1468), 1788 (Richart l'Angloix and Charles de Wignacourt, "archers de corps", 1468), 1897 (Gerardin Haguet, "archer de corps", 1468), 1898 (Guerre le Franconnier, "archer de corps", 1468), 1911 (Pierquin Malefault, "archer de corps", 1468) ; ADN, B 2124, fol. 258r (Massin Angot, "archer de corps," 1481) ; AGR, CC 1926, fol. 101v (Josse van Slosse, "hallebardier du roi," 1488) ; ADN, B 2173, fol. 174v (Hector Agaiche, "hallebardier de monseigneur," 1501).

dukes. For instance, Thierry de la Porte, a domestic servant in the ducal stables, received £4 16s. to heal from a facial injury incurred while tending to the duke's horses in 1468.[93] Similarly, in 1496, Alain Escharny, an officer in charge of the linen of the household's bread-department ("panneterie"), lost a finger and received £12 as a compensation to help him pay his surgeons.[94]

Reflecting an expected and theorized order of charity prioritising recipients according to their degree of closeness to the benefactor,[95] the predominance of members from the (extended) household among the beneficiaries of princely gifts did not, however, preclude other combatants from accessing ducal munificence. For some beneficiaries, information as to their affiliation to a household is lacking. This was the case of the bastard of Coulogne to whom the duke granted a monetary gift to recover ("guérir") from a gunshot incurred at the siege of Belleville (1434).[96] Similarly, the affiliations of Evrart de Neufve Roiche and Huguenin Guyart, both squires injured at Liege in 1468 and receiving £40 and £24 respectively, are unknown.[97] Strikingly, an unnamed archer from the company of Jean IV, lord of Auxy, also wounded at the taking of Liege in 1468, is given £6 in compensation for a disabled hand.[98] His anonymous presence in the alms chapter ("offrandes et aumônes"), rather than in the section relating to princely gifts, could reveal a strict distinction made to the detriment of those combatants who did not belong to the ducal household, all the more so as this archer appears to be the only combatant present in this section. However, one should probably not attribute too much significance to this isolated gift. Augustin de la Pierre, archer in the company of Gapennes, and Massin Angot, bodyguard archer to John II of Chalon, Prince of Orange, both benefitted from princely gifts in 1479 and 1481, respectively.[99] Whether their respective commanders interceded in their favour seems possible but must remain hypothetical. Nevertheless, it is worth noting that Hennequin de Fretin, a squire, was given a lump sum to distribute among the further unnamed archers of his company wounded at

---

**93** *Comptes de l'argentier*, vol. 1, art. 694.

**94** ADN, B 2155, fol. 175v.

**95** Miri Rubin, *Charity and Community in Medieval Cambridge* (Cambridge: Cambridge University Press, 1987), 68–74; Brodman, *Charity*, 33–35.

**96** ADN, B 1954, fol. 114r (cited in Ali Bacha, "Blessures," 253).

**97** *Comptes de l'argentier*, vol. 1, art. 1789, art. 1905.

**98** *Comptes de l'argentier*, vol. 1, art. 2088 ("affolé d'une main a ladicte prinse de Liege").

**99** ADN, B 2121, fol. 284v; B 2124, fol. 258r.

the Battle of Brouwershaven (1426), reflecting both widened access to the prince beyond the household *and* an order of charity whereby a company captain, remained, in principle, responsible for his men.[100]

As suggested above, subtle changes in princely policy appear for the first time under Charles the Bold, this prince's principate witnessing at least some degree of novelty in the form of pensions granted to physically harmed combatants henceforth considered unable to make a living. Indeed, beyond an exponential increase of gifts handed out to injured soldiers (no less than twenty-seven out of 138 recorded cases, i.e., 19.6 percent of the beneficiaries, a percentage even more impressive if we consider that sources only cover three years of this duke's ten-year-long principate), the duke provided at least three combatants with a lifelong pension.[101]

Although serving in the prince's wars, neither of these men were directly part of the duke's household when granted a pension. Whereas later sources mention Morenges and Caulier as "gunners of his lordship [the duke]," the first occurrence of their pension, usually referring to the original grant, just states their capacity as gunners. Similarly, Adrienet Denis' activity as an archer was not carried out within the ducal guard. Whether their pensions constituted the kick-start of a more systematically implemented policy in the later years of Charles the Bold's principate remains unknown in the absence of preserved account books between 1471 and 1477. As gunners, Morenges and Caulier may have benefitted from the duke's eagerness to attract rare and valuable technicians by offering them superior conditions.[102] Denis, however, was but an archer, and our information on his grant indicates that he petitioned for his pension himself, suggesting a shift in practice and expectations.[103]

In any case, both the exponential increase in gifts and the newly instated pensions are a testimony to an unprecedented degree of militarization of

**100** ADN, B 1933, fol. 97r.

**101** *Comptes de l'argentier*, vol. 2, art. 116, 117; *Comptes de l'argentier*, vol. 3, art. 118, 119; ADN, B 2085, no. 66115, cited in Ali Bacha, "Blessures," 258.

**102** On this policy: Michael Depreter, "Les canonniers-fondeurs des ducs de Bourgogne. Recrutement, implantation et rapports au prince (v.1450–1494)," in *Medieval Copper, Bronze and Brass: History, Archaeology and Archaeometry of the Production of Brass, Bronze and Other Copper Alloy Objects in Medieval Europe (12th–16th centuries)*, eds. Nicolas Thomas and Pete Dandridge (Namur: Agence wallonne du Patrimoine, 2018), 169–80.

**103** ADN, B 2085, no. 66115 (cited in Ali Bacha, "Blessures," 258: "receu avons l'humble supplicacion").

the ducal household and, more generally, a substantial increase in army size under this warmongering duke.[104] Noteworthily, both the gunners and the archer benefiting from a pension were professional soldiers, likely recognized as such. As suggested, their affiliation to the princely court is highly doubtful. However, rather than merely seeing these gifts and pensions as precursors of more systematic institutionalized policies towards care for wounded soldiers in state service, one must consider how these grants fitted into Charles the Bold's general policy. In increasing the number of beneficiaries from gifts and in offering pensions to those men who had suffered permanent physical injury while serving in his wars, the duke may, in fact, not so much have intended to instate a new welfare system for the professional soldiers of his standing army as to tie these men directly to him, aiming to supplant the social networks upon which they would customarily rely. Indeed, in replacing solidarities based upon traditional modes of recruitment (princely and other noble households, feudal levies, professional companies, urban militia) by reliance on the dynast's munificence, increased gift-giving and pensions would reflect Charles the Bold's overall aims to substitute a new form of loyalty, directly binding combatants to their sovereign, to the formerly existing military and socio-political hierarchy mediating soldiers' ties with the monarch.[105]

With the demise of Charles the Bold's army reforms, financial compensation to combatants seems to have reverted to earlier practices of gift-giving. Spread over four years for which accounts were preserved (1479–1482), fourteen cases of men compensated by monetary gifts for incurred injuries during Maximilian's joint rule with Mary of Burgundy can be counted, i.e., approximately half of the cases of compensation in the first three full years of Charles the Bold's principate despite a similarly permanent state of war. Many of these gifts are explicitly related to the Battle of Guinegatte, where the Habsburg prince was personally present to halt the French invasion of the Low Countries. The preserved accounts, however, testify to another

**104** On the intertwinement of court and army under Charles the Bold, Hans Cools, "The Burgundian-Habsburg Court as a Military Institution from Charles the Bold to Philip II," in *The Court as a Stage: England and the Low Countries in the Later Middle Ages*, eds. Steven Gunn and Antheun Janse (Woodbridge: Boydell, 2006), 156–68. On general army scale, see: Schnerb, *L'État bourguignon*, 269–74.

**105** On Charles the Bold's policies as disruptive of existing social bonds, see: Lecuppre-Desjardin, *The Illusion*, 53–69. For their significance within the Burgundian army: Michael Depreter, "Les armées 'bourguignonnes' après Nancy: Ruptures et continuités structurelles d'un instrument politique," in *Mary of Burgundy: Persona, Reign, and Legacy of Late Medieval Duchess*, eds. Michael Depreter et al. (Turnhout: Brepols, 2021), 251–74.

priority in gift-giving: to compensate combatants having lost horses and other military equipment to allow them to reequip themselves and to rejoin the battlefield as soon as possible at a time of foreign invasion and civil strife.[106] Although Maximilian held on to Charles the Bold's ambitions and policies in the Low Countries, it remains uncertain whether he reinstated pensions for combatants who had lost the ability to sustain their livelihood through combat. In 1488, the only year for which accounts are preserved in the decade between 1482 and 1492, just two combatants, both from the prince's household, received a gift upon having incurred an injury![107] Amidst the height of foreign and civil war, such parsimony towards injured combatants reflects both the dynasty's financial shortcomings and a military reorganization as the provincial States, whether siding against or with Maximilian, regularly took control over the armies through direct payment of the soldiers.[108] In these circumstances, and with a reduced princely household,[109] compensa-

**106** Among other gifts: ADN, B 2121, fol. 447r–v (£100 to Adrien Mamboide, man-at-arms in the company of Chanteraine, who affirmed having lost 2 horses and some equipment at Guinegatte), fols. 447v–448r (£100 to Philip of Burgundy, to rearm himself and the men of his company, 1480); ADN, B 2124, fol. 231v (£13 to Colinet Poulet, men-at-arms in the company of Corneille de Berghes, to help him pay his ransom), fols. 242v–243r (£120 to Guillaume de Saint-Andoiche, cupbearer and squire to Maximilian, to equip himself for war—"affin qu'il se puist de tant mieulx monter, armer et mectre empoint pour continuer sondit service"), fol. 255r (£400 to Anthoine Dyvaen, a German squire, to compensate for loss of horse and other military equipment; £410 to Henry Hoffer, German, to compensate for imprisonment, loss of horses and other military equipment), fol. 257r (£100 to three men-at-arms from the company of Mingoval, to compensate for ransom and loss of all horses and military equipment and rearm themselves); ADN, B 2127, fol. 190r (£300 to Martin Zwarts, German squire, to compensate loss of horses and other losses, and to be able to continue his service), fol. 193r (£60 to Jehan de La Haye, squire, to compensate for horses, prison, and other losses, and to buy a new horse to further serve the prince).

**107** AGR, CC 1926, fol. 101v, fol. 106r.

**108** Depreter, "Les armées bourguignonnes," 259–65; Jelle Haemers, *For the Common Good: State Power and Urban Revolts in the Reign of Mary of Burgundy (1477–1482)* (Turnhout: Brepols, 2009), 39–44; Jelle Haemers, *De strijd om het regentschap over Filips de Schone: Opstand, facties en geweld in Brugge, Gent en Ieper (1482–1488)* (Ghent: Academia, 2014), 288; Amable Sablon du Corail, *La guerre, le prince et ses sujets: Les finances des Pays-Bas bourguignons sous Marie de Bourgogne et Maximilien d'Autriche (1477–1493)* (Turnhout: Brepols, 2019), 92–100.

**109** Valérie Bessey, "L'hôtel de Marie de Bourgogne d'après l'ordonnance de cour du 26 mars 1477," in *Mary of Burgundy*, 211–23, at 214–15; *Les ordonnances de l'hôtel des ducs de Bourgogne*, vol. 3: *Marie de Bourgogne, Maximilien d'Autriche et Philippe le Beau 1477–1506*, eds. Valérie Bessey et al. (Berlin: Lang, 2019), 10, 17.

tion to injured combatants would mainly fall under the responsibility of the States' mandators, if not directly under that of the company captains.

Under the comparatively peaceful personal rule of Philip the Fair (1494–1506), two cases of injured pensioners reappear. Noteworthily, one of them is pensioned as he was unable to join the prince on his travels to the Spanish peninsula, once more underscoring the importance of the household and its treasury as a source of regular support.[110] After over a decade of constant warfare, however, one can only be struck by the relative absence of compensations for previously injured combatants in the central dynastic accounts: out of twenty-seven counted cases under Philip the Fair, twenty-two pertain to the Guelders campaign of 1505. By then, the balance of power within the Low Countries, and the responsibility towards one's soldiers, had been renegotiated and partly reverted to the prince who not only compensated two members of his household, but also twenty combatants whose personal affiliations remain unspecified.[111]

## Conclusion: The Wounded Soldier in Socio-Economic Perspective

Overall, gift-giving practice suggests that Burgundian princely authorities mainly recognized physical and mental injuries after combat when they threatened the means and livelihood of combatants and, potentially, their ability to carry on making a good living in accordance with their previous living standards. Whereas social status and type of injury could play a part in setting the amount granted to compensate for lesions incurred in military service, the dukes primarily intervened to prevent or mitigate financial hardship, offering a lump sum of cash or a periodically recurring pension. In doing so, they may also have prevented (former) combatants from resorting to more violent means of retrieving socio-economic status or, at least, livelihood, as occasionally mentioned among mitigating circumstances in letters of

**110** A first occurrence appears in 1497 as Henry Tamburin, a German soldier ("compagnon de guerre"), was granted a daily pension of 3s. after being "disabled in one arm by a serpentine [artillery] shot" ("afolé d'un bras d'un cop de serpentine"): ADN, B 2159, fol. 90r–v. A second occurrence appears in the early sixteenth century, when Michiel Carpentier, an archer from the ducal guard, receives a 4s. per diem pension due to "illness" ("maladie"). Payments to Carpentier in: ADN, B 2177, fol. 48r–v, 124v–125r; ADN, B 2181, fol. 43v; ADN, B 2185, fol. 41v.

**111** ADN, B 2191, fol. 287v, 291r, 296v, 307v–308r. On the new balance of power, including for war taxation: Cauchies, *Philippe le Beau*, 57–89, esp. 84; Sablon du Corail, *La guerre*, 289–90.

remission granted to disabled veterans and studied by Quentin Verreycken.[112] Of course, this perspective is highly influenced by the nature of our source material, namely account books. It did not prevent the Burgundian court from valuing injured combatants for their service or, indeed, for their bravery and sacrifice on the battlefield, sometimes hinted at in financial records when they had been at the forefront of an assault.[113] Nevertheless, although prowess and courage may have been emphasized and even promoted in literary works and chivalric culture,[114] they were never at the core of the prince's charitable generosity. In socio-economic terms, then, the perception of an injured combatant may not have differed too much from that of any other person incurring impairment leading to financial hardship, whether a craftsman, a day labourer or a clerk suffering an accident at work.

Consequently, and rather unsurprisingly, no single far-reaching or coherent policy targeted combatants suffering injuries in dynastic service. Individual combatants were handled on a case-by-case basis, most likely through petitioning the prince for gifts granted "by [his] singular grace" ("de grace especial"), echoing a language also used in granting pardons.[115] Even Charles the Bold's military reforms, instating a first Burgundian standing army, did not yet lead to systematic change in this area: despite the first appearance of pensions signalling a progressive shift in considering the long-term effects of combat wounds and caring for soldiers injured in dynastic service in the long run, Adrienet Denis still had to petition the duke for his pension in March 1472.[116] The absence of general policy should

**112** Compare, in this volume, Quentin Verreycken, "A Vulnerable Military Masculinity: Soldiers and Disability in Late Medieval Pardon Letters."

**113** For instance: *Comptes de l'argentier*, vol. 1, art. 812 ("bleschure qu'il ot a la prinse des faubours [sic] dudit Dynant"), 1909 ("la maladie qu'il a nagaires eue a prinse de Liege"); ADN, B 2191, fol. 291 ("certaines blessures et playes qu'ilz avoient eues en ung bolewerch devant la ville de Aernhem"), 307v–308r ("en consideracion des bons et aggreables services qu'ilz lui avoient faiz a la prinse du bollewerck de ladicte ville de Aernhem").

**114** Craig Taylor, *Chivalry and the Ideals of Knighthood in France during the Hundred Years War* (Cambridge: Cambridge University Press, 2013), 91–98; Rosalind Brown-Grant and Mario Damen, *A Chivalric Life: The Book of the Deeds of Messire Jacques de Lalaing* (Woodbridge: Boydell, 2022), 1–2, 17–26, and 34–36.

**115** ADN, B 2085, no. 66115; ADN, B 2115, fol. 273v; ADN, B 2121, fol. 379r–v, 479r. On the language for pardons: Claude Gauvard, *"De grace especial": Crime, État et société en France à la fin du Moyen Âge*, 2 vols. (Paris: Publications de la Sorbonne, 1991). See also Meyer-Schilf, "'dazu jch jedem raten wil,'" 116.

**116** ADN, B 2085, no. 66115 (cited in Ali Bacha, "Blessures," 258).

not, however, be understood as a lack of interest in the fate of the wounded combatants. Rather, it strongly indicates that financial support was first and foremost to be sought for in those familial and socio-professional units (the noble household, the military company, the guild in the case of urban militia) of which the prince's household, to which many beneficiaries of ducal gifts belonged throughout the fifteenth century, was just one.

Reliance on pre-existing military and extra-military networks would only gradually be replaced by stronger interventions from the dynastic State, a shift possibly observed for the first time under Charles the Bold, when the socio-economic status of Burgundian combatants progressively changed as the duke endeavoured to create a standing army. Whereas warfare certainly offered profitable opportunities through pay, ransoms, and loot, a medieval nobleman's sources of income would still largely have depended on landed property and the offices he held. Similarly, the livelihood of urban militiamen would have primarily been sustained through their guild's trade, not through warfare. Even combatants whose primary occupation had been to fight would have had to look for alternative occupations—or at least employers—beyond their period of employment in a dynast's campaign.[117] Increased professionalization of men-at-arms and archers integrated in standing armies and, hence, in theory entirely relying on a stipend (*soldus*) paid by the dynastic state now led to new responsibilities and forms of care, including pensioning, especially when a ruler desired to promote a soldier's direct loyalty to the dynasty as did Charles the Bold.[118] Assuredly, the transition was slow, the process irregular, and military companies would still serve as a chief unit to support socio-professional solidarities throughout

**117** On Burgundian army recruitment before Charles the Bold, see Schnerb, *L'État bourguignon*, 269–74. On the continued importance of feudal levies and non-professional troops in France, even beyond the instatement of a permanent royal army: Contamine, *Guerre*, 277–398. On typologies of late medieval combatants and their incomplete, aborted transition from socio-professional careerists to true professional soldiers, a transition which could only be sustained by a war of occupation (Normandy, 1420–1453), see Adrian R. Bell et al., *The Soldier in Later Medieval England* (Oxford: Oxford University Press, 2013), 260–70.

**118** On Charles the Bold's reorganization of the Burgundian army and ordinance companies to promote direct loyalty, see: Depreter, "Les armées 'bourguignonnes,'" 251–74. Noteworthily, the Byzantine Empire's veterans, as former soldiers within a branch of the state apparatus, could also benefit from allowances from the fifth to the mid-seventh century: John Haldon, *Warfare, State and Society in the Byzantine World, 565–1204* (London: University College London Press, 1999), 256–64.

the sixteenth century.[119] Only when, then, by the late sixteenth and in the seventeenth century, soldiering became a regular, professional occupation in large-scale standing armies in direct service of the dynastic state, less or un-mediated by other socio-professional organizational structures such as a lord's household, a town's guild or a captain's company, more systematic policies would lead to legally established pension schemes[120] and the foundation of institutions to take care of those men who, having incurred injuries leading to their unemployability as soldiers, would become *unable* to sustain themselves through their honest profession. Simultaneously, the standardization of soldiers' equipment and movements through drilling and tactical discipline, whereby each man was to be replaceable for an identical one within ever more uniform units of infantry and cavalry, must have put new limitations on the further participation of impaired soldiers, now *disabled* in increasingly "mechanical" warfare.[121]

**119** On the autonomy of German landsknecht companies, for instance, albeit progressively declining, see Erik Swart, "From 'Landsknecht' to 'Soldier': The Low German Foot Soldiers of the Low Countries in the Second Half of the Sixteenth Century," *International Review of Social History* 51 (2006): 75–92.

**120** See in particular Geoffrey L. Hudson, "Disabled Veterans and the State in Early Modern England," in *Disabled Veterans in History*, ed. David A. Gerber (Ann Arbor: University of Michigan Press, 2012), 154–85; Ismini Pells, "Petitioning Soldiers, the Power of the Patient and the Provision of Military Welfare in 17th-Century England," in *Petitions and Petitioning in Europe and North America*, 254–67.

**121** On overall tactical change, see Clifford Rogers, "Tactics and the Face of Battle," in *European Warfare, 1350–1750*, eds. Frank Tallett and David Trim (Cambridge: Cambridge University Press, 2010), 203–35.

# SELECT BIBLIOGRAPHY


Ali Bacha, Rabah. "Les blessures de guerre à la fin du Moyen Âge." 2 vols. PhD diss. Université Lille III–Charles de Gaulle, 2010.

Auge, Oliver. "So solt er im namen gottes mit mir hinfahren, ich were doch verderbt zu einem kriegsmann: Durch Kampf und Turnier körperlich versehrte Adelige im Spannungsfeld von Ehrpostulat und eigener Leistungsfähigkeit." *Medizin, Gesellschaft und Geschichte* 28 (2009): 21–46.

Barnes, Joseph K. *The Medical and Surgical History of the War of the Rebellion (1861–1865)*. 2 vols. Washington: Government Printing Office, 1870–1888.

Bowen, Lloyd. "Genre, Authorship and Authenticity in the Petitions of Civil War Veterans and Widows from North Wales and the Marches." In *The Power of Petitioning in Early Modern Britain*. Edited by Brodie Waddell and Jason Peacey, 33–60. London: University College London Press, 2024.

Clarke, Catherine. "Signs and Wonders: Writing Trauma in Twelfth-Century England." *Reading Medieval Studies* 35 (2009): 55–77.

Clasper, Jon C. "The Management of Military Wounds in the Middle Ages." In *Wounds in the Middle Ages*. Edited by Anne Kirkham and Cordelia Warr, 17–39. Farnham: Ashgate, 2014.

Crocker, Christopher. "Narrating Blindness and Seeing Ocularcentrism in *Þorsteins saga hvíta*." *Gripla* 31 (2020): 267–92.

Crocker, Christopher and Yoav Tirosh. "Health, Healing, and the Social Body in Medieval Iceland." In *Understanding Disability Throughout History: Interdisciplinary Perspectives in Iceland from Settlement to 1936*. Edited by Hanna Björg Sigurjónsdóttir and James G. Rice, 113–27. New York: Routledge, 2021.

Crocker, Christopher, Yoav Tirosh, and Ármann Jakobsson. "Disability in Medieval Iceland: Some Methodological Concerns." In *Understanding Disability Throughout History: Interdisciplinary Perspectives in Iceland from Settlement to 1936*. Edited by Hanna Björg Sigurjónsdóttir and James G. Rice, 12–28. New York: Routledge, 2022.

Cullum, Patricia H. *Cremetts and Corrodies: Care of the Poor and Sick at St. Leonard's Hospital, York, in the Middle Ages*. York: Borthwick Institute, 1991.

DeVries, Kelly R. "Military Surgical Practice and the Advent of Gunpowder Weaponry." *Canadian Bulletin of Medical History* 7, no. 2 (Fall 1990): 131–46.

——. "Medieval Warfare and the Value of a Human Life." In *Noble Ideals and Bloody Realities: Warfare in the Middle Ages*. Edited by Niall Christie and Maya Yazigi, 27–55. Leiden: Brill, 2006.

Dittmar, Jenna M. et al. "Caring for the Injured: Exploring the Immediate and Long-Term Consequences of Injury in Medieval Cambridge, England." *International Journal of Paleopathology* 40 (2023): 7–19.

Frohne, Bianca. "Performing Dis/Ability? Constructions of Infirmity in Late Medieval and Early Modern Life Writing." In *Infirmity in Antiquity and the Middle Ages: Social and Cultural Approaches to Health, Weakness and Care*. Edited by Christian Krötzl et al., 51–65. Farnham: Ashgate, 2015.

——. *Leben mit "kranckhait": Der gebrechliche Körper in der häuslichen Überlieferung des 15. und 16. Jahrhunderts. Überlegungen zu einer Disability History der Vormoderne*. Affalterbach: Didymos, 2014.

Gagné, John. "Emotional Attachments: Iron Hands, their Makers, and their Wearers, 1450–1600." In *Feeling Things: Objects and Emotions through History*. Edited by Stephanie Downes et al., 133–53. Oxford: Oxford University Press, 2018.

Hausse, Heidi. "The Locksmith, the Surgeon, and the Mechanical Hand: Communicating Technical Knowledge in Early Modern Europe." *Technology and Culture* 60, no. 1 (2019): 34–64.

——. *The Malleable Body: Surgeons, Artisans, and Amputees in Early Modern Germany*. Manchester: Manchester University Press, 2023.

Heebøll-Holm, Thomas Kristian. "Apocalypse Then? The First Crusade, Traumas of War and Thomas de Marle." In *Denmark and Europe in the Middle Ages c. 1000–1525: Essays in Honour of Professor Michael H. Gelting*. Edited by Kerstin Hundahl et al., 237–54. London: Routledge, 2014.

Heide, Mareike. *Holzbein und Eisenhand: Prothesen in der Frühen Neuzeit*. Frankfurt: Campus, 2019.

Heiniger, Anna Katharina. "The Silenced Trauma in the *Íslendingasögur*." *Gripla* 31 (2020): 233–65.

Hodges, Kenneth. "Wounded Masculinity: Injury and Gender in Sir Thomas Malory's 'Le Morte Darthur.'" *Studies in Philology* 106, no. 1 (2009): 14–31.

Hsy, Jonathan et al., eds. *A Cultural History of Disability in the Middle Ages*. London: Bloomsbury, 2020.

Hudson, Geoffrey L. "Arguing Disability: Ex-Servicemen's Own Stories in Early Modern England, 1590–1790." In *Medicine, Madness and Social History*. Edited by Roberta Bivins and John V. Pickstone, 105–17. London: Palgrave, 2007.

Jakobsson, Ármann et al. "Disability Before Disability: Mapping the Uncharted in the Medieval Sagas." *Scandinavian Studies* 92, no. 4 (2020): 440–60.

Kafer, Alison. *Feminist, Queer, Crip*. Bloomington: Indiana University Press, 2013.

——. "Un/Safe Disclosures: Scenes of Disability and Trauma." *Journal of Literary & Cultural Disability Studies* 10 (2016): 1–20.

Kerth, Sonja. "Die letzten taflrunder? Krieg in adligen Autobiographien des 15. und 16. Jahrhunderts." In *Dulce bellum inexpertis: Bilder des Krieges in der deutschen Literatur des 15. und 16. Jahrhunderts*, 175–245. Wiesbaden: Reichert, 2002.

——. "Narratives of Trauma in Medieval German Literature." In *Trauma in Medieval Society*. Edited by Wendy J. Turner and Christina Lee, 274–97. Leiden: Brill, 2018.

Kjellström, Anna A. "Sixteenth-Century Warrior Grave from Uppsala, Sweden: The Battle of Good Friday." *International Journal of Osteoarchaeology* 15 (September 2005): 23–50.

Knüsel, Christopher J. "Courteous Knights and Cruel Avengers: A Consideration of the Changing Social Context of Medieval Warfare from the Perspective of Human Remains." In *The Routledge Handbook of the Bioarchaeology of Human Conflict*. Edited by Christopher J. Knüsel and Martin J. Smith, 263–81. London: Routledge, 2014.

——. "Orthopaedic Disability: Some Hard Evidence." In "Disability and Archaeology." Edited by Nyree Finlay. Special issue, *Archaeological Review from Cambridge* 15, no. 2 (January 1999): 31–53.

——. "The Physical Evidence of Warfare: Subtle Stigmata?" In *Warfare, Violence, and Slavery*. Edited by Michael Parker Pearson and I. J. Nick Thorpe, 49–65. Oxford: Archaeopress, 2005.

——. "The Unwritten History of Medical Treatment: Evidence for Ritual-healers and their Activities in the Pre-literate Past." *International Journal of Paleopathology* 34 (September 2021): 206–16.

Knüsel, Christopher J. and Anthea Boylston. "How has the Towton Project Contributed to Our Knowledge of Medieval and Later Warfare?" In *The Archaeology of a Mass Grave from the Battle of Towton AD 1461*. Edited by Veronica Fiorato et al., 169–88. Oxford: Oxbow, 2000.

——, and Martin Smith, eds. *The Routledge Handbook of the Bioarchaeology of Human Conflict*. London: Routledge, 2013.

Künzler, Sarah. *Flesh and Word: Reading Bodies in Old Norse-Icelandic and Early Irish Literature*. Berlin: de Gruyter, 2016.

Lawing, Sean. "Perspectives on Disfigurement in Medieval Iceland: A Cultural Study Based on Old Norse Laws and Icelandic Sagas." PhD diss., University of Iceland, 2016.

Metzler, Irina. *Disability in Medieval Europe: Thinking about Physical Impairment during the High Middle Ages c. 1100–1400*. London: Routledge, 2006.

——. *A Social History of Disability in the Middle Ages: Cultural Consideration of Physical Impairment*. Routledge Studies in Cultural History. New York: Routledge, 2013.

Meyer-Schilf, Karolina. "'Dazu jch jedem raten wil / er buw vff kriegen nit zu vil': Grundüberlegungen und Forschungsperspektiven zum Umgang mit Kriegsinvalidität im Spätmittelalter." In *Phänomene der "Behinderung" im Alltag: Bausteine zu einer Disability History der Vormoderne*. Edited by Cordula Nolte, 113–23. Affalterbach: Didymos, 2013.

Mitchell, David T. and Sharon L. Snyder. *Narrative Prosthesis: Disability and the Dependencies of Discourse*. Ann Arbor: University of Michigan Press, 2000.

Morosini, Giulia. "Manly Virtues, Emotions, and Scars: Competition among Italian Renaissance Soldiers through Bodily Practices." In *Gender and Status Competition in Pre-Modern Societies*. Edited by Martha Bayless et al., 79–107. Turnhout: Brepols, 2021.

Mounier-Kuhn, Alain. "Les blessures de guerre et l'armement au Moyen Âge dans l'Occident latin." *Médiévales* 39 (2000): 112–36.

——. *Chirurgie de la guerre: Le cas du Moyen Âge*. Paris: Economica, 2006.

Novak, Shannan A. "Battle Related Trauma." In *Blood Red Roses: The Archaeology of a Mass Grave from the Battle of Towton AD 1461*. Edited by Veronica Fiorato et al., 90–102. Oxford: Oxbow, 2000.

Ott, Katherine. "Material Culture, Technology, and the Body in Disability History." In *The Oxford Handbook of Disability History*. Edited by Michael Rembis et al., 125–35. Oxford: Oxford University Press, 2018.

Otte, Andreas. "Christian von Mechel's Reconstructive Drawings of the Second 'Iron Hand' of Franconian Knight Gottfried (Götz) von Berlichingen (1480–1562)." *Prosthesis* 3 (2021): 105–9.

Patsavas, Alyson. "Recovering a Cripistemology of Pain: Leaky Bodies, Connective Tissue, and Feeling Discourse." *Journal of Literary & Cultural Disability Studies* 8 (2014): 203–18.

Patzuk-Russell, Ryder and Yoav Tirosh. "Icelandic Hospitals, Clergy, and Disability in the *Saga of Bishop Lárentíus*." *Mirator* 24, no. 1 (2024): 1–17.

Pearman, Tory V. *Disability and Knighthood in Malory's Morte Darthur*. London: Routledge, 2019.

——. *Women and Disability in Medieval Literature*. New York: Palgrave, 2010.

Pfau, Aleksandra. "Warfare, Trauma, and Madness in French Remission Letters of the Hundred Years War." In *The Hundred Years War (Part III): Further Considerations*. Edited by L. J. Andrew Villalon and Donald J. Kagay, 437–54. Leiden: Brill, 2013.

Quayson, Ato. *Aesthetic Nervousness: Disability and the Crisis of Representation*. New York: Columbia University Press, 2007.

Rees, Owen et al., eds. *Combat Stress in Pre-Modern Europe: Mental Health in Historical Perspective*. London: Palgrave, 2022.

Sayers, Edna Edith (published as Lois Bragg). *Oedipus Borealis: The Aberrant Body in Old Icelandic Myth and Saga*. Madison: Fairleigh Dickinson University Press, 2004.

Sexton, John P. "Atypical Bodies: Seeking after Meaning in Physical Difference." In *A Cultural History of Disability in the Middle Ages*. Edited by Jonathan Hsy et al., 19–34. London: Bloomsbury, 2020.

——. "Difference and Disability: On the Logic of Naming in the Icelandic Sagas." In *Disability in the Middle Ages: Reconsiderations and Reverberations*. Edited by Joshua R. Eyler, 149–63. London: Ashgate, 2010.

Skinner, Patricia. "Visible Prowess? Reading Men's Head and Face Wounds in Early Medieval Europe to 1000 CE." In *Wounds and Wound Repair in Medieval Culture*. Edited by Larissa Tracy and Kelly DeVries, 81–101. Leiden: Brill, 2015.

Stiker, Henri-Jacques. *A History of Disability*. Translated by William Sayers. Ann Arbor: University of Michigan Press, 1999.

Talhoffer, Hans. *Medieval Combat: A Fifteenth-century Manual of Swordfighting and Close-quarter Combat*. Edited and translated by Mark Rector. London: Greenhill, 2000.

Tracy, Larissa, and Kelly DeVries, eds. *Wounds and Wound Repair in Medieval Culture*. Leiden: Brill, 2016.

Turner, Wendy J. *Care and Custody of the Mentally Ill, Incompetent, and Disabled in Medieval England*. Turnhout: Brepols, 2013.

——. "Mental Incapacity and the Financing of War in Medieval England." In *The Hundred Years War (Part II): Different Vistas*. Edited by Andrew L. Villalon and Donald J. Kagay, 387–466. Leiden: Brill, 2008.

Turner, Wendy J. and Christina Lee, eds. *Trauma in Medieval Society*. Leiden: Brill, 2018.

Villalon, L. J. Andrew and Donald J. Kagay, eds. *The Hundred Years War (Part II): Different Vistas*. Leiden: Brill, 2008.

——. *The Hundred Years War (Part III): Further Considerations*. Leiden: Brill, 2013.

Walker, Katie K. "Peril, Flight and the Sad Man: Medieval Theories of the Body in Battle." In *War and Literature: Essays and Studies*. Edited by Laura Ashe and Ian Patterson, 21–37. Cambridge: Brewer, 2014.

Woosnam-Savage, Robert C. and Kelly R. DeVries. "Battle Trauma in Medieval Warfare: Wounds, Weapons and Armor." In *Wounds and Wound Repair in Medieval Culture*. Edited by Larissa Tracy and Kelly R. DeVries, 27–56. Leiden: Brill, 2015.

# INDEX

agency, 12, 57, 68–69, 215
Ambroise Paré.
  *See* Paré, Ambrose
amputation/limb loss, 7, 14, 63–64, 67, 69–71, 77, 165, 180–81, 184, 188, 197, 201–2, 223, 227
analgesic/pain relief, 153, 172, 176, 181–82
Andreas Vesalius.
  *See* Vesalius, Andreas
antemortem (healed) trauma.
  *See* wounds
Arthurian romance, 7, 27, 30, 77, 79–98, 109.
  *See also under* Malory, Sir Thomas
artisans, 60, 196, 200–202, 204
authenticity and authorship, 104, 115, 120, 180
autobiographies/autobiographical writing, 15, 27, 167, 169–70, 180, 183–85, 187

barber/surgeons, 31, 48–50, 109, 118, 148, 154, 162, 164
Beris, Johannes (fl. 15th century), 165, 173–74, 176, 189
Berlichingen, Gottfried (Götz) von.
  *See* Gottfried (Götz) von Berlichingen
biographies/biographical writing.
  *See* autobiographies/autobiographical writing
Burgundian Low Countries.
  *See* Low Countries

charity, 104, 111, 113–14, 220–21, 225, 229–31, 235
Charny, Geoffroi de.
  *See* Geoffroi de Charny
Chauliac, Guy de.
  *See* Guy de Chauliac
collecting, 196, 204, 207
compensation, 13, 24, 33, 67–69, 73, 100, 122, 162, 201, 215–19, 222–30, 232–34
courtly eating.
  *See under* dining
crimes, 80, 100–103, 108, 110–14, 117, 121, 125, 133–35, 137–39, 184
criminal archives, 27, 106, 119, 133

debridement/debriding.
  *See under* wounds
dining
  courtly eating, 83, 86–87, 90, 96, 152
*Diagnostic and Statistical Manual of Mental Disorders* (*DSM*), 73, 144, 155
disabilities
  mental disabilities, 1, 3, 5–7, 12, 14, 17–18, 27, 32, 38, 45, 52, 54–56, 60, 62, 73, 76–77, 79, 81–85, 87, 89, 94–98, 105, 132–33, 135–36, 140–42, 143–44, 152, 154–60, 163–64, 186, 189–91, 214–16, 220, 223, 228, 234

ecclesiastical households.
  *See* households, princely/ecclesiastic
embodiment, 8, 57, 60–65, 72, 77, 184, 195, 208
England, 26, 31, 35, 49, 101, 110–15, 117, 120, 125, 132–33, 142, 143, 146, 148, 157, 161, 163, 220

fight manuals, 32, 145
France, 6, 9, 49, 99, 101–2, 110–11, 113, 115, 117, 120, 121, 124–25, 131–33, 135, 137–38, 148, 159, 187, 193, 216, 236
fright (shock), 173, 177, 189–90

gender
masculinity, 4, 21, 72, 77, 84–85, 109, 124, 134, 191
*See also* masculinity/masculinities
Geoffroi de Charny (ca. 1300–1356), 22, 177–79, 184, 189
Gersdorff, Hans von.
*See* Hans von Gersdorff
gifts, 13, 160, 201, 214–16, 218, 220–25, 227–28, 230–36
Gottfried (Götz) von Berlichingen (ca. 1480–1562), 63, 180–81, 183–85, 187, 190–91, 201, 205
gunners, 26, 36, 196, 201–2, 218–19, 226–28, 231–32
Guy de Chauliac (ca. 1300–1368), 48–49, 147

Hans von Gersdorff (ca. 1455–after 1529), 40, 151, 165, 170–71, 174–77, 181–82, 189
Heinrich von Pfalzpaint (ca. 1400–ca. 1464), 171–73, 176, 182, 189
honour, 2, 10, 59, 70–72, 81, 83, 93, 97–98, 103, 105, 118–19, 161, 178–79, 187, 202
households, princely/ecclesiastic, 48, 218–19, 223–24, 229–34, 236–37

Iceland, 15, 21, 27, 46, 58–78, 83
identity, 4, 15, 17, 21, 27, 53, 60, 63, 70, 74, 77, 82, 89–91, 95, 97, 103–4, 112, 114–15, 120, 128, 186, 189, 191, 220
illness, 24, 52, 83, 85, 95–96, 122, 128, 131, 135, 144, 147, 154–55, 167–70, 177, 179, 188–89, 217–18, 221–22, 226, 234,
intersectional concerns, 11, 17, 23, 43, 47, 49, 61, 81, 106, 162–63, 186, 221–23, 229, 234–36
*Íslendingasögur* (sagas of early Icelanders), 58, 61–62

Johannes Beris.
*See* Beris, Johannes
justice, 102–3, 113, 137, 207

knowledge, 4, 9, 67, 170, 188, 191, 196, 202

Launcelot, 81, 84–86, 89–98.
*See also* Malory, Sir Thomas: *Le Morte Darthur*
love-madness, 17, 79, 83–85, 87–89, 95, 97–98
love-sickness, 83–85, 88, 95, 97–98
Low Countries, 101–2, 110–11, 115, 117, 213–14, 232–34
Burgundian, 14, 16, 25–27, 36, 48–49, 55, 101–3, 107, 111, 113–14, 116, 120, 125, 130, 132, 136, 138, 201, 212–16, 219–21, 223–26, 228, 232–36

madness, 6, 18, 52, 82, 84–95, 123–24, 126–35, 137–38, 140–42, 160, 219, 226
Malory, Sir Thomas (ca. 1405–1471), 7, 30, 79–98
*Le Morte Darthur*, 30, 79–98
*See also* Launcelot; Tristram
masculinity/masculinities, 16, 22, 65, 67, 76, 85, 102, 104–5, 109–10, 115, 119, 124, 191.
*See also under* gender
mechanisms, 22, 185, 195–201, 204, 207, 237
mental disabilities.
*See under* disabilities.
*See also Diagnostic and Statistical Manual of Mental Disorders*
mercy, 101–2, 105, 111, 113–14, 117, 133, 139, 178
metalwork, 197, 200–201
metaphors, 72, 196, 207–8

*Ómagi* (dependent), 60–61, 77

pain, 7, 12, 16–17, 54–55, 109, 134, 140, 153, 165, 168–91
chronic, 75, 167–69, 187–89
pardon/remission/abolition letters, 6, 13–14, 16–17, 19, 21, 24–25, 99–103, 105–11, 113–20, 121–22, 132–35, 137–42, 219, 235

Paré, Ambroise (ca. 1510–1590), 31, 48, 176, 184–85, 193–95, 198–99, 204
pensions/corrodies, 25–26, 32, 54–55, 110, 120, 160–61, 214–15, 226–28, 231–37
petitions, 14, 24, 55, 100–108, 111–19, 201, 215, 221, 231, 235
Pfalzpaint, Heinrich von. *See* Heinrich von Pfalzpaint
physiognomy, 71
policies, 142, 213–15, 228, 232–33, 237
post-traumatic stress disorder (PTSD), 6, 17, 34, 73–76, 95, 105, 131, 143–44, 148, 153, 155, 189, 220
poverty, 4, 54, 56, 105, 110, 119, 221,
princely households. *See* households, princely/ecclesiastical
prosthesis, 11, 16, 21–22, 64, 67–68, 71, 150, 193
  prosthetic hand, 27, 63, 152, 180, 184–85, 193–208

recidivists, recidivism, 45–46, 225

scars, 41, 53, 69–71, 81, 105, 108–9, 115, 118, 219. *See also* wounds
service, 11, 16, 25, 48, 54–55, 73, 76, 99–100, 105, 107–8, 111–15, 119, 131, 147, 158, 160–61, 167, 187, 201, 208, 212, 215, 220–24, 227, 229, 232–35, 237
socio-economic support networks, 7, 11–12, 14, 25–27, 73, 97, 139, 160–61, 180, 186–87, 215, 222, 224, 228, 234, 236–37
starvation, 79, 83, 87–88, 89, 91, 93, 95–98
state formation, 11, 18, 25–26 213, 233, 236–37
surgery manuals, 170, 19. *See also* Paré, Ambroise; Guy de Chauliac; Hans von Gersdorff; Heinrich von Pfalzpaint

Talhoffer, Hans (master of arms, ca. 1420–1490), 32, 145
theory of humours, 71, 172
trauma
  physical, 6, 12, 29, 33–34, 36–39, 43–47, 49–52, 55, 61, 108, 110, 143, 147, 150, 159, 167, 169–70, 179, 189–91, 214, 227
  psychological/emotional, 6, 12, 34, 46, 53, 61, 73–77, 82, 110, 123, 131, 135–37, 142, 143–44, 147–48, 155–57, 159, 167, 169, 187, 189–91, 214, 219–20, 227
trepanation, 40, 174
Tristram, 84–86, 89–98. *See also* Malory, Sir Thomas: *Le Morte Darthur*

Vesalius, Andreas (1514–1564), 202–4
vulnerability, 71, 105–6, 110, 113–14, 119, 191

wound man (surgical diagram), 150–51, 165–66
wounds
  debridement/debriding, 40
  perimortem (unhealed), 29, 31–32, 34, 41–46, 53
  survival of, 29, 39–40, 45, 47, 49, 52–53, 147, 222
  treatment, 20, 23, 30–33, 39–41, 45, 48–54, 144, 162, 164, 168, 170–72, 176–77, 180–82, 213, 223

Printed and bound by CPI Group (UK) Ltd, Croydon, CR0 4YY

13/09/2026

14961066-0001